MARMA CHIKITSA: The Hidden Science of Ayurvedic Energy Healing for Pain Relief, Disease Reversal, and Vitality Restoration Across Asia

Published by Meta Journal Press: BeardedMedia.Com, 8491 Central Ave. Brooksville, Fl 34613

For general information on our products and services or for technical support, please contact our customer care Department within the United States at 1(706) 358-8646.

- **Cover Art Credits**

Cover concept and indigenous motif design by Dr. Anthony B. James.
Base imagery generated using artificial intelligence tools including Grok4 AI
Final composition © 2025 Dr. Anthony B. James.

AI-generated elements used under license with OpenAI-Grok4, in accordance with its commercial use policy. All design, prompt creation, modification, and post-production editing were executed by the author to ensure originality and cultural integrity.

This cover is a human-authored, derivative work incorporating AI-assisted components, and is protected under U.S. copyright law.

Contributor: Dr. Benoit Tano

- **Library of Congress Control Number:** 2025915089
- **ISBN:** 978-1-886338-42-5

ISBN-13: 978-1-886338-42-5
54995
9 781886 338425

- **Country the book is printed in United States of America**

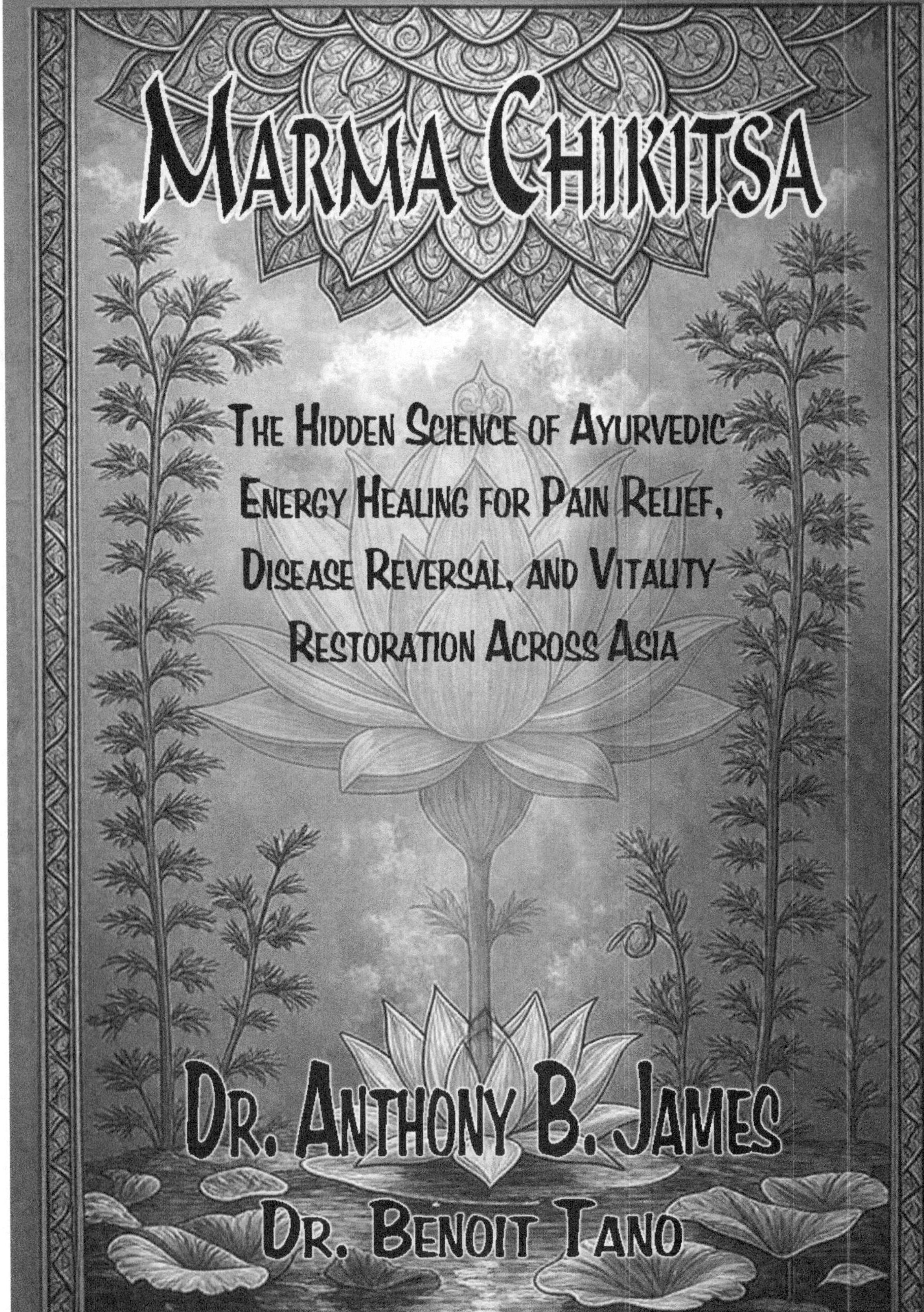
MARMA CHIKITSA
THE HIDDEN SCIENCE OF AYURVEDIC ENERGY HEALING FOR PAIN RELIEF, DISEASE REVERSAL, AND VITALITY RESTORATION ACROSS ASIA
DR. ANTHONY B. JAMES
DR. BENOIT TANO

Disclaimer

This book, 'MARMA CHIKITSA™: The Hidden Science of Ayurvedic Energy Healing for Pain Relief, Disease Reversal, and Vitality Restoration Across Asia', authored by Dr. Anthony B. James and Dr. Benoit Tano, explores the traditional healing method known as Marma Chikitsa. While extensive efforts have been made to ensure the accuracy and reliability of the information contained herein, the authors and publisher, Integrative Medical Press, make no representation, warranty, or guarantee as to the content's accuracy, reliability, or completeness. The information provided in this book is intended to serve as an educational resource and not as a substitute for professional medical advice. Readers are encouraged to consult healthcare professionals before adopting any practices, especially those with pre-existing health conditions. The treatments and methodologies discussed in this book are based on traditional knowledge and may not have undergone thorough testing using modern scientific methods. Moreover, variations in individual responses to treatments are common, and what may be effective for one person may not work for another. Marma Chikitsa, as represented here, showcases a wide-ranging cultural perspective and should not be viewed as a universal solution applicable outside its cultural and traditional context. Any application of the ideas contained here is at the reader's sole discretion and risk. Neither the authors nor the publisher shall be liable for any damages or injuries arising from the interpretation or application of the book's contents. The depiction of Marma practices across different regions of Asia represents a broad overview and may not entirely reflect all the nuances specific to local practices. The case studies included are illustrative examples and not prescriptive guidelines. The book also contributes to the academic examination of Marma Chikitsa by offering a comprehensive insight that encourages further research and discussion. It is a crucial contribution to both historical knowledge and contemporary practice, bridging the gap between ancient wisdom and its modern application.

Table of Contents

Preface

Welcome to the profound world of Marma Chikitsa, an ancient Ayurvedic practice heralded for its extraordinary healing potential. Traditionally steeped in the mysticism and holistic philosophy of Vedic sciences, Ayurveda's Marma Chikitsa serves not only as a therapeutic intervention but as a narrative of interconnectedness between the body, mind, and cosmos. In ***'MARMA CHIKITSA: The Hidden Science of Ayurvedic Energy Healing for Pain Relief, Disease Reversal, and Vitality Restoration Across Asia'***, we embark on an explorative journey that unearths the age-old secrets and modern applications of Marma therapy. As dedicated researchers and practitioners of alternative medicine, we aim to bridge indigenous knowledge and contemporary science, making credible healing techniques accessible. This book distills centuries of practices from across Asia, explored through comprehensive academic and clinical perspectives.

The initial chapters delve into the very essence of Marma points, vital energy spots on the human body influencing physical health and energetic well-being. Through a meticulous examination, we chart the anatomical, physiological, and energetic dimensions of these points, underpinned by both classical Ayurvedic texts and modern scientific investigations. As the narrative unfolds, we delve into the profound philosophical and esoteric frameworks that offer deeper insights into the subtler aspects of Marma Chikitsa, including its integration with spiritual practices and psychological well-being. Designed for both novices and seasoned practitioners, the chapters progressively introduce practical techniques, step-by-step applications, and case studies, demonstrating the efficacy of Marma in addressing a range of health conditions, from chronic pain to psychological disorders. Special focus is placed on how Marma therapy can be integrated with other healing disciplines, enhancing its scope and effectiveness. This book also provides aspiring practitioners with a blueprint for professional development, addressing educational pathways, certification, and ethical practice, setting the stage for Marma Chikitsa's integration into global healthcare paradigms. The book, 'MARMA CHIKITSA' is more than a manual; it is a gateway to transformative health, offering a compass for those who seek to restore vitality, alleviate suffering, and transcend the conventional limits of healing.

Foreword

It is with great reverence and excitement that we introduce 'MARMA CHIKITSA: The Hidden Science of Ayurvedic Energy Healing for Pain Relief, Disease Reversal, and Vitality Restoration Across Asia.' This book marks a pivotal moment in the world of holistic healing and Ayurveda. Marma Chikitsa, a profound yet often overlooked discipline within Ayurvedic medicine, offers not just insights into the ancient practice of energy healing but also a systematic approach tailored for contemporary application.

The practice of Marma Chikitsa, a primary therapeutic practice derived from Classical Indian Ayurveda, a national heritage of Indian culture and traditional medicine, which relies on strategic points in the human body like acupuncture's meridians, is a testament to Ayurveda's holistic vision of health. This art, documented by ancients such as Sushruta and further elaborated in our text, captures a comprehensive mapping of these vital points, promising significant relief from pain, expedited recovery from chronic ailments, and an overall enhancement of vitality. This book canvases extensive ground from the basic anatomy of Marma points through their physiological impacts, onto philosophical and spiritual bases, to provide a rounded perspective on the subject. Moreover, through modern clinical studies and practical guidance on techniques, our compilation connects timeless wisdom with concrete evidence, making it not only a rich academic resource but also a practical guide for practitioners and enthusiasts alike.

A significant effort has been made to include practical case studies, reflecting real-world applications and the effectiveness of Marma therapies across a range of ailments. Dr. Anthony B. James and Dr. Benoit Tano, having dedicated decades to the study and practice of Ayurvedic medicine, Traditional Thai Ayurveda and "*Ryksaa Thaang Nuad Phaen Boran Thai*" bring forward this ensemble of knowledge, aiming to bridge the gap between traditional and modern medical practices.

As a practice, "Ayurveda "Marma Chikitsa" is practiced therapeutically in every country or region worldwide as a vital and functional practice of Ayurveda Medicine. This classical therapeutic is not limited to practice in India nor to "Indian" Ayurveda practitioners. It is practiced by Hindu, Buddhist and Christian communities as primary care. These countries include India, Sri Lanka, Pakistan, Bangladesh, Tibet, Nepal, Bhutan, Myanmar, Thailand, Laos, Cambodia, Malaysia, Indonesia, Philippines and the USA, North and South America. Our endeavor is shared by our publisher, Meta Journal Press, to whom we extend our profound thanks for their meticulous assistance and guidance. We trust that this book will serve not merely as a text but as a vital instrument to those seeking holistic paths to health and well-being, thus continuing the venerable tradition of Marma Chikitsa across new generations and geographies.

CHAPTER ONE: Introduction to Marma Chikitsa – The Ancient Energy Science of Healing

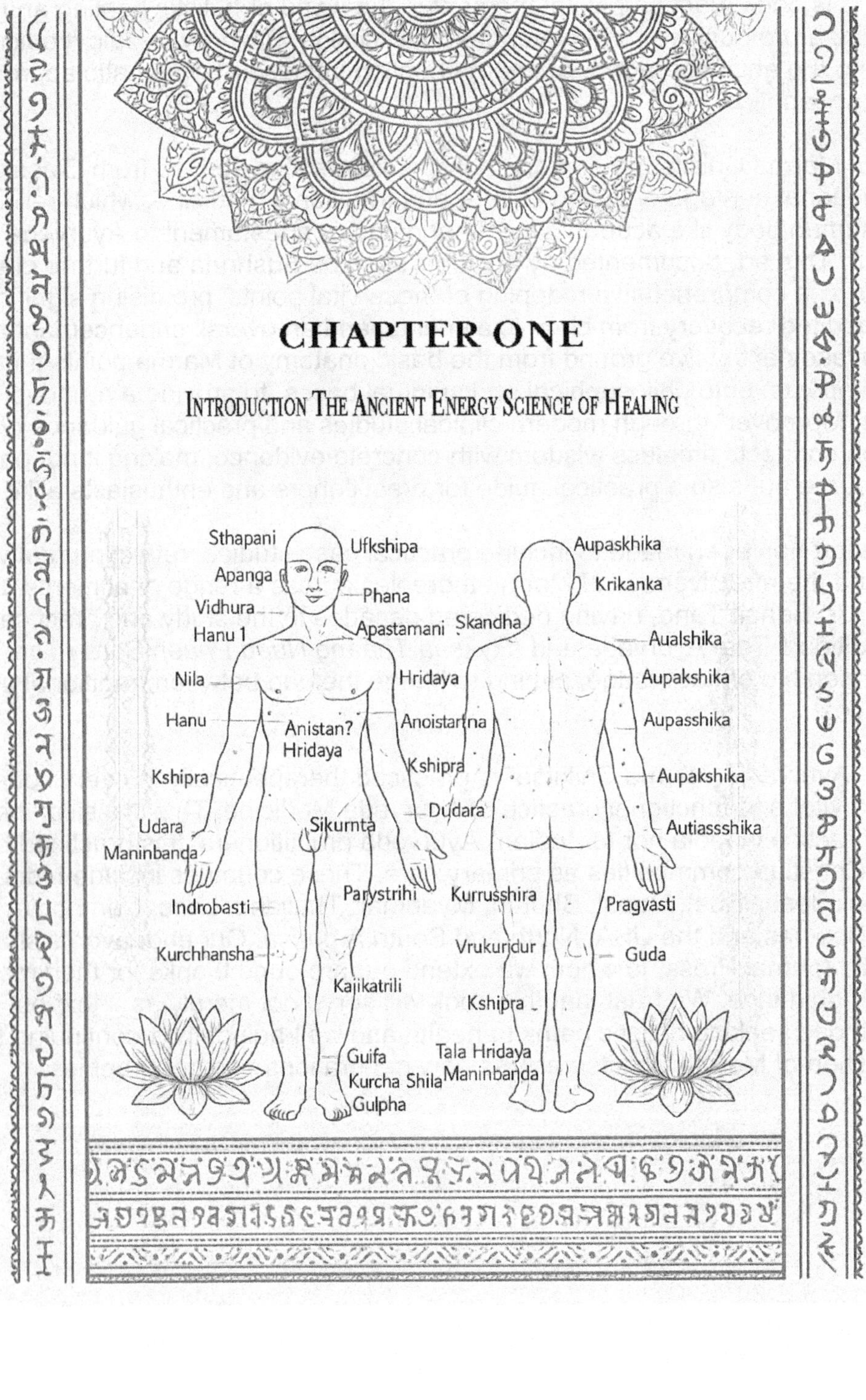

Definition and Meaning of Marma Chikitsa

Marma Chikitsa, an integral facet of Ayurvedic medicine, revolves around the ancient practice of energy healing, founded on the manipulation of specific points and skeletal segments or specific regions on the body termed 'Marma points'. These strategic points, segments, or regions are considered vital energy intersections where flesh, veins, arteries, bones, and joints converge, serving not only the physical body but also influencing the subtle energy flows responsible for our vitality and overall well-being.

The practice involves gentle pressure or stimulation to these points to unblock, balance, and direct energy flows, thereby fostering healing and rejuvenation. Rooted deeply in the traditions of Classical or Indigenous Traditional Ayurveda medicine, Marma Chikitsa is viewed as a holistic approach to health, addressing not only physical ailments but also emotional and spiritual imbalances.

In its essence, Marma Chikitsa transcends mere physical treatment, venturing into the realms of energy healing by influencing Prana. This life force governs biological functions and is a key to maintaining health equilibrium. Thus, this traditional practice holds significant promise as a complementary therapeutic discipline, merging ancient wisdom with the pursuit of modern well-being.

Historical Origins in Vedic and Ayurvedic Texts

The roots of Marma Chikitsa are deeply embedded in the ancient Vedic and Ayurvedic scriptures, marking its significance as far back as the dawn of Indian civilization. These texts, particularly the Vedas, serve as the earliest records, referencing the usage of Marma points in the context of healing and spiritual practices. The connection is made more evident in the subsequent Ayurvedic compendiums, which detail the application and theory behind this profound medical system.

Foremost among these are the writings of Sushruta and Charaka, whose works, dating back to the 1st millennium BCE, codified the knowledge of Marma therapy. Sushruta, in his seminal text 'Sushruta Samhita', outlined the locations and functions of 107 Marma points, integrating them into surgical practices and therapeutic interventions. This documentation not only preserved the knowledge but also laid down guidelines for future practitioners, ensuring the methods were passed through generations.

As Marma Chikitsa as one of the primary disciplines of classical Indian Ayurveda was shared and traveled across East Asia (Tibet, India, Pakistan, Sri Lanka, Nepal, Bhutan, Myanmar, Burma, Thailand, and South to the Philippines), adapting to different cultural contexts, its foundational theories remained firmly rooted in these ancient texts. This origin in sacred literature highlights its dual role as both a physical and spiritual healer, revered not just for its efficacy in bodily ailments but also for its capacity to align the life energies of spirit, mind and body.

The Role of Sushruta and Charaka in Documenting Marma Science

Sushruta and Charaka, towering figures in Ayurvedic medicine, played pivotal roles in defining and documenting Marma Chikitsa. Sushruta, often hailed as the 'Father of Surgery', integrated Marma knowledge into his surgical techniques. His 'Sushruta Samhita' meticulously describes 107 Marma points, specifying their anatomical positions and potential impacts when injured.

This detailed exposition has been crucial in safeguarding Marma Chikitsa's surgical relevance over the centuries.
Charaka's contributions, centered around internal medicine in his 'Charaka Samhita', complement Sushruta's surgical focus. He provides insight into the therapeutic manipulation of Marma points, emphasizing their utility in non-invasive treatment. Charaka's texts underscore the preventive and curative aspects of Marma points, highlighting their importance in holistic healing practices.
Together, these seminal works form the backbone of traditional Ayurvedic medicine, ensuring that Marma therapy's practices are not only preserved but also scientifically validated. Their writings continue to inspire and inform contemporary interpretations and applications of Marma Chikitsa.

Geographical Spread of Marma Chikitsa Across Asia

As Marma Chikitsa evolved within the Indian subcontinent, its healing wisdom spread far beyond its Vedic birthplace, permeating various cultures across Asia. Influential monks and Ayurvedic practitioners carried these practices to the Buddhist monasteries of Nepal and Sri Lanka, integrating them into local medicinal systems. This diffusion was particularly pronounced along the trade routes, where cultural interchange was rampant.
In Tibet, the principles of Marma Chikitsa merged with Tibetan healing arts, giving rise to unique hybrid practices that catered to the high-altitude condition's characteristic of the region. Further east, through the influence of both trade and conquest, Marma principles were subtly integrated with traditional Chinese medicine, adding depth to acupuncture techniques.
Today, the legacy of Marma Chikitsa's geographical spread is evident in its practice in Asian wellness centers and its recognition in global holistic health circles. It stands as a testament to the enduring appeal and adaptability of this ancient science, gaining new adherents and evolving forms that continue to soothe modern ailments.

Integration of Marma Therapy with Other Traditional Systems

Marma Chikitsa, deeply anchored in the Ayurvedic system, has found remarkable integration with other traditional healing systems across Asia, transcending boundaries and enriching diverse cultural medical practices.
In Tibet, for instance, Marma therapy merged seamlessly with Tibetan Bon medicine, creating a robust framework for healing that emphasizes the balance of body energies through the stimulation of specific points. This convergence not only bolstered local medicinal techniques but also infused Marma practices with unique Tibetan spiritual philosophies, thereby enhancing the holistic approach to healthcare.
Similarly, in traditional Thai medicine, elements of Marma Chikitsa have been observed in therapeutic techniques like Traditional Thai Ayurveda, Thai Yoga (Traditional Thai Medical Massage), which utilize energy lines (Thai Sen lines) comparable to Marma lines. This synthesis has given rise to a unique therapeutic hybrid that capitalizes on the strength of both systems, providing a comprehensive method of treatment that addresses both physical alignment and energy flow rejuvenation.
Through these integrations, Marma Chikitsa has not only sustained its relevance but also expanded its therapeutic reach, proving its adaptability and enduring influence in the realm of traditional medicine.

Classification of Marma Points According to Ancient Texts

The classification of Marma points, as delineated in ancient Ayurvedic texts, reveals a structured approach to understanding human anatomy and its intricate energy systems. These texts categorize Marma points into various types based on anatomical location, functional significance, and therapeutic potential. The primary classifications include Mamsa Marma (muscle), Asthi Marma (bone), Sira Marma (blood vessel), Snayu Marma (ligament), and Sandhi Marma (joint). Each category encompasses specific points that correspond to crucial bodily structures and functions.

Moreover, these classifications are not merely anatomical but are imbued with profound therapeutic insights. For instance, stimulating the Sira Marma can influence the circulatory system, promoting enhanced blood flow and toxin removal, which is essential for health rejuvenation. Similarly, Snayu Marma manipulation aids in alleviating musculoskeletal pain and enhancing flexibility.

Ancient practitioners strategically utilized this knowledge, designing targeted treatments to harness the body's innate healing capabilities. By meticulously documenting these classifications, texts such as 'Sushruta Samhita' provided a roadmap not just for treatment but for a comprehensive understanding of body energy dynamics crucial for holistic healing.

Physiological and Pranic Foundations of Marma Points

Marma Chikitsa's effectiveness stems from its dual reliance on physiological and Pranic (energy) systems, building a comprehensive framework for healing. The physiological aspect involves bodily structures such as muscles, joints, and organs, where Marma points are believed to be located. Stimulating these points can influence bodily functions, aiding in pain relief and promoting recovery from ailments.

On the energetic front, Marmas play a pivotal role in controlling the flow of Prana, or the life force, throughout the body. This concept parallels the circulatory system for Prana, akin to veins and arteries for blood. Disturbances in Prana flow are perceived as blockages that lead to health issues, and Marma therapy aims to clear these blockages, thereby restoring energy balance and enhancing vitality.

Such dual interplay between the tangible and intangible underscores Marma Chikitsa's holistic approach. The balance achieved through aligning physical functions with energy pathways paves the way for profound health transformations, embodying the essence of Ayurvedic healing principles.

The Five Categories of Marma Points Based on Tissue Type

The categorization of Marma points into five distinct groups based on tissue type reflects the profound understanding of human anatomy inherent in ancient Ayurvedic wisdom. These categories are Mamsa (muscle), Asthi (bone), Sira (blood vessels), Snayu (ligaments), and Sandhi (joints). Each type plays a specialized role in bodily healing and energy regulation, emphasizing the holistic approach of Marma Chikitsa.

Mamsa Marma points, associated with muscles, are targeted to enhance muscular health and to alleviate pain, aiding in the recovery of muscle-related injuries. Asthi Marma points safeguard bone health, which is vital for maintaining structural stability. Sira points, linked with blood

vessels, facilitate better blood circulation, significantly impacting detoxification and nutrient distribution throughout the body.
Snayu and Sandhi points, connected to ligaments and joints, respectively, are crucial for maintaining mobility and flexibility. Manipulating these Marma points helps reduce joint stiffness and enhance connective tissue health, highlighting the intricate synergy between physical and energetic healing in Marma therapy.

Vital Marma (Sadyapranahara) vs. Non-Vital Marma Points

Marma Chikitsa distinguishes between Vital (Sadyapranahara) and Non-Vital Marma points, a classification critical to both therapeutic techniques and the training of practitioners. Vital Marmas are points where life energies are concentrated and, when stimulated or injured, can have profound effects on the body and consciousness. These points are integral not just for healing, but also historically, in martial applications where precise strikes could incapacitate an opponent.
Non-vital Marmas, while necessary, do not hold the same potential for a dramatic impact on life force or bodily function. Their stimulation promotes overall health and well-being, facilitating more gradual healing processes. They are typically used for routine therapy and are safer for less experienced practitioners to handle.
Understanding the differences between these Marmas is crucial for effective treatment. Knowledge of the specific properties and impacts of each point allows therapists to tailor their approach to meet individual patient needs, ensuring both safety and the efficacy of the therapeutic interventions.

Understanding the Prana-Vayu Pathways

The ancient science of Marma Chikitsa intricately entwines the Prana-Vayu, the vital life forces that govern physiological activities and emotional states. Within this traditional practice, understanding the prana-vayu pathways is paramount to mastering energy manipulation for healing and revitalization. These pathways serve as channels for the flow of energy, connecting the physical body to the subtle energetic structures within.
Prana-Vayu is primarily responsible for inhalation and the downward flow of life energy, directing vitality throughout the body's core. By skillfully stimulating specific Marma points, a practitioner can influence this energy, optimizing the body's innate healing capacity. The pathways are viewed not just as conduits of breath or air, but as ethereal streams that carry the life force, instrumental in maintaining physiological balance and health.
Effective Marma therapy relies on a profound understanding of these pathways, enabling the redirection of Prana to alleviate ailments, enhance vitality, and sustain physiological harmony. This conceptual framework serves as the cornerstone of Marma Chikitsa, enabling a holistic approach to health that integrates the body, mind, and spirit.

Comparison of Marma with Chinese Acupuncture and Acupressure

Marma Chikitsa and Chinese Acupuncture and Acupressure, while originating from distinct ancient traditions, share fundamental principles centered around the body's energy systems.

Marma, derived from Ayurveda, identifies energetic and physical junctions on the body, aiming to enhance Pranic flow and thereby facilitate healing and vitality. Similarly, Acupuncture and Acupressure from Traditional Chinese Medicine (TCM) focus on meridians or channels that carry 'Qi' or life force, targeting specific points to balance energy flow.
The methodologies, however, exhibit unique approaches. Marma therapy incorporates not only the stimulation of specific points but also considers the holistic integration with Ayurvedic practices, such as the use of herbal oils and lifestyle adjustments. In contrast, Acupuncture uses needles and Acupressure employs physical pressure, focusing mainly on the rebalancing of Qi without the extensive holistic lifestyle integration seen in Marma Chikitsa.
Both systems see the human body as a network of interconnected energy pathways that, when blocked, lead to disease. By understanding and comparing these modalities, practitioners can leverage the strengths of each, promoting greater health and well-being across diverse patient populations.

Why Marma is Considered the Mother of All Manual Therapies

Marma Chikitsa is often revered as the mother of all manual therapies, holding a profound position due to its comprehensive approach to healing. This ancient practice transcends mere physical manipulation, integrating a profound understanding of physiological and energetic systems. By activating specific points that control the flow of Prana, or life force, Marma therapy influences both body and mind, paving the way for transformative health interventions.
The primacy of Marma in the realm of manual therapies arises from its holistic inclusivity. Unlike other therapies that often target isolated symptoms or areas, Marma Chikitsa addresses the integral unity of the body's systems. Such comprehensive care promotes the optimal redistribution of energy, which is essential for curing ailments and bolstering vitality. This distinctive approach not only relieves pain but also revitalizes life energies, setting Marma apart as a foundational therapeutic technique.
Moreover, the historical depth and extensive documentation by ancient scholars, such as Sushruta, lend Marma Chikitsa a credibility that is both profound and enduring. Practitioners have, for centuries, leveraged this wisdom to master the art of healing, making it a cornerstone of traditional medicine across Asia. Its influence permeates various healing practices today, underscoring its title as the progenitor of manual healing therapies.

The Esoteric Nature of Marma Knowledge and Its Oral Transmission

Delving into the core of Marma Chikitsa reveals a rich reservoir of esoteric knowledge, traditionally passed down through generations by word of mouth. This oral transmission mirrors the sacred rituals of ancient mentors instructing disciples, ensuring the purity and sanctity of the practice remained uncorrupted by the written word. Such transmission emphasizes the mystical dimensions of Marma, steeped in spiritual reverence and experiential learning.
The guardians of this knowledge, usually seasoned practitioners or gurus, selected disciples who exhibited not only a keen intellectual grasp but also the requisite spiritual maturity. This method of teaching preserved the inner sanctum of Marma wisdom from dilution, often reserving the deeper secrets for those initiated into higher levels of understanding and trust. It created a lineage of healers whose insights into human anatomy and energetics were profoundly intimate.
Thus, the esoteric nature of Marma is closely tied to its method of sharing—oral and experiential rather than purely theoretical. This approach has kept Marma Chikitsa vibrant and evolving,

bridging ancient insights with contemporary practices seamlessly while maintaining the integrity of its profound healing capabilities.

Ancient Warriors and the Use of Marma in Kalari Payattu

In the ancient martial art of Kalari Payattu, practitioners harnessed the profound knowledge of Marma Chikitsa to gain an upper hand in combat. This formidable technique enabled warriors to target specific Marma points, which could incapacitate opponents by disrupting vital energy flows or Prana. The strategic application of Marma strikes in warfare highlights the dual nature of this science, which can both heal and harm, depending on the user's intent.

Training in Kalari not only involved physical prowess but also an intricate understanding of the human body's energy channels. Warriors were trained to see beyond mere physical forms, perceiving opponents in terms of Marma points and energy pathways. This profound insight allowed them to execute strikes with surgical precision, exploiting vulnerabilities in the body's energy network.

Hence, Marma Chikitsa within Kalari Payattu was not just a form of healing but also a crucial element of martial strategy, embodying the synthesis of body, energy, and mind. The use of Marma demonstrates a sophisticated integration of anatomical, energetic, and spiritual wisdom, deeply rooted in the traditions and combat lore of ancient India.

How Marma Points are Linked to Chakras and Nadis

The intricate relationship between Marma points and the subtle energy systems of chakras and Nadis is foundational in Marma Chikitsa. Chakras, the central nodes of spiritual power within the human body, are intimately connected to the network of Nadis, the channels through which prana, or life energy, flows. Marma points serve as critical junctures on these pathways, regulating the movement and health of Pranic energy.

Stimulation of Marma points can directly influence the corresponding chakras, promoting the balance of energies that govern physical and emotional states. For instance, stimulating Marma points near the heart chakra can enhance cardiac function and emotional well-being. This is due to the direct impact on the Anahata Nadi, which governs the flow of energy through the heart region.

Similarly, specific Marma points along the spine align with the Sushumna Nadi, critical for Kundalini activation, highlighting their role in spiritual awakening and healing. This essential connectivity underscores the holistic nature of Marma therapy, integrating physical, emotional, and spiritual health.

Relationship Between Marma Points and the Endocrine System

The intricate interplay between Marma points and the endocrine system represents a pivotal aspect of Marma Chikitsa's therapeutic prowess. These points, strategically located on the body, act as gateways influencing hormone secretion, which in turn regulates a myriad of bodily functions. Manipulation of specific Marma points can stimulate corresponding glands, promoting the release of hormones that facilitate healing and maintain physiological balance.

For instance, stimulating the 'Adhipati Marma' located on the crown is believed to affect the pituitary gland, the master gland that governs other glands in the endocrine system. This action can help synchronize hormone output, impacting everything from growth to metabolism. Similarly, the 'Hridaya Marma', located over the heart area, may influence the thymus gland, which is crucial for immune response mechanisms.

By integrating endocrinological knowledge with Marma Chikitsa, practitioners can offer targeted interventions that aim not only at symptomatic relief but also at restoring the body's intrinsic health equilibrium. This synergy highlights Marma's role in holistic health, serving as a compass for navigating the complex biochemistry of the human body.

Scientific Research on Marma Stimulation and Nervous System Effects

Recent scientific inquiries into Marma Chikitsa have shed light on its significant impact on the nervous system, underscoring its potential as an integrative therapeutic modality. Studies indicate that stimulation of Marma points triggers neural responses that can modulate pain perception, potentially offering pathways to non-pharmacological pain management.

Neurological research has also explored how Marma therapy influences autonomic nervous functions, which include the regulation of heart rate and blood pressure. Data suggest that Marma practices may foster a state of relaxation and decrease stress responses by activating the parasympathetic nervous system. This effect not only aids in stress management but also enhances overall physiological resilience to stressors.

Moreover, preliminary electroencephalogram (EEG) studies reveal changes in brainwave patterns during Marma point manipulation, suggesting enhancements in alertness and mental clarity. These findings pave the way for further exploration into how Marma Chikitsa can be systematically integrated into holistic health regimes, potentially improving cognitive functions and emotional well-being.

Modern Evidence Supporting Marma Therapy in Pain Management

Contemporary research into Marma Chikitsa unveils promising findings, underscoring its efficacy in pain management. Accumulated evidence through clinical experiments suggests Marma therapy can significantly mitigate chronic pain. This is particularly observed in musculoskeletal conditions, where targeted stimulation of Marma points appears to alleviate discomfort and enhance mobility.

Moreover, the non-invasive nature of Marma practice offers a safe alternative to conventional painkillers, potentially reducing the dependency on pharmaceuticals. Pain relief outcomes recorded in these studies suggest that Marma therapy has a profound effect on the body's pain perception pathways, facilitating a more natural approach to pain management. Trials incorporating Marma therapy have shown lower pain scores and improved patient satisfaction, reinforcing its role in therapeutic pain interventions.

This growing body of evidence not only validates the historical assertions regarding Marma's effectiveness but also cements its place within the modern integrative medicine paradigm. As research expands, health professionals increasingly advocate for integrating Marma techniques into holistic health strategies, advocating for a balance between traditional wisdom and contemporary clinical practice.

Review of Published Studies on Marma and Physiological Health Benefits

Scholarly examinations have corroborated the physiological benefits of Marma Chikitsa, emphasizing its efficacy across various health domains. Published studies document notable improvements in circulatory and respiratory functions, demonstrating that Marma therapy can significantly enhance blood flow and oxygen saturation within the body.

Research also highlights the role of Marma Chikitsa in boosting immunity and enzymatic activity, which can lead to improved disease resistance and enhanced metabolic rates. Such studies consistently indicate an improved quality of life for individuals who regularly undergo Marma treatments. Additionally, the influence of Marma therapy on serotonin and other neurotransmitter levels has been studied, linking it to mood enhancement and a reduction in anxiety levels.

With its roots deeply entrenched in traditional wisdom, Marma Chikitsa's modern scientific backing opens the potential for its broader application in non-traditional settings, aligning ancient practices with contemporary health needs. These studies help bridge the ancient art with modern health practices, substantiating traditional claims with empirical evidence.

Marma Therapy as a Bridge Between Ayurveda and Modern Integrative Medicine

Marma Therapy, rooted in ancient Ayurvedic science, emerges as a promising bridge to modern integrative medicine, reveling in a holistic approach that caters to individualized patient care. The therapy's grounding in both spiritual and physical healing parallels the biopsychosocial models used in contemporary medicine, where treatment is targeted at the intersection of body, mind, and socio-environmental factors.

The scientific validation of the influence of Marma points on physiological and neural pathways has caught the attention of the modern medical community. Marma's techniques for managing pain, improving circulatory function, and enhancing neurological health dovetail neatly with integrative strategies that seek non-pharmacological alternatives. This symbiosis provides a comprehensive healing blueprint that transcends the limitations of conventional methods.

As healthcare leans towards more sustainable practices, Marma Therapy's non-invasive nature and emphasis on restoring natural balance present a viable adjunct or alternative in modern treatment plans. This integration signifies a growing acceptance and revaluation of historical wisdom within contemporary curative frameworks.

Basic Terminologies Every Student of Marma Chikitsa Should Know

Embarking on the study of Marma Chikitsa requires familiarity with its specialized vocabulary, which forms the foundation of this ancient therapeutic practice. Key terms include 'Marma' (vital points), 'Prana' (life force), and 'Agni' (digestive fire), each encapsulating unique concepts integral to treatment effectiveness. Understanding these terms not only enhances comprehension but also deepens the student's ability to engage proficiently with the therapy's principles.

Further, 'Doshas' (biological energies: Vata, Pitta, Kapha) represent fundamental theories in Ayurvedic medicine, influencing Marma practice. Knowledge of these terms enables practitioners to tailor treatments to individual constitutional needs, thereby optimizing healing outcomes. Additionally, 'Ojas' (vital essence for strength and immunity) is crucial, as Marma

therapies often aim to preserve and enhance this essence.
Lastly, 'Chikitsa' itself means treatment or therapy, underscoring the practice's goal of restoring balance and health. Mastery of these terms is foundational, illuminating the path towards competent practice and profound understanding of Marma Chikitsa.

Common Misconceptions and Misuse of Marma Therapy

Despite the potent benefits of Marma Chikitsa, misconceptions and misuse often shadow its practice. A prevalent misconception is that Marma therapy can be self-taught from books or online resources without comprehensive training. Such an approach is fraught with risks, as incorrect application may lead to adverse effects rather than healing. This non-traditional learning bypasses the intricate knowledge of Marma points and their precise stimulation, which is crucial for safe practice.
Moreover, some practitioners claim exaggerated benefits, like instant cures for chronic ailments, which undermines the therapy's credibility and historical significance. Authentic Marma practice is not a quick fix, but rather a component of a holistic approach to health that integrates well with other medical treatments.
Additionally, the commercialization of Marma therapy has led to inappropriate adaptations, which dilute its true essence. Workshops promising certification in just a few hours misrepresent the depth and dedication required to master this ancient art, potentially compromising patient health and the integrity of the therapy. Quality programs of study that emphasize traditional and proven methodologies for focused treatment are now found worldwide, from India to Thailand, as well as in the USA. Wherever there are conventional or professional schools, colleges, or programs with an emphasis on Ayurveda, there will be an emphasis on the use and treatment of Marma Chikitsa. It is a fundamental practice of Classical and modern Indian Ayurveda, Traditional Thai Ayurveda, and Yoga Therapy as well.

How Marma Therapy Differs from Massage or Reflexology

Marma Therapy, often likened to massage and reflexology due to its manual stimulation of body points, stands distinct in its approach and philosophical underpinnings. Unlike massage, which involves manipulating broad muscle groups, Marma focuses on specific points that channel Pranic energy—the vital life force in Ayurveda—throughout the body. This targeted stimulation is designed to unlock energy pathways and restore balance in health.
Reflexology targets reflex points primarily in the hands and feet, reflecting the body's entire organ system. In contrast, Marma points are distributed throughout the body and are considered intersections of flesh, veins, arteries, tendons, bones, and joints. Each Marma point serves as a conduit for bioenergy, or 'Prana,' and its stimulation affects the body's spiritual, emotional, and physiological health.
The technique used in Marma therapy also contrasts with that of reflexology and massage. Marma involves gentle touches that are not necessarily rhythmic or deep, but are precise in terms of location and duration, to influence energy flow significantly. This deliberate and minimalist approach underscores Marma's complex theoretical basis, rooted in Ayurvedic texts, which links body and consciousness more closely than its counterparts.

Cultural Significance of Marma Points in Daily Indian Life

In the tapestry of Indian culture, Marma Chikitsa weaves a narrative of holistic well-being, embedding itself in the daily rituals and healthcare practices of its people. Traditionally, these vital points are not merely seen as therapeutic tools but as integral to daily spiritual and physical maintenance. Every morning, many Indians engage in self-massage, unknowingly stimulating Marma points that enhance the flow of prana, setting a vibrant tone for the day.
This practice extends into the realm of Indian athletics, particularly in disciplines such as wrestling and martial arts, where knowledge of Marma points is utilized both to enhance performance and to treat injuries. The ancient martial art of Kalari Payattu, for example, teaches the warriors both the application and defense against Marma point strikes, showcasing the depth of knowledge and its practical relevance.
Culturally, Marma therapy is often incorporated in spiritual practices linked to yoga and meditation, further emphasizing its role in fostering an internal balance. Festivals and traditional dances also subtly incorporate Marma principles, ensuring participants' energy levels remain high and their bodily systems harmonious. Thus, Marma Chikitsa is not just a medical practice but a living aspect of cultural identity, shaping health, spirituality, and communal activities within Indian society.

Summary

Marma Chikitsa, rooted in Ayurvedic tradition, focuses on the manipulation of Marma points—vital energy spots on the body where key biological structures converge. These points are crucial for the flow and regulation of Prana, the life force essential to health and vitality. The practice, deeply embedded in ancient Vedic and Ayurvedic texts, is particularly highlighted in the works of Sushruta and Charaka, who detailed the locations and therapeutic uses of Marma points, integrating them into holistic healing practices. Marma Chikitsa addresses not only physical ailments but also emotional and spiritual imbalances, offering a comprehensive approach to wellness. Through centuries, this practice has traversed across Asia, influencing and integrating with other traditional healing systems, thereby enriching and maintaining its relevance in contemporary holistic medicine. Practitioners strategically stimulate Marma points to unblock and redirect energy flows, enhancing bodily functions and promoting healing. The nurturing of these points influences both the physiological and energetic systems of the body, emphasizing the interconnectedness of physical and subtle body structures. The classification of Marma points into types such as Mamsa (muscle) and Asthi (bone) further illustrates their specific roles in therapeutic interventions. Modern research supports the benefits of Marma Chikitsa in areas such as pain management and psychological well-being, bridging traditional practices with contemporary medical understanding. The therapy's adherence to holistic principles, which align body, mind, and spirit, positions it as a valuable integrative medical practice, respected in both traditional and modern health discourses.

References

[1] Autonomic responses to breath holding and its variations following pranayama. http://www.ncbi.nlm.nih.gov/pubmed/21598116

[2] Neurophysiological effects of stimulation of trigger points in patients with chronic Lower back

pain. http://www.ncbi.nlm.nih.gov/pubmed/21595999

[3] Traditional Medicine in Asia. http://apps.who.int/medicinedocs/en/d/Jh2943e/

[4] The Concept of Marma: A Traditional Background. https://www.nih.gov/

[5] Evaluation of Ayurvedic Diagnosis and Management of Chronic Disorders. https://www.researchgate.net/profile/

Case Study: Revitalizing Holistic Health: A Marma Chikitsa Intervention

Anita, a 45-year-old software developer, sought to address her chronic neck pain and pervasive anxiety through holistic therapies. After exhausting various medical treatments with minimal relief, her encounter with Marma Chikitsa offered a new avenue of hope. The treatment was centered on a series of sessions targeting specific Marma points to alleviate physical and emotional issues.

During her initial assessment, the practitioner identified key Marma points along Anita's cervical spine and shoulders implicated in her discomfort. These points, known for their convergence of nerve pathways and muscular junctions, were believed to be blocked, stifling the flow of Prana, contributing to her physical and mental distress. The practitioner employed gentle, precise manipulation techniques aimed at restoring energy balance and enhancing physiological health. This was complemented by the application of herbal oils, believed to penetrate deeply into the tissue and amplify the healing process.

Her sessions were scheduled bi-weekly, and after the first month, Anita reported a significant reduction in her neck pain. By the third month, not only had her pain diminished, but she also experienced enhanced mental clarity and reduced anxiety levels. Concomitant lifestyle advice, including dietary changes and yoga, reinforced the effects of Marma Chikitsa, offering her a holistic revitalization.

This case illustrates the intricate interplay between physical and energetic systems addressed by Marma Chikitsa. It underscores the therapy's capacity to impact multi-dimensional health concerns, extending beyond mere symptomatic relief to foster overall well-being and vital energy balance. Significantly, as seen in Anita's case, the therapy's efficacy is enhanced through individual assessment and comprehensive lifestyle integration, embodying the holistic essence of Marma therapy.

Case Study: Enhancing Athletic Performance through Marma Chikitsa: The Case of a Professional Runner

Rahul, a 30-year-old professional marathon runner, faced a significant challenge with recurring hamstring injuries and sluggish recovery rates that threatened his athletic career. Desperate for a solution that transcended conventional medical treatments, which had provided only temporary relief, Rahul turned to Marma Chikitsa, intrigued by its promise of enhancing physical vigor and accelerating recovery processes.

A seasoned Marma therapist assessed Rahul's condition, pinpointing several vital Marma points along his lower limbs and back that were deemed crucial for muscular strength and injury recovery. These included specific points, such as the Gulpha (ankle) Marma, which enhances joint mobility, and the Urvi (thigh) Marma, vital for strengthening the muscles and ligaments around the thigh and knee. The therapeutic sessions focused on gently stimulating these points to enhance the flow of Prana, aiming not just to alleviate pain but to invigorate the healing and strengthening of tissues.

Each session began with a thorough application of herbal oils specifically designed to reduce inflammation and promote tissue regeneration. This was followed by a precision-driven technique to activate the targeted Marma points, intended to rebalance the vital energies (tri-dosha) specific to Rahul's bodily constitution. The therapy was supplemented with nutritional guidance and yoga postures selected to bolster the effects of the Marma treatments and support overall muscle flexibility and joint health.

After several weeks of consistent Marma therapy, Rahul observed a notable improvement not only in his injury recovery rate but also in his performance endurance and agility during runs. His susceptibility to injuries decreased, and his recovery times improved remarkably, letting him maintain a more rigorous training schedule. These results underscore the efficacy of Marma Chikitsa in bridging the gap between traditional healing wisdom and modern athletic performance demands, effectively enhancing both physical health and energy dynamics that are crucial for high-level sports.

Case Study: Comprehensive Healing through Marma Chikitsa: Case Study of a Stroke Recovery

Ravinder, a 60-year-old retired schoolteacher, suffered a mild stroke that left him with partial paralysis on his right side and significant depression due to his sudden loss of independence. Traditional rehabilitation therapies provided only marginal improvements. Seeking a more holistic approach, his family turned to Marma Chikitsa, intrigued by its potential for integrating physical and emotional healing.

An expert in Marma Chikitsa first conducted a thorough assessment of Ravinder, identifying not only the physical deficits caused by the stroke but also the psychological impact. The therapist developed a treatment plan that targeted specific Marma points related to motor control and emotional regulation. Points such as Kshipra Marma, located at the base of the thumbs and big toes, were targeted to enhance motor function, while Anahata Marma, located on the chest, was treated to alleviate emotional distress and improve heart function.

The sessions involved gentle stimulation of these points with appropriate herbal oils, which are believed to penetrate deep into the tissues and aid in healing and energizing the body. The treatment was complemented with tailored dietary recommendations to optimize neurological health and exercises that were synchronized with the energy treatments to enhance overall coordination and strength.

After several months of consistent therapy, Ravinder exhibited remarkable improvements. Not only did his motor skills improve, allowing him more physical independence, but his mood and outlook on life also transformed significantly, demonstrating reduced symptoms of depression and increased vitality. This recovery journey highlighted the effectiveness of Marma Chikitsa in addressing both physical and subtle energy levels, promoting recovery by balancing and enhancing life energies (Prana), which proved vital in managing post-stroke conditions effectively.

Case Study: Restoring Equilibrium: Marma Chikitsa in Managing Hormonal Imbalances

Simran, a 38-year-old marketing executive, struggled with symptoms of hormonal imbalance, including irregular menstrual cycles, severe mood swings, and persistent acne. Traditional treatments with hormone therapy provided only temporary relief and often came with undesirable side effects. In search of a more holistic and sustainable solution, Simran turned to Marma Chikitsa, influenced by its reputed efficacy in balancing the body's natural energies and enhancing overall well-being.

An experienced Marma therapist began by assessing Simran's overall health, lifestyle, and specific symptoms to tailor a treatment plan. The focus was on Marma points that correspond with the endocrine system, which controls hormonal emissions. Key points targeted included the Adhipati Marma, located on the crown of the head, and the Hridaya Marma, situated over the heart area. These points are thought to influence the pituitary and thymus glands, key regulators of hormonal activity. The treatment involved gentle stimulation of these points combined with the application of specially prepared herbal oils to maximize penetration and therapeutic effects.

Each session was accompanied by dietary recommendations to support hormonal balance and reduce systemic inflammation, along with yoga routines designed to align and strengthen the body's energy pathways. Over several weeks, Simran experienced a noticeable improvement in her symptoms. Her menstrual cycles became more regular, mood swings were less intense, and her skin started to clear up. Further, she reported enhanced energy levels and a greater sense of emotional stability.

This case highlights the potential of Marma Chikitsa to not only alleviate physical symptoms related to hormonal imbalances but also to contribute to emotional and psychological health by restoring the body's natural balance. The therapy's approach in addressing the root causes of hormonal disturbances illustrates its comprehensive impact on health, positioning Marma Chikitsa as an effective integrative treatment within the broader scope of holistic medicinal practices.

Case Study: Cultural Relevance and Modern Adaptation: The Role of Marma Chikitsa in Treating Chronic Stress in Urban Populations

Deepak, a 52-year-old urban planner, approached a well-known Marma Chikitsa practitioner to manage his chronic stress and fatigue, which he attributed to the demanding nature of his job and the pressures of city life. The practitioner evaluated Deepak's lifestyle and stress levels and proposed a comprehensive treatment plan focusing on the Prana-Vayu pathways to address not only the physical but also psychological components of his condition. The treatment began with the identification of significant Marma points known to alleviate stress, specifically the Manya Marma, located near the neck, to relieve tension, and the Hridaya Marma, located over the heart area, to calm emotional disturbances.

Each session included targeted stimulation of these points through gentle pressure and the application of specially formulated herbal oils crafted to penetrate deeply and foster relaxation.

The practitioner also advised Deepak on dietary changes, emphasizing foods that pacify (balance) the Vata dosha—traditionally associated with nervous system activity and the stress response—while recommending daily meditation and yoga exercises tailored to enhance the grounding and calming effects of the treatment. This holistic approach not only addressed the energetic disturbances identified through Marma Chikitsa but also integrated lifestyle modifications essential for sustained relief from stress.

Over several months, Deepak reported a notable decrease in stress symptoms and an improved sense of well-being. The consecutive sessions paved the way for a deeper understanding of his body's energy systems, highlighted by an increased awareness of how environmental and lifestyle factors influenced his Prana distribution. His ability to manage stress improved considerably, which he credited to the personalized nature of the treatment that adeptly combined ancient techniques with modern lifestyle needs. He became an advocate for Marma Chikitsa, highlighting its relevance and adaptability to contemporary health challenges common in urban living. His experience underscored the potent capabilities of Marma Chikitsa in navigating the complexities of modern stressors through a framework that respects both cultural heritage and the necessity for modern scientific approaches.

Case Study: Integrating Marma Chikitsa in Post-Surgical Recovery: A Path to Enhanced Healing

Vikram, a 58-year-old retired army officer, underwent knee replacement surgery following years of debilitating arthritis. Post-surgery, Vikram faced significant challenges in regaining full mobility and managing post-operative pain, common complications that can impede recovery. To complement his conventional rehabilitation, Vikram's physiotherapist suggested integrating Marma Chikitsa into his recovery regimen, intrigued by its potential to accelerate healing and reduce pain.

The Marma therapist conducted a detailed assessment, focusing on points that could potentially enhance joint function and alleviate pain. Key Marma points around the knee and lower leg, such as Janu Marma at the knee and Gulpha Marma at the ankle, were targeted to improve circulation and reduce stiffness. Each session involved gentle stimulation of these points using specific herbal oils known for their anti-inflammatory properties. This approach aimed not only at physical healing but also at restoring the flow of Prana, believed to be crucial in speeding up the recovery process.

In addition to the Marma therapy, Vikram was advised on dietary modifications to reduce inflammation and support joint health. This holistic treatment plan was further supplemented with gentle yoga exercises tailored to his condition, focusing on enhancing joint flexibility and muscle strength. Over the course of several weeks, Vikram observed a notable improvement in his knee flexibility and a substantial reduction in pain levels. His recovery was noticeably quicker compared to his previous orthopedic surgeries, particularly after incorporating Marma Chikitsa.

This case exemplifies how Marma Chikitsa can play a pivotal role in post-surgical contexts, enhancing conventional medical treatments. It illustrates the power of integrating traditional healing practices with modern medicine, offering a comprehensive and multidimensional approach to recovery that addresses both the physiological and energetic aspects of healing.

Case Study: Navigating Mental Health Challenges: A Journey with Marma Chikitsa

Mira, a 34-year-old journalist, found herself grappling with the daunting challenges of anxiety and recurrent mild depressive episodes, particularly exacerbated by the high-pressure environment of her profession. Her journey through various therapies had brought negligible relief, leading her to explore alternative solutions. She was introduced to Marma Chikitsa by a colleague who had seen significant improvements in a similar situation. Fueled by curiosity and the hope of finding a lasting solution, Mira committed to a comprehensive treatment plan with a seasoned Marma therapist.

Initial consultation revealed that Mira's symptoms might be associated with disruptions in her Prana flow, specifically around the heart (Anahata) and head (Adhipati) Marma points, known to influence emotional regulation and mental clarity. The therapist devised a schedule that included bi-weekly sessions focusing on these critical points. Each session began with a gentle cleansing ritual followed by the application of specific herbal oils formulated to calm the mind and balance emotional energy. Through precise stimulation of the Marma points, along with guided breathing exercises to enhance Prana's receptivity, the therapy aimed to restore Mira's emotional and psychological equilibrium.

Several weeks into the treatment, Mira reported a noticeable decrease in her anxiety levels. She observed that her episodes of depression were becoming less frequent and less intense, attributing this change to the newfound balance in her body's energy systems. The therapist also integrated dietary consultations and lifestyle adjustments to support the treatment, focusing on Sattvic foods that promote mental clarity and emotional stability.

By the third month, Mira had developed an enhanced ability to manage stress and experienced a significant improvement in her overall mood and outlook on life. Her journey with Marma Chikitsa was transformative, demonstrating the therapy's profound impact on mental health, beyond just symptom management, to fostering a resilient and balanced emotional state. This case accentuates the integral role of energy balance in mental health and the potential of Marma Chikitsa to serve as a powerful tool in managing complex mental health conditions holistically.

Case Study: Strategic Intervention in Corporate Wellness: Marma Chikitsa for Managing Executive Burnout

Samira, a 42-year-old senior executive at a multinational corporation, had reached the pinnacle of her career, but at the expense of her health. Facing severe burnout, insomnia, and relentless anxiety, she sought a comprehensive, non-pharmacological approach to regain her health and vitality. She was introduced to Marma Chikitsa as part of a corporate wellness initiative aimed at supporting high-performing executives experiencing similar conditions.

The Marma practitioner assigned to Samira conducted an in-depth assessment focusing on her lifestyle, work environment, and specific symptoms. The assessment revealed significant disruptions in Samira's Prana flow, especially within the pathways related to stress response and relaxation. The practitioner pinpointed several critical Marma points, including the Brahmarandhra (the crown of the head) and the Hridaya (the heart area), which are key in regulating emotional balance and circadian rhythms.

Therapy sessions were scheduled twice a week, incorporating the gentle stimulation of identified Marma points using special herbal oils known for their calming properties. Each session included a personalized routine emphasizing the relaxation of the nervous system and rebalancing of Samira's Doshas, particularly addressing the aggravation of Vata, which in Ayurveda is often linked to stress and anxiety.

Parallel to the Marma treatments, the wellness program incorporated Ayurvedic nutrition counseling aimed at strengthening Samira's Agni (digestive fire) and promoting Ojas (vital essence), both of which are deemed essential for combating stress and enhancing overall resilience. Gentle Yoga Asanas and guided meditation practices were also recommended to complement the Marma therapy and facilitate more profound relaxation and mindfulness.

After three months of consistent Marma Chikitsa and adherence to the holistic recommendations, Samira reported a marked improvement in her sleep patterns, a significant reduction in anxiety, and an increased ability to manage workplace stress. Additionally, her overall energy levels improved, which she attributed to the better alignment of her body's natural rhythms and energy flows, highlighting the profound impact of Marma Chikitsa in a corporate wellness context.

Case Study: Revitalizing Fertility and Emotional Well-being: A Case Study on Marma Chikitsa's Holistic Impact

Sunita, a 33-year-old HR professional, had been struggling with fertility issues for several years, which had also led to severe emotional distress and depression. Conventional medical treatments had not yielded successful results, and the side effects compounded her emotional turmoil. Feeling disillusioned and physically drained, she turned to Marma Chikitsa as a last resort, hopeful for a holistic remedy.

An experienced Marma Chikitsa practitioner, Dr. Nanda, first conducted a thorough assessment of Sunita's overall health, lifestyle, medical history, and specific symptoms. He pinpointed that her issues might be linked to an imbalance in the sacral and heart chakras (Muladhara and Anahata), affecting her reproductive health and emotional state. Sunita's treatment plan was designed to stimulate specific Marma points associated with these chakras, notably the Basti (bladder) Marma, which influences the reproductive organs, and the Anahata (heart) Marma, used for emotional healing.

Each treatment session involved precise stimulation of these points followed by the application of herbal oils tailored to enhance reproductive health and soothe the nervous system. Alongside physical Marma therapy, Sunita was prescribed a diet rich in fertility-enhancing foods, stress management techniques including yoga and meditation, and lifestyle changes to support hormonal balance.

After months of dedicated treatment, Sunita reported not only a significant improvement in her emotional state but also welcomed the news of her pregnancy. Her case highlights how Marma Chikitsa addresses the interconnectedness of physical and emotional health, providing a comprehensive approach to treating complex health issues, such as fertility.

The holistic philosophy of Marma Chikitsa recognizes the intricate interplay of physiological, psychological, and spiritual factors that contribute to an individual's overall well-being. In Sunita's scenario, balancing the energy flow not only facilitated her physical healing but also restored her emotional and psychological well-being, illustrating the profound capabilities of Marma Chikitsa.

Case Study: Harmonizing Prana for Enhanced Creativity: The Case of a Visual Artist

Maya, a 40-year-old accomplished visual artist, encountered a significant creative block that was impacting her ability to produce innovative work. This challenge coincided with bouts of insomnia and an overall lack of vitality, which she believed were disrupting her creative flow. In pursuit of a remedy, Maya was introduced to Marma Chikitsa by a fellow artist who credited the practice for revitalizing his own creative energies.

Upon consulting a renowned Marma practitioner, Maya underwent a comprehensive evaluation, which revealed a disbalance in her Vata Dosha, predominantly affecting her mental clarity and the air element, which is crucial for artistic thinking and execution. The practitioner tailored a treatment plan that focused on the Brahmarandhra (crown) and Ajna (forehead) Marma points, which are crucial for enhancing mental focus and imagination. The strategy was to stimulate these points to harmonize the flow of Prana, thereby facilitating cognitive functions and emotional well-being.

Each session began with a calm setting, ensuring Maya was relaxed, followed by the application of softly scented herbal oils. The practitioner delicately stimulated the specific Marma points with gentle pressure, aiming not only for physical relief but also to release energy blockages that were impacting her mental state. This treatment was accompanied by soothing Vedic chants believed to enhance the therapy's effects by resonating with the body's energy vibrations.

As the weeks progressed, Maya reported a noticeable improvement in her sleep patterns and a renewed sense of emotional stability. The continuous Marma Chikitsa sessions evidently enhanced her mind-body connection, leading to bursts of creative insights and an enriched artistic expression evident in her recent works. Her restored creativity was not merely suggestive of a returning artistic acumen but pointed towards a larger, holistic enhancement of her personal and professional life.

This case highlights how Marma Chikitsa's focus on vital points can decisively influence mental faculties and emotional equilibrium, illustrating the utility of traditional practices in addressing challenges of modern professional lives. Maya's journey reaffirms the relevance of Marma Chikitsa in fostering not only physical and emotional health but also enhancing cognitive and creative capacities essential in artistic domains.

Review Questions

1. A 55-year-old woman has been experiencing chronic joint pain and stiffness. She seeks a holistic and non-pharmacological treatment and decides to try Marma Chikitsa. Which category of Marma points should be the focus of her treatment to alleviate her joint-related symptoms, potentially?

A) Mamsa Marma (muscle)
B) Asthi Marma (bone)
C) Sandhi Marma (joint)
D) Sira Marma (blood vessel)

Answer: C

Explanation: For joint pain and stiffness, focusing on Sandhi Marma, which specifically relates to joints, would be most pertinent. Sandhi Marma points are located around joints and help improve joint mobility and reduce stiffness by facilitating the flow of energy, potentially reducing energy blockages that may contribute to pain and restricted movement.

2. During a session of Marma Chikitsa, a practitioner targets the Adhipati Marma located on the crown of the head. What could be the potential impact of stimulating this Marma point?
A) It may enhance digestive functions
B) It might improve respiratory efficiency
C) It could influence the hormonal balance by affecting the pituitary gland
D) It may directly heal muscle injuries
Answer: C
Explanation: The Adhipati Marma, situated at the crown of the head, is closely associated with the pituitary gland, often referred to as the 'master gland' of the body. Stimulating this Marma point could potentially influence the hormonal activities controlled by the pituitary gland, thereby affecting overall hormonal balance and indirectly impacting various physiological functions across the body.

3. A researcher is studying the effects of Marma Chikitsa on the autonomic nervous system. What outcomes might they expect to observe if the therapy is effective?
A) Increased sympathetic nervous system activity
B) Reduction in cognitive functions
C) Activation of the parasympathetic nervous system leading to relaxation
D) Heightened pain sensitivity
Answer: C
Explanation: Marma Chikitsa, through gentle stimulation of specific points, may primarily activate the parasympathetic nervous system. This system is responsible for the body's 'rest and digest' responses. An effective session can lead to a state of relaxation, decreased stress responses, and an overall calming effect on the patient, as opposed to increasing sympathetic activity, which corresponds to the 'fight or flight' response.

4. Comparing Marma Chikitsa with Chinese acupuncture, which statement correctly reflects a difference between these two practices?
A) Marma Chikitsa uses needles while acupuncture does not
B) Acupuncture targets the rebalancing of Qi, while Marma Chikitsa does not involve energy work
C) Marma Chikitsa often includes herbal oils and lifestyle adjustments, unlike acupuncture
D) Acupuncture is limited to physical healing, whereas Marma Chikitsa includes spiritual healing
Answer: C
Explanation: While both Marma Chikitsa and Chinese acupuncture focus on the body's energy systems (Qi in acupuncture and Prana in Marma Chikitsa), a key difference lies in the holistic approach of Marma Chikitsa. It not only involves the stimulation of points but also integrates herbal oils and lifestyle adjustments to enhance treatment efficacy, a component not typically found in acupuncture practices.

5. Considering the role of Marma Chikitsa in traditional Indian culture, which activity might inadvertently involve the stimulation of Marma points?
A) Daily morning self-massage practices
B) Regular consumption of spicy food
C) Listening to classical music
D) Reading traditional Vedic texts
Answer: A

Explanation: In traditional Indian culture, daily self-massage is a common practice that can inadvertently involve stimulating Marma points. The Marma point self-treatment is often incorporated into a daily Yoga practice. This not only enhances prana flow but also sets a vibrant, health-promoting tone for the day. While other options, such as food, music, and reading, have cultural significance, they do not directly involve physical interaction with Marma points.

CHAPTER TWO: Anatomy and Physiology of Marma Points

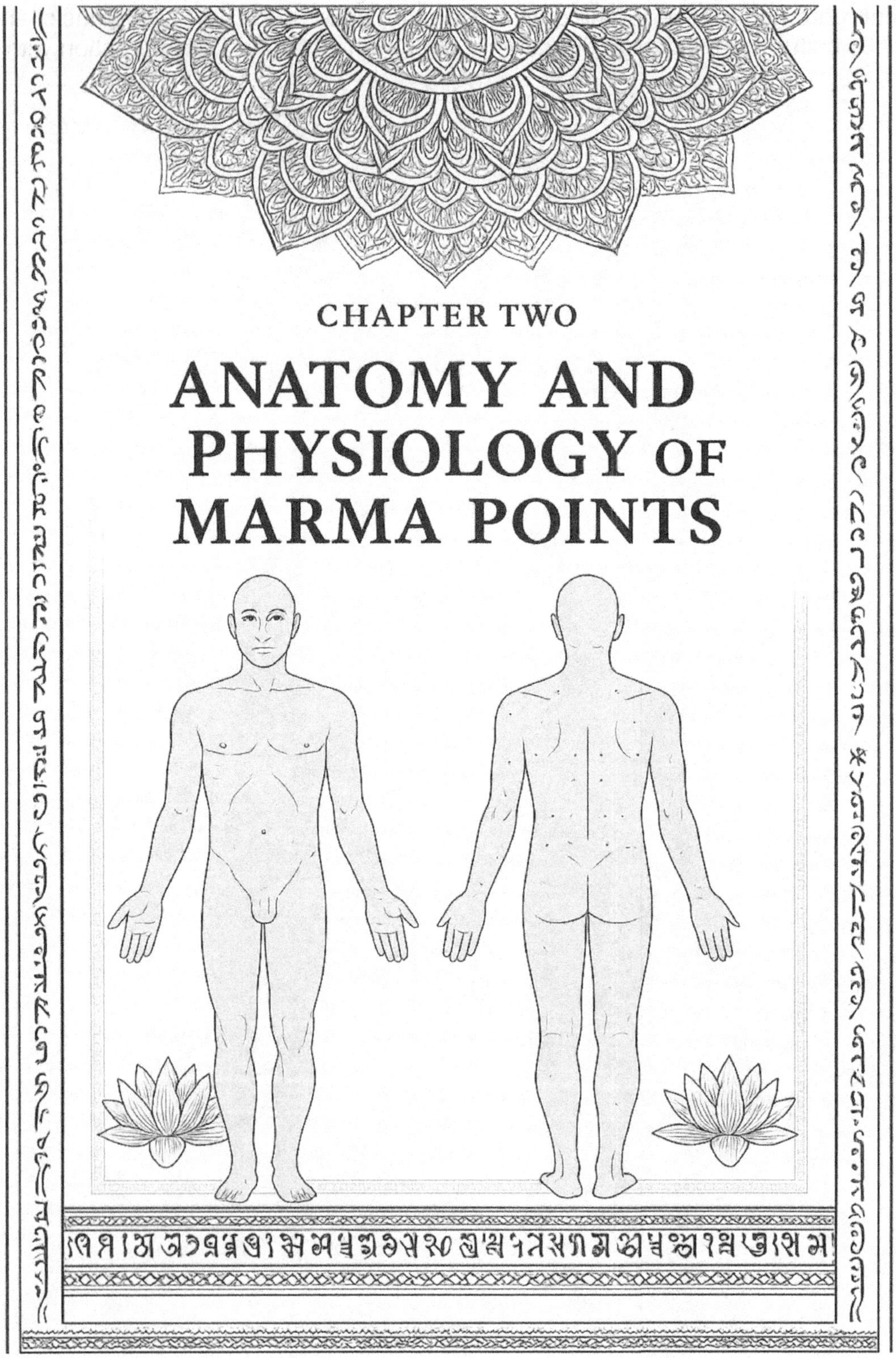

Definition of Marma According to Ayurvedic Physiology

In the realm of Ayurvedic medicine, Marma points are defined as critical life centers or junctures where flesh, veins, arteries, bones, and ligaments converge. Originating from the Sanskrit word 'Marm', meaning mortal, vulnerable, or secret, these points are vital to the body's energetic and physiological well-being.

The Ayurvedic texts, including the Sushruta Samhita, describe these sites not only as physical entities but as pivotal zones of Prana, the life force that circulates through the body, governing psychological and spiritual health. Activation or healing of these points can significantly affect the body's healing processes and overall vitality. Manipulation of these Marmas can free blocked energy, stimulate internal organs, enhance the immune system, and detoxify the body. Appropriately practiced, Marma Chikitsa facilitates the deepest level of healing, integrating the physical, mental, and emotional dimensions of health. Each Marma holds the potential to dramatically shift the body's energy landscapes, offering pathways to profound health improvements and energetic rejuvenation.

Marma Points as Vital Life Junctions

Marma points, the vital life junctions within the Ayurvedic healing system, act as critical nodes where the body's fundamental energies intersect. As junctions, these points are more than mere physical locations; they are pivotal energetic gateways influencing the flow of Prana, or life force, embodying Ayurveda's holistic approach to health and vitality.

Each Marma serves as a nexus for the intersection of muscular, vascular, ligamentous, and bony tissues, integrating these diverse anatomical features to facilitate complex physiological functions. Think of them as circuit breakers in the body's bioelectrical system, where a precise touch can reboot health and restore functional harmony. Their strategic activation can profoundly impact bodily functions, governing everything from hormonal secretions to the functioning of major organ systems. "Marma" as an Ayurvedic Medical term also refers to the segmental construction of the skeleton. The segment between the hip and the knee is a "Marma," and the path is analogous to the length of the Femur bone.

Furthermore, by addressing both the physical and subtle energy bodies, Marma therapy harnesses the potential for deep, integrative healing. This multi-dimensional approach positions Marma points as essential elements in the prevention and treatment of illnesses while promoting an all-encompassing sense of well-being.

Detailed Tissue Classification of the 107 Classical Marma Points

The classification of the 107 classical Marma points in Ayurveda extends beyond mere anatomical locations to encompass detailed insights into various tissue types. Every Marma point intersects specific tissues, including muscles, ligaments, bones, veins, and joints, each contributing to its unique therapeutic properties.

For instance, muscle (Mamsa) Marmas are predominantly involved in movement and force generation, making them crucial in treatments targeting strength and mobility. In contrast, ligaments (Snayu Marmas) aid in joint stabilization and are often the focus in managing flexibility and structural integrity. Bone (Asthi) Marmas resonate particularly with issues of structural support and are vital in addressing postural imbalances.

Adding depth to this understanding, each type of Marma is linked to different bodily functions and energy flows, thereby presenting a holistic approach to treatment. Such detailed classification not only enhances the practitioner's ability to diagnose and treat but also furthers our understanding of the body's interconnected nature.

Sira (Veins) Marma: Vascular Significance and Therapeutic Use

Within the intricate web of Marma points, the Sira (Veins) Marma stand out for their pivotal role in vascular health and energy circulation. These points are strategically positioned to influence the venous system, crucial for the return of deoxygenated blood to the heart, and their stimulation can engender profound shifts in the body's energetic and circulatory dynamics. Therapeutic manipulation of Sira Marmas is used primarily to enhance blood flow, reduce venous congestion, and facilitate the removal of metabolic waste. This is particularly beneficial in conditions like varicose veins and deep vein thrombosis. By enhancing venous return and improving circulation, Marma therapy helps in detoxifying and rejuvenating the body, thereby boosting vitality and energy levels.

The therapeutic applications extend beyond mere physical ailments; they also encompass psycho-emotional benefits such as alleviating stress and anxiety, which are often linked to circulatory issues. Therefore, Sira Marmas serve as crucial junctures for both physical and emotional healing, aligning with the holistic principles of Ayurvedic medicine.

Snayu (Ligament) Marma: Structural Stability and Healing

In Ayurvedic healing, the Snayu (Ligament) Marma points are pivotal in maintaining structural stability and facilitating healing. These specialized points are strategically located at key ligament sites across the body, serving as essential connectors that reinforce joint stability. The health and functionality of ligaments are crucial, as they support and bind joints, ensuring smooth and safe movement patterns.

When these Marma points are stimulated, they enhance the inherent healing capabilities of ligaments, promoting quicker recovery from injuries and strengthening the connective tissues. Ayurvedic practices, such as applying herbal oils and gentle pressure, stimulate these points to decrease inflammation and alleviate pain, which is often linked to ligament strains or sprains. Furthermore, this stimulation helps to balance the flow of Prana, aiding in the overall vitality and functionality of the musculoskeletal system. One way to think of the term “balance” is that it is defined as a functional homeodynamic equilibrium or stasis.

Moreover, through the lens of Ayurveda, Snayu Marmas play a crucial role in preventing joint stiffness and maintaining flexibility. Regular Marma therapy can profoundly impact not only physical health but also enhance the body's resilience to stress and fatigue. These practices are integral to a holistic approach, emphasizing not only recovery but also sustained health and the prevention of further injuries. It is also thought to reduce the inclinations that lead to such injuries in the first place. These inclinations or oversights could be mental, emotional or spiritual in origin.

Asthi (Bone) Marma: Role in Postural Alignment and Pain

Beneath the intricate system of Marma points, the Asthi Marmas (Bone Points) emerge as crucial components for structural alignment and pain modulation. These unique Marma sites are located at strategic points on the skeleton, exerting a potent influence over skeletal stability and posture. The accurate stimulation of these points can correct misalignments and alleviate pain, providing a foundation for improved bodily function and enhanced movement efficiency.
In-depth knowledge of Asthi Marmas helps Ayurvedic practitioners harness the flow of energy through skeletal structures. This facilitates not only physical alignment but also alleviates compressive stress on bones, often a hidden contributor to chronic pain scenarios. The interplay between bone Marmas and the body's weight-bearing capabilities illuminates pathways for mitigating discomfort and enhancing endurance.
Moreover, engagement with these Marma points fosters a renewed synergy between the musculoskeletal system (maha Nadi) and the broader network of bodily energies (prana nadi and Chakra). This alignment is pivotal not only in addressing immediate structural and pain issues but also in ensuring long-term health and vitality.

Sandhi (Joint) Marma: Mobilization, Arthritis, and Flexibility

The Sandhi (Joint) Marma points are pivotal sites for enhancing joint mobility and addressing ailments such as arthritis. These points, located at junctions where two or more bones meet, play a critical role in the Ayurvedic practice of ensuring smooth and flexible movement. Stimulation of these Marma points can lead to significant improvements in joint health, promoting flexibility and easing the stiffness associated with arthritic conditions.
Through purposeful manipulation of the Sandhi Marma, practitioners facilitate the movement of Vata energy, which is often implicated in joint diseases. This energetic modulation helps lubricate and nourish the joints, thereby reducing pain and enhancing range of motion. Such treatments not only target the physical symptoms but also aim to rectify energetic imbalances, contributing to overall joint health and functionality.
Moreover, regular Marma therapy, focusing on these joint points, can help prevent the degeneration of joint tissues and maintain long-term mobility and joint integrity. By incorporating Marma therapy into their regular health routines, individuals can achieve a more dynamic and pain-free life, aligning with Ayurveda's holistic approach to wellness.

Mamsa (Muscle) Marma: Muscle Healing and Strength Recovery

Mamsa (Muscle) Marma points are integral to Ayurvedic therapies aimed at enhancing muscle healing and recovery of strength. These points, strategically distributed within the muscle tissue, serve as catalysts for enhancing muscular health and vitality. Being central to locomotion and bodily strength, these Marmas are often targeted in Ayurvedic practices to hasten recovery from muscle strains or injuries.
When stimulated, Mamsa Marmas facilitate the natural healing process by enhancing blood circulation and promoting the removal of toxins. This not only helps in repairing damaged muscle fibers but also accelerates the recovery of muscular strength. Additionally, such stimulation supports the restoration of Prana (life energy), which is crucial for muscle function and resilience.

Furthermore, regular Marma therapy that targets these muscular points can prevent muscle atrophy and fatigue, significantly enhancing an individual's physical capabilities. This is particularly beneficial for athletes or those engaged in physically demanding jobs. By maintaining muscle integrity and energy flow, Mamsa Marma therapy plays a pivotal role in holistic health and sustained physical wellness.

Marma Points and the Tridosha Theory

In Ayurvedic medicine, the intersection of Marma points and the Tridosha theory encapsulates a profound layer of healing intelligence. The three doshas — Vata, Pitta, and Kapha — govern physiological activity and are believed to be influenced through specific Marma points. Stimulating these Marma points can effectively balance Vata, which regulates movement; Pitta, which oversees metabolism and energy production; and Kapha, which sustains fluid balance and physical structure.

The three doshas originate on a spiritual plane from the basic mental confusion that produces subject-object dualism. The main concept of "what is health" is seen as one of balance, balance within the physical body and balance between it and its corresponding aspects in the outer world. This balance is seen and expressed in the harmonious relationship of and between the three doshas. This subject /object dualism produces the karmic force necessary to manifest life and the perceived universe.

The literal translation of the word Dosha can be a constitution. According to Ayurvedic physician Dr. Sharadini Dahanukar in his book "Ayurveda Unveiled", states "The word dosha is derived from the root "dus", like the English prefix 'dys' (as in dysfunctiona, dysmeorrhoea). If directly translated, the word dosha would mean fault, stain, transgression against the cosmic rhythm, or an inaccuracy that leads to chaos. However, in the context of Ayurvedic philosophy, the doshas are not inherently harmful. Rather, they seem to be called doshas, for they can cause chaos or disease under certain circumstances... It is this intricate relationship between the troika-dosha-dhatu-mala that constitutes the foundation for the principles of Ayurvedic physiology, pathology, and therapeutics." (Ayurveda Unveiled, Dr. Sharadini Dahanukar & Urmilla Thatte, National Book Trust, India, 1996, p. 14)

It can also be wind, thus making your Dosha your Humor (Wind) type, or how the elements manifest as wind in you. The ultimate origin of the dosha is the encapsulated ego or the Ahamka, manifesting as three personalities, personality inclinations, or ego constructs. The dominance of these elements determines, literally, our mechanical faults or our inherent inclination towards strength or weakness.

Each Marma point is viewed as a conduit for the Doshi energies, where targeted therapy can help amend dosha imbalances, thereby fostering the prevention, management, or reversal of disease. For instance, Marma points correlated with Vata are crucial in treating neurological and movement disorders. Similarly, points associated with Pitta can be utilized to optimize digestion and metabolic processes, while Kapha-linked points enhance respiratory and structural functions.

One perspective is that the body surface itself is viewed as a "touch screen," where energy, attention, consciousness, breath, and pressure on Marma points cause changes in the state of spirit, mind, and body, specifically according to the location and combination of specific points. This viewpoint or philosophy of practice found in Ayurveda views the person holistically, as part of the environment, and considers all the energies and their influence. Every part of the person is seen to connect inextricably with every other part. This is one of the theories that justify a

particular type of stimulation being able to positively affect the function of all body systems, including the functions of the mind and emotions.
This synergy between Marma points and the Tridosha theory enhances the holistic nature of Ayurveda, allowing for nuanced interventions tailored to individual health needs. Through this intricate understanding, Marma Chikitsa not only addresses symptoms but also deeply nurtures the root causes of health issues, aligning body, mind, and spirit.

Mapping Marma Points Along Major Organ Systems

Marma points, integral to Ayurvedic anatomy, strategically interface with major organ systems, orchestrating a comprehensive modulation of physiological functions. These points, identified in classical texts, serve not merely as physical entities but as dynamic energy portals that influence organ health.
The mapping of Marma points is meticulously aligned with the layout of vital organs, including the heart, lungs, liver, and kidneys. This strategic placement ensures that each point, when stimulated, exerts a direct influence over the corresponding organ, thereby enhancing its function and resilience. For instance, heart-related Marma points aid in regulating cardiovascular activities, whereas those linked to the liver support detoxification processes. The holistic approach fosters an environment that is conducive to healing and restoring vitality. Furthermore, integrating this mapping with traditional practices amplifies its therapeutic potency. Techniques such as precise pressure application and herbal medicaments tailored to specific organs through their respective Marma points optimize health outcomes and fortify the body's natural defenses against ailments.

Correlation of Marma with Endocrine Glands and Neurocenters

The subtle and intricate relationship between Marma points and the body's endocrine glands and neurocenters unveils a profound avenue for therapeutic interventions in Ayurveda. These Marma points, serving as vital energy junctions, interact closely with the hormonal and nervous systems, influencing physiological and emotional states.
For example, specific Marma points located near the pituitary and pineal glands can modulate hormonal activities that govern growth, metabolism, and sleep cycles. Stimulation of these points can lead to the enhanced secretion of vital hormones, thereby fostering overall health and balance. Similarly, Marma points in proximity to major neural pathways can help regulate neuronal activity and response, offering benefits for neural health and cognitive functions. Such therapeutic approaches underscore the capacity of Marma Chikitsa to integrate bodily functions at a systemic level. By bridging the gap between physical touch and biochemical responses, these treatments promote healing and vitality, aligning the endocrine and nervous systems in a harmonious operational flow. This holistic interaction magnifies the scope of Marma therapy, positioning it as a keystone in the intricate architecture of Ayurvedic healing.

Anatomical Layers and Depth of Each Marma

Marma points, nestled at varying depths within the anatomical layers, offer a window into the Ayurvedic secrets of energy flow and therapeutic touch. Delving into these depths reveals how each Marma interacts across the skin, fascia, muscles, and bones, residing sometimes superficially and at times more deeply, near vital organs. The profundity of placement is key, dictating the specificity and effectiveness of Marma therapy.

Understanding these layers concerning each Marma point is vital for effective stimulation, ensuring that therapeutic maneuvers reach the intended depth. Practitioners are trained to discern the subtle differences in tissue resistance, which guides them in applying the correct pressure and enhancing healing efficacy. This deep engagement not only targets the physical manifestation of imbalances but also aligns the Pranic flow, essential for holistic healing.

Moreover, the strategic depth of Marmas correlates with their physiological influence—superficial Marmas tend to affect skin and blood flow, while deeper points impact organs and structural integrity. This nuanced comprehension enables the development of tailored therapeutic strategies, harnessing the full potential of Marma Chikitsa.

When considering the potential impact of stimulating Maram points, there is modern Western scientific research and understanding mainly located in the “neuroscience” fields that support the profound implications of the effects of Marma Therapy. The neurological connections between superficial skin points and underlying tissues involve a complex interplay of sensory, autonomic, and neuroimmune mechanisms. Here is a structured analysis of these principles:

1) Cutaneous Innervation and Neuropeptide Signaling
2) The epidermis and dermis contain a dense network of sensory nerves (unmyelinated C-fibers and thinly myelinated Aδ fibers) that release neuropeptides like substance P and calcitonin gene-related peptide (CGRP). These nerves:
    a) Terminate as free nerve endings in the epidermis, directly interacting with keratinocytes, Langerhans cells, and melanocytes.
    b) Modulate local immune responses, inflammation, and cell growth via neuropeptide release.
    c) Activate axon reflexes, where collaterals from sensory nerves innervate blood vessels and appendages (e.g., sweat glands), enabling rapid communication between skin layers.
3) Dermal-Hypodermal Connections
4) In the deeper dermis and hypodermis:
    a) Sympathetic autonomic nerves regulate blood flow via arteriovenous plexuses and control thermoregulation through sweat glands and arrector pili muscles.
    b) Sensory nerves extend into subcutaneous fat, forming a three-dimensional network that responds to mechanical and chemical stimuli.
5) Bone and Periosteal Innervation
6) Bone tissue receives innervation via:
    a) Sensory nerves expressing TrkA receptors, which respond to nerve growth factor (NGF) and cluster near remodeling surfaces in the periosteum and bone marrow.
    b) Sympathetic nerves that influence bone metabolism and vascular tone.
    c) Neuropeptides (e.g., CGRP) that regulate osteoblast and osteoclast activity, linking cutaneous signals to bone adaptation.
7) Systemic Neuroimmunoendocrine Integration
    a) The skin-bone axis is part of a broader neuroendocrine network:
    b) Cutaneous nerves communicate with the central nervous system (CNS) via spinal pathways, modulating systemic inflammation and pain perception.
    c) Stress-induced neuropeptides (e.g., cortisol, catecholamines) from the adrenal glands or immune cells can affect both skin homeostasis and bone remodeling.
    d) Sensory neurons in the skin interact with stem cells (e.g., hair follicle stem cells) and immune cells (e.g., mast cells), coordinating tissue repair and immune surveillance.

8) Clinical Implications
    a) Inflammatory skin diseases (e.g., psoriasis) show increased epidermal nerve density and neuropeptide-driven inflammation, which may exacerbate bone loss in conditions like osteoporosis [1][4].
    b) Small fiber neuropathies disrupt intraepidermal nerve fibers, impairing wound healing and altering bone turnover.
9) This multilayered connectivity underscores the skin's role as a neuroimmunoendocrine interface, bridging superficial stimuli to deep tissue responses through neural pathways, signaling molecules, and systemic feedback loops.

Neurovascular Bundles and Marma Location Accuracy

Understanding the meticulous placement of Marma points in relation to neurovascular bundles is crucial for maximizing therapeutic efficacy in Marma Chikitsa. These bundles, composed of nerves and blood vessels, are significant conduits of energy and information throughout the body. Accurate localization of Marma points near these bundles enhances the stimulation's impact on the nervous and circulatory systems.

This precision yields more effective therapeutic outcomes, including improved blood circulation and enhanced nerve function, which are crucial for overall health and recovery. Expert practitioners of Marma Chikitsa employ various techniques, including palpation and anatomical mapping, to locate these critical points with high accuracy. Their skill ensures that the applied therapy directly interfaces with the neurovascular architecture, amplifying the treatment's effectiveness.

Furthermore, the integration of modern imaging techniques, such as MRI scanning, with traditional knowledge refines the accuracy of Marma point localization. This synergy between ancient wisdom and contemporary technology not only bolsters the confidence in Marma therapy but also expands its application in modern therapeutic contexts, potentially offering new avenues for pain management and neurovascular health.

Marma Zones: Head, Neck, Chest, Abdomen, Limbs

Marma Zones categorize the body into regions, each harnessing pivotal Marma points critical for administering energy and therapeutic interventions. The head zone, encompassed by points that concentrate on cognitive and sensory functions, provides pathways for alleviating mental stress and enhancing sensory perceptions. These are traditionally stimulated to relieve headaches, improve vision, and balance cerebral functionalities.

The neck and chest zones encapsulate Marma points that oversee respiratory and cardiovascular functions. Stimulating these zones can help alleviate throat discomfort, improve lung capacity, and stabilize heart rhythms. Practices in these zones are integrated into routines aimed at strengthening the voice, ensuring efficient breathing, and toning the heart.

In contrast, the abdomen zone focuses on digestive health, with Marma points that are meticulously targeted to optimize gastrointestinal functions and strengthen the core vitality. Limb zones address mobility and structural health, influencing everything from joint function to muscular recovery, crucial for physical stability and movement efficacy. These delineated zones collectively form a comprehensive map for Marma Chikitsa practitioners, embodying the quintessence of therapeutic precision and holistic treatment.

External and Internal Marmas: Functional Differentiation

Marma points, integral elements of Ayurvedic medicine, are categorized into external and internal types, each serving distinct functional purposes. External Marmas are accessible on the body's surface and are primarily engaged for immediate relief of pain and to enhance blood circulation. These points are frequently targeted in therapeutic massages and are easier to manipulate due to their superficial location, making them pivotal in daily Ayurvedic practice for quick and effective treatment.

In contrast, internal Marmas are situated deeper within the body and are associated with the vital organs and deeper bodily functions. Their stimulation affects the body's core systems, including digestive, respiratory, and neurological functions. The treatment of internal Marmas requires greater precision and a deeper understanding of the body's anatomy, as improper handling can lead to adverse effects.

Thus, the differentiation in the functionality and handling of external and internal Marma points underscores their significance in Ayurvedic therapy. By addressing both the superficial and profound layers of human physiology, Marma Chikitsa provides a comprehensive approach to healing and well-being.

Precise Coordinates and Palpation of Marma Sites

Unlocking the precision in Marma Chikitsa requires a deep understanding of the exact coordinates and palpation techniques for Marma sites. These ancient points, pivotal in Ayurvedic healing, are meticulously mapped to ensure that each therapeutic touch resonates deeply with the body's innate energy circuits, thereby optimizing healing and revitalization. Skilled practitioners employ palpation, a touch-based technique, to identify the subtle energies and locate these points with high accuracy.

The act of palpation not only affirms the position but also gauges the energetic condition of the Marma site, enabling tailored treatments that are coherent with the individual's unique bodily and energetic constitution. Each point's precise coordinates are based on traditional Ayurvedic anatomical knowledge, which has been refined in conjunction with contemporary practices to ensure the efficacy and safety of treatments.

Through focused palpation, practitioners can manipulate these coordinates, fostering a profound interaction between their touch and the body's energy pathways. This interaction is crucial for ameliorating ailments and restoring vitality, making the precision of these practices essential for effective Marma Chikitsa.

Charts describing the locations of the Marma points on the Pranic pathways, Prana Nadis (Sip Sen in Thai Ayurveda), have been published and distributed among Ayurveda practitioners for centuries.

Role of Connective Tissue Fascia in Marma Activation

In Marma Chikitsa, the connective tissue fascia plays a critical role in the activation and efficacy of Marma therapy. This extensive network of fibrous tissue envelops and connects muscles, bones, and organs, providing both structural support and a conduit for vital energies. When Marma points are stimulated, the fascial pathways facilitate the spread of therapeutic effects across the body's systems.

The manipulation of Marmas influences the fascial tension and relaxation, thereby modulating the physiological functions linked through this intricate web. As practitioners apply targeted pressure, the responsive fascia can transmit healing signals deeper into the body, impacting well beyond the immediate location of the Marma point. This is crucial for addressing systemic imbalances and promoting overall well-being.

Additionally, the dynamic nature of fascia as a sensory organ allows it to respond uniquely to different pressures and stimuli applied during Marma therapy. This responsiveness is crucial for developing customized treatment approaches that adapt to individual patient needs and enhance overall therapeutic outcomes.

Somatic-Emotional Holding Patterns in Marma Regions

Marma Chikitsa not only addresses physical ailments but also delves into the somatic-emotional landscape of an individual, where emotional traumas and psychological stresses manifest physically in specific Marma regions. These holding patterns are zones where emotional tensions accumulate, causing blockages in the flow of prana, or life energy, which can result in pain or dysfunction.

The body's response to emotional stress can be observed as stiffness or discomfort at these Marma points. Practitioners of Marma Chikitsa apply techniques to release these blockages, thereby facilitating emotional release and alleviating related physical symptoms. This approach integrates the understanding of the neurovascular and fascial interactions discussed in previous sections, providing a holistic treatment that addresses both mind and body.

In modern Ayurveda and Yoga Therapy practices, such as those seen in SomaVeda Integrated Traditional Therapies® and Thai Yoga Therapy, Marma Points associated with specific emotional, psychological, mental, or physical distress or illness are referred to as "Armored Points." These "Armored Points" are local storage or focal points relating to specific historical traumas inculcated in the tissue, which are layered into the tissue over time. By bringing a practical focus to these local or specific points, relief occurs. As the points soften, the symptoms of psychological trauma and distress reduce. Systems such as Emotional Liberation Technique, EFT, SomaVeda® BET, and Energy Psychology are using point stimulation protocols successfully as functional alternatives to conventional drug-based therapies.

Identifying and treating somatic-emotional holding patterns requires a nuanced understanding of the interconnectedness of emotions and physical health. By applying targeted pressure to these critical points, Marma therapy facilitates a release, promoting healing and emotional well-being.

Surface Anatomy and Palpation Techniques

Exploring the surface anatomy within Marma Chikitsa involves mastering the art of palpation—a tactile method essential for accurately locating vital Marma points on the body's landscape. By delicate palpation, practitioners discern the subtle contours and textures of the skin and underlying structures, an expertise that facilitates the precise application of therapeutic techniques. This sensitivity enables the recognition of nuanced variations in tissue resilience, which reflect the health and energetic status of the Marma points.

The technique of palpation is not merely about physical touch but involves a synchronized dance of perception and response: the hands listen to the body's silent language, interpreting whispers of distress or harmony within the tissues. Each Marma site, when palpated correctly, reveals its unique texture, temperature, and tissue response, guiding the practitioner's actions to

promote healing and pain relief.
Accurate palpation is crucial for targeted Marma therapy, ensuring that interventions are not only safe but also effectively tailored to individual physiological and energetic needs. Training in these techniques allows practitioners to engage deeply with the physical and subtle energies of the body, channeling through Marma points, to restore balance and revitalize health.

Common Injuries Involving Marma Locations

Marma points, crucial nodes within the Ayurvedic therapeutic system, are not just centers for healing but also susceptible zones for injuries. Common injuries involving these vital points often stem from physical trauma, repetitive stress, or inadvertent intense pressure during activities.
Physical impacts, such as falls or direct blows, can disrupt the energy flow at these sites, leading to pain, swelling, or decreased function. Similarly, repetitive activities that strain the local Marma points, like those in the wrists or shoulders, can lead to conditions akin to carpal tunnel syndrome or rotator cuff injuries. These injuries are particularly challenging as they involve essential nodes of energy and physical function intersecting.
Treatment of such injuries through Marma Chikitsa not only focuses on alleviating localized pain but also aims to restore the systemic balance disrupted by the trauma. Proper stimulation of the affected Marma points can hence expedite healing, reduce pain, and restore functionality, emphasizing the interconnectedness of body energies in maintaining overall health.

MRI and Imaging Correlation with Marma Mapping

The integration of modern imaging technologies, such as MRI (Magnetic Resonance Imaging), with the ancient practice of Marma mapping offers a revolutionary perspective in Ayurvedic medicine. By employing MRI, practitioners can now visualize the anatomical precision of Marma points, verifying their locations against the classical texts. This correlation not only confirms the ancient wisdom embedded in Marma Chikitsa but also enhances the accuracy of diagnoses and therapeutic interventions.
MRI provides a detailed view of the internal structures surrounding the Marma points, including muscles, bones, nerves, and blood vessels. This capability is crucial for understanding the complex interactions at these energy junctions, particularly in terms of how they influence physiological and energetic pathways. Imaging studies help in identifying the impact of Marma manipulation on these structures, leading to more targeted and effective treatments.
Furthermore, the use of imaging establishes a bridge between traditional practices and contemporary medical science, fostering a deeper acceptance and integration of Marma Chikitsa within modern healthcare paradigms. This symbiosis not only enhances the credibility of Marma therapy but also expands the scope of its application in pain management, rehabilitation, and holistic wellness.

Brain-Marma Integration: Points on the Head and CNS

In the intricate realm of Marma Chikitsa, the Brain-Marma Integration focuses on the head and central nervous system (CNS), areas rich with vital Marma points that are instrumental in governing physiological and psychological functions. These points act as bridges, linking the central nervous system (CNS) with the body's subtle energy channels, influencing everything from cognitive processes to emotional stability.

Stimulation of these head-centered Marma points affects neurotransmitter production, neural pathways, and systemic circulation, which in turn can enhance mental clarity, relieve stress, and even mitigate neurological symptoms. Techniques used in their activation vary from gentle touches to specific pressures, designed to initiate healing responses not only within the central nervous system (CNS) but throughout the entire body.

Understanding and applying Brain-Marma integration involves a deep dive into neuroanatomy and energy pathways, enabling practitioners to skillfully influence the complex systems of the central nervous system (CNS). This knowledge allows for the development of targeted therapies that are finely tuned to promote overall neurological health and emotional well-being, making this practice a cornerstone of holistic healing in Ayurveda.

Heart-Marma Points and the Cardiovascular Interface

Heart-Marma Points represent a critical aspect of Marma Chikitsa, directly influencing cardiovascular health. These specific points are strategically located to modulate cardiac function, enhancing blood circulation and stabilizing heart rhythms. Activation of these points is believed to invoke subtle energy shifts, which facilitate the heart's energetic balance and physiological performance.

Traditional practices describe the heart as not only a physical entity but also an emotional and spiritual center. Therefore, Marma therapy targeting heart points integrates physical treatments with emotional healing, aiming to release emotional blockages that may manifest as cardiovascular ailments. This approach aligns with the holistic nature of Ayurveda, viewing the heart as pivotal to overall vitality.

Clinically, stimulating Heart-Marma points can lead to improved myocardial efficiency and reduced cardiac stress. This is complemented by a decrease in emotional stress, further promoting cardiovascular health. The delicate application of Marma techniques at these points thereby supports both the emotional state and the physical heart, illustrating the profound integration of body and mind within Ayurvedic medicine.

Gut-Brain Axis and Abdominal Marma Points

The fascinating interplay between the gut and the brain, mediated through Abdominal Marma points, highlights a cornerstone of Marma Chikitsa. These points, located strategically around the abdomen, facilitate communication pathways between the digestive system and the central nervous system (CNS), embodying the Ayurvedic principle that the gut acts as a 'second brain'.

Stimulation of these Marma points can influence gastrointestinal functions, modulate stress responses, and enhance overall emotional well-being. The technique not only supports digestion but also leverages the gut-brain axis to address issues such as anxiety and depression, which are often correlated with gastrointestinal disturbances. This holistic approach views the abdomen not merely as a site of physical processes but as a pivotal arena for psycho-physiological health.

Integrating gut-centric Marma therapy within broader treatment protocols may help synchronize the gut flora and CNS activities, promoting a balanced mental state and efficient digestive health. Such practices underscore the profound interconnectedness of human physiology in

Marma Chikitsa, reiterating its relevance in contemporary holistic healthcare.

Reproductive Health and Marma Activation in the Pelvic Region

Marma Chikitsa's enhancement of reproductive health through activation in the pelvic region represents a profound utilization of ancient Ayurvedic practices in maintaining wellness. The points located in this area, such as the Basti Marma, directly influence reproductive organs, facilitating hormonal balance and promoting fertility. Their stimulation supports the body's natural cycles and healing capacities, offering a non-invasive pathway to enhance reproductive function.

The techniques employed to activate these Marma points include gentle pressure, massage, and the application of medicated oils, each method tailored to the individual's specific needs. This personalized approach is crucial in addressing reproductive health issues such as menstrual irregularities, impotence, and pelvic pain. Furthermore, these practices are not solely about physical health but also involve the emotional and spiritual well-being of the individual, recognizing the interconnectedness of all these aspects in reproductive fitness.

By integrating the Marma knowledge with modern holistic care, therapies targeting pelvic Marma points serve not only as interventions but as preventive measures. This underscores their role in a comprehensive health strategy, optimizing not just reproductive health but overall vitality.

Hormonal Modulation via Marma Point Therapy

Marma Chikitsa provides a unique therapeutic approach to regulating hormonal health through specific Marma points. These points, strategically located throughout the body, serve as gateways to directly influence endocrine function. By applying targeted pressure or manipulation, Marma therapy can stimulate organs to optimize their hormonal outputs. This natural regulation plays a crucial role in maintaining homeostasis and supporting overall vitality.

Hormonal imbalances are often at the root of various health issues such as stress, diabetes, and thyroid problems. Marma point therapy addresses these disruptions by enhancing the body's innate ability to balance hormone production and secretion. For instance, stimulating points near the thyroid may help modulate thyroxine levels, aiding in the treatment of hypothyroid or hyperthyroid conditions.

Furthermore, the integration of Marma therapy into daily wellness routines is considered a preventive measure to maintain hormonal balance. It is a subtle yet powerful complement to conventional treatments, offering a holistic approach to health that aligns with the principles of Ayurveda. By fostering a deeper connection between body and mind, Marma point therapy enhances the systemic harmony essential for optimal health.

Nerve Plexuses and Marma Overlap

The intersection of Nerve Plexuses and Marma points unveils another profound layer of Ayurvedic healing, showcasing how these vital energy spots are intrinsically linked to the complex network of nerves. By aligning Marma therapy with the anatomical positioning of nerve plexuses, practitioners can access deeper physiological responses and promote nerve health,

thereby enhancing overall body function.
Interestingly, Marma points situated near major nerve junctions serve as gateways for manipulating bodily energies. Activation of these points can alter neural signals, potentially alleviating pain and improving neuromuscular coordination. This strategic engagement with nerve plexuses underlines the capability of Marma Chikitsa to impact the nervous system through both direct and indirect stimulation.
With a holistic approach, interventions focus not only on symptom relief but also on underlying nerve health, fostering a better connection between nervous and energetic systems. Such practices reinforce the body's resilience, attuning the flow of life energy to sustain wellness.

Myofascial and Musculoskeletal Marma Interactions

The interconnection between the myofascial and musculoskeletal systems with Marma points forms a fascinating sphere of Ayurvedic practice. These Marma points, pivotal in their role, integrate deeply with the myofascial tissues, illustrating a direct pathway to influence musculoskeletal health. Activation of these points can alleviate musculoskeletal strain and improve structural alignment, thereby enhancing overall physical stability and mobility.
By targeting myofascial structures connected to these specific Marmas, therapists can manipulate bioenergetic and biomechanical dynamics across the musculoskeletal system. This method effectively addresses chronic pain, enhances muscle recovery, and promotes joint health. It is rooted in the comprehensive understanding that Marma distinctly bridges the physical and subtle energy realms, profoundly influencing bodily functions.
Moreover, these interactions highlight the therapeutic potential of Marma Chikitsa in treating sports injuries and addressing postural corrections. It provides a non-invasive alternative, significant for rehabilitation and preventive care, enriching modern holistic health paradigms with ancient wisdom.

Comparison with Myotherapy and Trigger Points

Marma Chikitsa, while deeply rooted in Ayurvedic traditions, shares intriguing parallels with modern therapeutic approaches such as Myotherapy and the use of trigger points. Both methodologies emphasize the significance of specific points on the body for pain relief and healing, yet they originate from vastly different medical philosophies and historical contexts.
In Myotherapy, trigger points are perceived as tight areas within muscle tissue that cause pain in other parts of the body. These are often treated through techniques such as massage, needling, or the application of pressure, which aim to release these points to alleviate pain and improve functional movement. Conversely, Marma Chikitsa involves not only the physical aspect but also considers the flow of life energy (Prana) through these critical junctions, aiming to restore balance across physical and subtle body layers.
Despite these differences, both approaches effectively address musculoskeletal pain and enhance mobility. An understanding of these techniques reveals how ancient wisdom and modern practices can converge, providing a holistic approach to health that transcends cultures and centuries.

Summary Table: 107 Marma Points and Their Biophysical Role

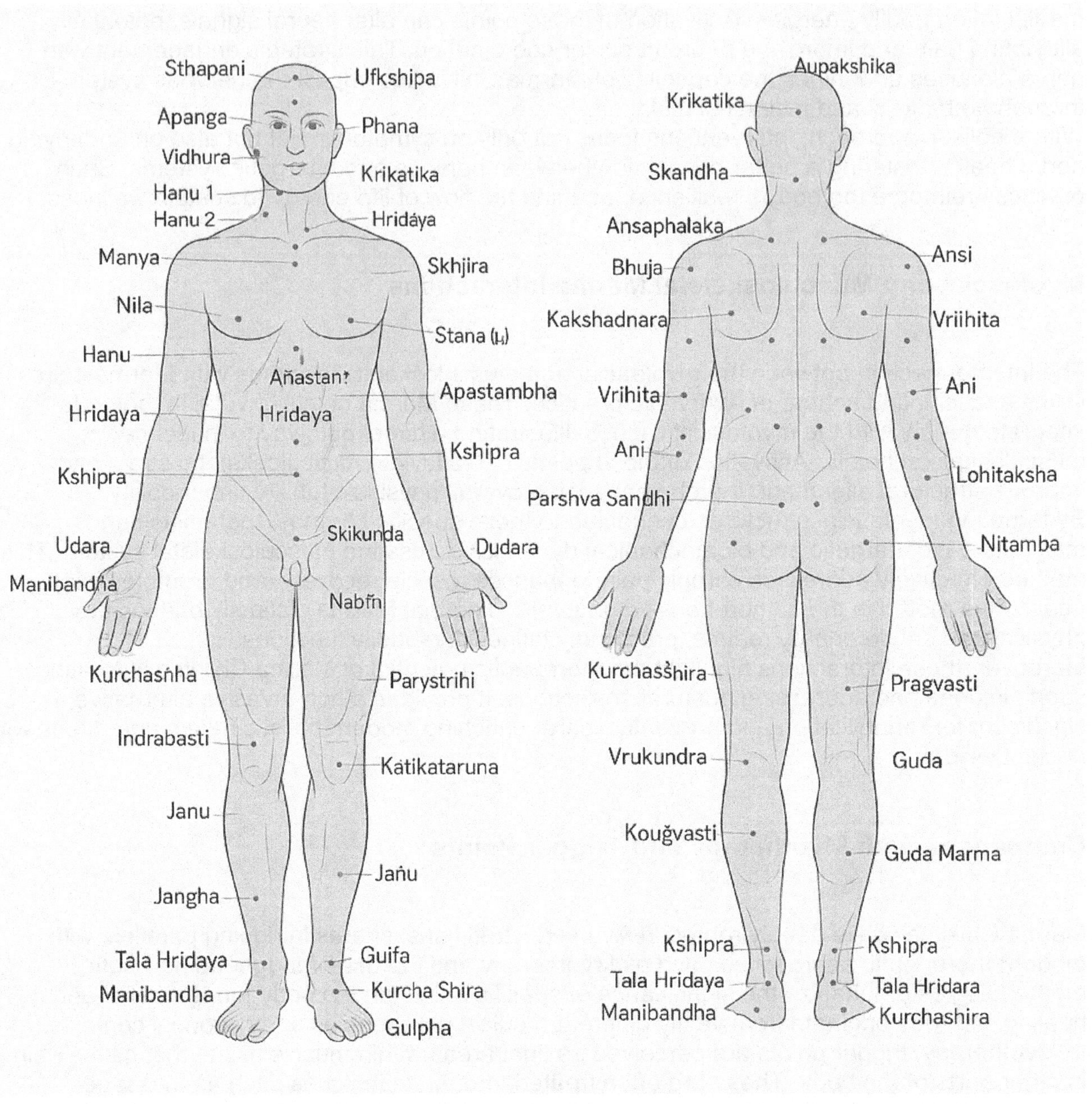

The Summary Table encapsulates the essence of the 107 classical Marma points, each of which is detailed in terms of its physiological and therapeutic significance. Organized meticulously, the table serves not only as a reference but as a profound insight into the biophysical roles that these points play in Marma Chikitsa. Each entry combines anatomical precision with the subtle nuances of energetic influence, highlighting how these points interact with the body's doshas and dhatus, thereby revealing the intricate relationship between the two. Intended as both a practical guide and an educational resource, this table bridges traditional knowledge with modern investigative findings, such as those from MRI imaging studies, which confirm the specific locations and effects of Marma applications. This integration provides practitioners and learners alike with a robust framework for understanding and effectively applying Marma therapy.

Reflecting the comprehensive scope of previous chapters, the table delineates the interconnectedness of systems, such as the neurovascular, musculoskeletal, and endocrine, through the lens of Marma therapy. Ultimately, it underscores a holistic approach to healing and wellbeing, ensuring a balance across bodily systems through precise, non-invasive techniques.

Summary

Marma points, central to Ayurvedic medicine, are vital energy centers where key structural components converge, including muscles, ligaments, bones, veins, and arteries. These points are not only physical junctures but also pivotal zones for the flow of 'Prana', the life energy essential for physical, psychological, and spiritual health. Activation or manipulation of these points can enhance the body's healing processes, boost immune response, stimulate internal organs, and promote overall detoxification and vitality. The practice of Marma Chikitsa, or therapy, involves precise stimulations of these points to unblock energy, facilitating deep, integrative healing across the body's physical and emotional dimensions. There are 107 classical Marma points, each associated with distinct tissues, including muscles, ligaments, bones, and veins, that contribute uniquely to overall health. For instance, muscle Marmas deal with movement and strength, while ligament Marmas focus on joint stability, and bone Marmas on structural support. This classification aids in precise diagnostic and therapeutic processes, ensuring customized treatment that aligns with individual health needs. Some Marma points are particularly noted for their influence on vascular health, targeting issues like varicose veins and enhancing blood circulation by activating specific vein (Sira) Marmas. Other points impact the nervous system and hormonal balance, illustrating the comprehensive nature of Marma therapy, which extends beyond mere physical healing to encompass emotional and mental health. Additionally, the anatomical depth of each Marma point varies, which is crucial for the effectiveness of the therapeutic techniques used. The precision in their stimulation is essential, guided by palpation techniques that help in identifying the exact location and state of each Marma point. Ultimately, the integration of these points in therapy highlights a holistic approach in Ayurveda, aiming not just to cure symptoms but to nurture the root cause of diseases, thereby aligning and harmonizing the body, mind, and spirit.

References

[1] Frawley, D., & Ranade, S. (2001). Ayurveda Nature's Medicine. https://example.com/frawley-ranade-ayurveda

[2] Lad, V. (1998). Marma Points of Ayurveda: The Energy Pathways for Healing Body, Mind, and Consciousness with a Comparison to Traditional Chinese Medicine. https://example.com/lad-marma

[3] Tripathi, R. M. (2012). Ayurveda and Marma Therapy: Energy Points in Yogic Healing. https://example.com/tripathi-marma-therapy

[4] John Douillard's LifeSpa. https://lifespa.com/marma-points

[5] International Journal of Yoga. https://example.com/international-journal-of-yoga

[6] Yoga Journal - Understanding Marma Points. https://example.com/yoga-journal-marma-points

Case Study: Enhancing Recovery in Post-Stroke Patients Through Marma Therapy

The application of Marma therapy in post-stroke rehabilitation provides a distinctive perspective on the adaptability of Ayurvedic practices in contemporary therapeutic settings. Consider the case of Sunita, a 58-year-old woman who suffered an ischemic stroke, leading to partial paralysis of her right side and mild speech impediments. Traditional rehabilitation strategies focused on physical therapy, speech therapy, and occupational therapy proved beneficial yet progressed slowly, prompting her medical team to integrate Ayurvedic Marma therapy into her treatment plan.

Under the supervision of a certified Ayurvedic practitioner, Sunita began Marma therapy, focusing on specific points believed to improve neurological function and energy flow. Points like Brahmarandhra and Apanga, located on the head, were targeted to enhance cognitive processes and nerve rejuvenation. Additionally, her treatment included stimulation of the Gandha Marma, an essential point on the neck that influences the throat and voice box, aimed at assisting her speech recovery.

The Marma therapy was conducted in conjunction with her conventional treatments, with each session lasting approximately 30 minutes, twice a week. After three months of integrated therapy, Sunita showed remarkable improvements. Her speech clarity improved, and the muscle strength on her affected side increased more rapidly than before. These enhancements were not just physical; Sunita reported feeling less anxious and more positive, highlighting the holistic impact of Marma therapy.

The significant improvements in Sunita's recovery illustrate the potential of incorporating Marma therapy into post-stroke rehabilitation. By focusing on neurovascular bundles and key Marma points, the therapy effectively complements medical treatments, facilitating faster and more comprehensive recovery. This case highlights the importance of interdisciplinary approaches in healthcare, where traditional practices like Marma therapy can play a vital role in modern medical settings, offering a more comprehensive spectrum of care that addresses both physiological and psychological dimensions.

Case Study: Revitalizing Endocrine Health through Marma Therapy

Exploring the efficacy of Marma therapy in addressing hormonal imbalances, we examine the case of Anil, a 42-year-old executive experiencing chronic fatigue, stress, and pre-diabetic symptoms. Despite following a medically recommended lifestyle and medication regimen, Anil's conditions showed minimal improvement, leading his endocrinologist to suggest an integrated approach including Marma therapy.

Anil's treatment began with an assessment by a skilled Ayurvedic practitioner who identified key Marma points related to endocrine function. Special focus was given to the Indrabasti and Nabhi Marmas, which are central to influencing pancreatic function and insulin regulation. Sessions included gentle pressure and specialized herbal oils applied at these points to stimulate and balance his endocrine system. Over eight weeks, Anil received bi-weekly sessions, each complemented by dietary adjustments and stress-reduction techniques based on Ayurvedic principles.

The results were compelling. Within four weeks, Anil reported increased energy levels and a noticeable reduction in stress. Blood tests conducted eight weeks later showed a significant improvement in his blood sugar levels, indicating enhanced pancreatic function and improved glucose management. Additionally, his cortisol levels had stabilized, indicating an improved stress response.

This case illustrates how Marma therapy, when used in conjunction with conventional medical treatments, can significantly enhance endocrine health and overall well-being. By targeting specific Marmas, the treatment addresses both the physical and subtle aspects of health, promoting a comprehensive recovery that encompasses the body's energetic and hormonal landscapes. It suggests an expanded role for Marma therapy in the management of chronic conditions often associated with hormonal imbalances, offering a holistic alternative or complementary option to conventional endocrine treatments.

Case Study: Integrative Marma Therapy for Enhanced Musculoskeletal Recovery

In the holistic practice of Ayurvedic medicine, Marma therapy serves as a critical tool for addressing musculoskeletal ailments, offering an integrative approach to healing and recovery. This case study focuses on Rohan, a 35-year-old software engineer who developed chronic lower back pain, which was diagnosed as lumbar spondylosis. Traditional treatment modalities, including physical therapy and medication, provided only temporary relief. This led his healthcare providers to explore complementary therapies, introducing Marma therapy into his regimen.

An experienced Ayurvedic practitioner identified specific Marma points along Rohan's lower back and legs that correspond to the vertebral column and musculature, which were affecting his condition. These included Kukundara Marma in the pelvic region and Katikataruna Marma near the lumbar area. The therapy sessions involved gentle manipulation of these points with herbal oils, aimed at reducing pain and inflammation while promoting the flow of energy and nerve function.

Over twelve weeks, Rohan underwent weekly Marma therapy sessions, in addition to his ongoing physical therapy. Each session focused on the precise application of pressure and herbal formulations known for their efficacy in treating musculoskeletal disorders. As the weeks progressed, Rohan noted significant reductions in pain and improvements in mobility. His follow-up assessments revealed noticeable improvements in spinal alignment and muscle tension, which contributed to his overall recovery.

The success of Rohan's case underscores the potential of Marma therapy as a complementary strategy in musculoskeletal rehabilitation. By targeting specific Marma points associated with the affected anatomical structures, the treatment not only addressed the physical symptoms but also worked to realign Rohan's energy pathways, leading to sustained improvements. This case reinforces the argument for a multidisciplinary approach to managing chronic conditions, where traditional and modern practices are integrated to achieve optimal health outcomes.

Case Study: Reviving Digestive Health with Targeted Marma Therapy

This case study delves into the application of Marma therapy in treating chronic digestive disorders, using the example of Priya, a 47-year-old woman who suffered from Irritable Bowel Syndrome (IBS) and associated symptoms such as bloating, constipation, and abdominal pain. Despite conventional treatments including medications and dietary modifications, Priya's symptoms persisted, affecting her quality of life and overall well-being. Upon referral to an Ayurvedic practitioner, a holistic approach involving Marma therapy was employed to address her condition.

The practitioner identified specific Marma points that influence the digestive system, primarily the Nabhi (located around the navel) and Annavaha Srotas (along the intestines), which are crucial in regulating gastrointestinal functions. The therapy sessions involved gentle stimulation of these points using herbal oils known for their digestive properties, along with mild pressure techniques to restore the balance of the Vata dosha, which in Ayurvedic medicine is often linked to digestive irregularities. Priya received treatment twice per week for ten weeks, accompanied by Ayurvedic dietary advice tailored to pacify her aggravated Vata.

As the weeks progressed, Priya reported a noticeable decrease in bloating and abdominal pain, with improved bowel regularity. Not only did the Marma therapy help alleviate her physical symptoms, but it also had a calming effect on her emotional state, reducing anxiety and stress, which are known aggravators of IBS. The improved Vata balance also enhanced Priya's energy levels and overall vitality, demonstrating the body's interconnected response to holistic treatments.

This case study exemplifies how Marma therapy can effectively integrate into treatment plans for digestive health, offering a non-invasive option that complements conventional medical practices. By focusing on the energy pathways related to digestive organs and the nervous system, Marma therapy addresses both the symptoms and root causes of digestive disorders, providing a comprehensive approach to health and recovery. This integrative method illustrates the depth of Ayurvedic treatment strategies and their relevance in managing chronic health issues.

Case Study: Strategic Marma Therapy for Chronic Migraine Management

Chronic migraines present a significant challenge in medical management, often requiring a multifaceted treatment approach. This case study explores the impact of Marma therapy on 40-year-old Meera, who has been suffering from chronic migraines for over a decade. Traditional methods, including pharmacological treatments and lifestyle modifications, provided her only partial relief, leading her to seek alternative therapies.

An experienced Ayurvedic practitioner assessed Meera's condition and identified specific Marma points related to the cerebral and neurological subsystems. Points such as Shivarandhra (the top of the head) and Sthapani (the forehead) were targeted, which are traditionally believed to regulate cerebral circulation and alleviate stress, respectively. Each session involved gentle activation of these points with therapeutic oils, thought to release blocked Prana (energy) affecting her head region.

Therapy sessions were scheduled twice weekly and were complemented with Ayurvedic dietary recommendations aimed at pacifying Pitta dosha, commonly associated with heat and believed to trigger or exacerbate migraine symptoms in Ayurvedic medicine. Over three months, Meera experienced a significant reduction in migraine frequency from multiple episodes per week to a couple per month. Additionally, the intensity of pain during each migraine was reported to be notably less severe.

The marked improvement in Meera's condition emphasizes the potential of Marma therapy in managing chronic migraines, suggesting that strategic stimulation of key Marma points may modify the neurovascular functions contributing to migraine pathophysiology. This case serves as a testament to the efficacy of integrating traditional Ayurvedic practices, such as Marma therapy, into modern clinical settings to provide a holistic approach to healthcare, specifically for conditions inadequately controlled by mainstream medicine.

Case Study: Revitalizing Respiratory Health through Marma Therapy in Chronic Asthma Management

Exploring the potential of Marma Therapy in managing chronic respiratory disorders, this case study examines the treatment of Leela, a 54-year-old schoolteacher with a long-standing history of asthma, which commonly manifested in recurrent wheezing, shortness of breath, and reliance on inhaled corticosteroids and bronchodilators. Despite conventional respiratory therapies and medications, Leela's symptoms remained poorly controlled, affecting her quality of life and daily functioning.

Upon discussing integrative treatment approaches with her pulmonologist, Leela was referred to an Ayurvedic practitioner specializing in Marma Therapy. Initial assessments focused on identifying distinct Marma points that could potentially revitalize her respiratory health. Specific attention was given to the Kshipra Marma points located between the thumb and index finger, the Urvi Marma in the thigh region, and the Anahata Marma around the chest area—all believed to directly influence respiratory dynamics and energy pathways.

Treatment sessions were conducted weekly, involving gentle stimulation of these Marma points with therapeutic oils conducive to respiratory health. Leela's treatment plan also incorporated breathing exercises designed to complement the Marma stimulation, aiming to improve lung capacity and alleviate breathing difficulties. Over the course of ten weeks, Leela reported marked improvements in her breathing patterns, reduction in asthma attacks, and a decreased dependence on her inhaler.

By addressing both the physical and the subtle energy aspects of respiratory health, Marma Therapy provided Leela with a holistic treatment option that complemented her conventional medical treatments. This integrative approach not only improved her respiratory function but also positively impacted her emotional and psychological well-being, reducing anxiety linked to her asthma symptoms. Leela's case highlights the potential of Marma points in managing chronic conditions by enhancing bodily functions and vitality, thereby promoting a broader spectrum of well-being that transcends conventional treatment limitations.

Case Study: Alleviating Chronic Pelvic Pain Through Targeted Marma Therapy

Chronic pelvic pain (CPP), a complex ailment often entwined with both physical and psychological components, presents a significant challenge in healthcare. Marma therapy, with its unique approach to pain and systemic healing, offers a promising adjunct to conventional pain management strategies. This case study explores the treatment of Tara, a 33-year-old female diagnosed with CPP, whose symptoms persisted despite various medical interventions, including medication and pelvic physiotherapy.

An experienced Ayurvedic practitioner, introduced to her by her primary care physician, decided to integrate Marma therapy into her treatment regimen. Initial assessments focused on identifying crucial Marma points that correlated with her pain sites and underlying physiological imbalances. Key points, such as the Basti Marma in the pelvic region and the Nabhi Marma around the navel area, were targeted, considering their pivotal roles in reproductive and digestive health, respectively. This therapy aimed not just at alleviating pain but also at addressing digestive irregularities and menstrual dysfunctions often associated with CPP.

Twice weekly sessions were initiated, utilizing gentle stimulation with herbal oils renowned for their anti-inflammatory and pain-relieving properties. Additionally, Tara received guidance on dietary adjustments to support the therapy. Over three months, Tara reported significant reductions in pelvic pain and noticeable improvements in her menstrual cycle regularity and bowel movements. The Marma therapy appeared to promote an enhanced flow of Prana, balancing Tara's bodily functions and enhancing her overall quality of life.

This case study highlights the potential synergy between Marma therapy and conventional medical treatments in managing complex conditions, such as CPP. By focusing on specific Marma points, the therapy effectively addresses the multifaceted nature of pain, promoting a holistic recovery path. It also illustrates the broader applicability of Ayurvedic practices in contemporary medical settings, enhancing outcomes through integrative approaches.

Case Study: Restoring Neurovascular Harmony in Parkinson's Disease through Marma Therapy

Parkinson's disease (PD), characterized by progressive neurological degeneration resulting in motor and non-motor symptoms, presents substantial challenges in clinical management. This case study explores the integrative use of Marma therapy for improving the quality of life in Raj, a 65-year-old retired teacher diagnosed with PD. Despite conventional treatments employing medications such as Levodopa and physical therapy, Raj experienced persistent tremors, rigidity, and emotional disturbances like anxiety and depression, which are common in PD patients.

An Ayurvedic practitioner introduced Marma therapy as a complement to his existing treatment regimen. The practitioner focused on specific Marma points, which are believed to influence neurological functions and mental health. Points such as Brahmarandhra (the top of the head) and Adhipati (the crown) were stimulated to alleviate stress and enhance cerebral circulation. At the same time, Manibandha (the wrist) and Kshipra (the hands) were targeted to address Raj's motor symptoms. The dual approach of activating both central and peripheral Marmas aimed to harmonize the neurovascular and Pranic flows, which are often disrupted in PD.

Over a series of bi-weekly sessions lasting three months, Raj noted a noticeable improvement in his tremor control and rigidity. Additionally, the sessions seem to have a tranquilizing effect, helping reduce his anxiety levels. His sleep quality improved, and he reported feeling more emotionally balanced. Raj's case illustrates how Marma therapy, by targeting specific neurological and systemic points, can potentially modulate neurovascular functions crucial in diseases like Parkinson's.

The extended impact of Marma therapy in this integrative treatment approach for PD supports the neuroprotective role suggested in Ayurvedic texts, promoting not only symptomatic relief but also contributing to neuro-regenerative processes. Raj's improved motor function and emotional well-being reflect the holistic benefits achieved by integrating traditional Ayurvedic practices with modern medical treatments, providing a promising avenue for enhancing care in neurodegenerative diseases.

Case Study: Optimizing Cardiovascular Health through Strategic Marma Therapy

This case study explores the application of Marma therapy in the comprehensive management of cardiovascular health, particularly focusing on the treatment of a 55-year-old male patient named Arjun, who was experiencing early stages of hypertension and stress-related palpitations. Despite adherence to prescribed antihypertensive medications and lifestyle modifications including diet and exercise, Arjun's blood pressure remained marginally above normal, and he frequently reported episodes of anxiety and palpitations, especially under stress.

Upon consulting an Ayurvedic practitioner, Arjun was introduced to Marma therapy as an adjunct treatment to his conventional regimen. The practitioner identified key Marma points that correlate with cardiovascular and emotional health, particularly the Hridaya Marma (located in the heart region) and the Anahata Marma (on the chest), which are known for their roles in regulating heart function and emotional balance. Each session involved gentle stimulation of these points with herbal oils renowned for their calming properties, accompanied by rhythmic breathing exercises to enhance relaxation and circulatory efficacy.

The therapy sessions were scheduled twice weekly, and detailed attention was given to the precise manipulation of the Marma points to ensure optimal energy flow and physiological responses. Over a period of twelve weeks, Arjun observed a significant reduction in his blood pressure readings and a decrease in the frequency of palpitations. Moreover, he reported improved sleep quality and lower levels of anxiety, suggesting a beneficial modulation of his overall autonomic functions and stress response.

This case illustrates how Marma therapy, by targeting specific points that affect both the physical and emotional aspects of cardiovascular health, can be a valuable component in the holistic management of cardiac conditions. By integrating traditional Ayurvedic practices with modern medical treatments, patients like Arjun can achieve a more stable and comprehensive health outcome, address not only symptoms but also enhance the quality of life through improved physiological and emotional well-being.

Case Study: Cognitive Enhancement and Stress Reduction through Marma Therapy

This case study explores the application of Marma therapy for cognitive enhancement and stress reduction, focusing on 50-year-old Vishal, a senior software engineer facing significant stress and cognitive decline, which affected both his personal and professional life. Over time, Vishal experienced a marked decrease in memory retention, difficulty in concentrating, and elevated stress levels, which prompted his search for non-pharmacological interventions to aid his condition.

An Ayurvedic practitioner was consulted, who recommended a tailored Marma therapy regimen. Marma points, such as Brahmarandhra (the top of the head) and Ajna (the forehead), known for their influence on cognitive functions, were identified for treatment. Alongside, Anahata (chest area) Marma was selected to address his emotional and stress-related issues. Each session involved gentle stimulation of these points using specific herbal oils that are believed to enhance cognitive function and alleviate stress.

The therapy sessions were conducted twice a week over a three-month period. Vishal's treatment plan was complemented by dietary advice rich in brain-boosting nutrients and yoga practices designed to promote mental clarity and stress relief. After the first month, Vishal reported noticeable improvements in his stress management and a slight improvement in memory. By the end of the third month, he had exhibited significant improvement in cognitive functions, including memory, attention span, and problem-solving skills. Additionally, he experienced a profound reduction in stress and anxiety levels, attributing this to the integrated approach of Marma therapy with his lifestyle modifications.

This case highlights how Marma therapy can effectively enhance cognitive functions and manage stress, underscoring its potential as a complementary therapeutic strategy alongside conventional methods. The strategic stimulation of cognitive and stress-related Marma points, combined with holistic lifestyle practices, showcases the comprehensive approach of Ayurveda in treating modern-day ailments associated with mental health.

Review Questions

1. A 55-year-old male patient with a history of type 2 diabetes and hypertension comes to an Ayurvedic clinic complaining of chronic lower back pain and reduced mobility. He has tried various conventional treatments with minimal relief. The Ayurvedic physician decides to focus on Marma therapy, targeting specific points. Which Marma points should be considered for his condition based on Ayurvedic physiology, and what is the primary goal of this treatment?

A) Kati and Nitamba Marma points, to restore energy flow and relieve pain
B) Hridaya and Talahridaya Marma points, to enhance cardiovascular function
C) Sthapani and Adhipati Marma points, to address headaches
D) Guda and Basti Marma points, primarily for reproductive health enhancement

Answer: A

Explanation: Kati and Nitamba Marma points are strategically located in areas that relate to the lower back and pelvic regions, crucial for addressing issues of pain and mobility, especially in patients with chronic conditions like diabetes and hypertension. Marma therapy at these points aims to release blocked Prana (life force) and ensure smoother Vata flow, which in Ayurveda is associated with movement and pain management. The primary goal of targeting these points is to alleviate the patient's pain and improve functional mobility by restoring energy pathways.

2. A practitioner of Marma Chikitsa is planning a therapeutic session for a patient suffering from frequent headaches and stress accumulation. Referring to the Ayurvedic classification of Marma points, which Marma points should be the focus to alleviate her symptoms, and why?
A) Basti and Guda Marma points, to improve digestive health
B) Shankha and Sthapani Marma points, to relieve headaches and reduce mental stress
C) Indrabasti and Janu Marma points, to address knee pain
D) Phana and Kurcha Marmas, to support liver detoxification
Answer: B
Explanation: Shankha (located around the temple) and Sthapani (forehead region) Marma points are integral in managing symptoms above the neck. These points are known to have a profound impact on reducing mental stress and alleviating headache symptoms, which is consistent with the patient's complaints of stress accumulation and frequent headaches. By targeting these Marma points, the therapy focuses on balancing Pranic flow in the head region, offering relief from pain and enhancing mental clarity and relaxation.

3. An elderly female patient with arthritis and limited joint mobility visits an Ayurvedic practitioner. The practitioner decides to use Marma Chikitsa to enhance her joint mobility and reduce pain. Which Marma category should be the focal point for her treatment, and what is the expected outcome of stimulating these, Marmas?
A) Asthi (Bone) Marma, for structural support and pain modulation
B) Mamsa (Muscle) Marma, for enhancing muscle healing
C) Sandhi (Joint) Marma, to mobilize joints and alleviate arthritis
D) Sira (Veins) Marma, to improve vascular health
Answer: C
Explanation: Sandhi Marma points, situated at the junctions of bones, play a crucial role in maintaining joint health. This choice is particularly relevant for a patient with arthritis and limited mobility. By focusing on Sandhi Marmas, the therapy aims to facilitate the movement of Vata energy, which is crucial for joint functions and maintenance. The expected outcomes of this treatment include improved flexibility, reduced stiffness, and alleviation of pain, making daily movements more effortless and less painful for the patient.

CHAPTER THREE: The Philosophy and Esoteric Foundations of Marma Chikitsa

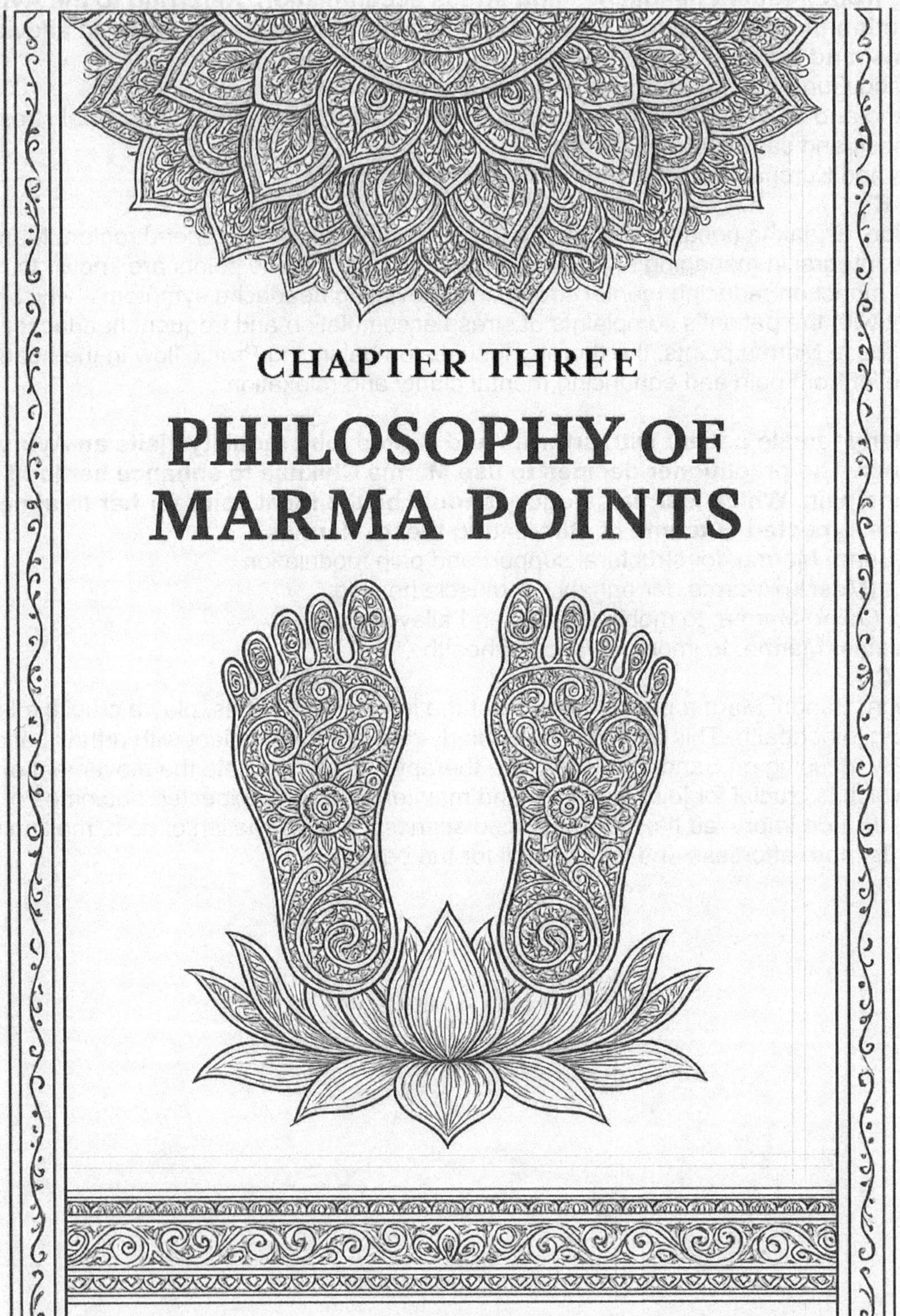

The Concept of Prana and Marma: Flow of Life Force

Marma Chikitsa encapsulates the profound integration of the body's vital energy, prana, with points known as Marmas, where this life force is believed to converge and flow. These points act as crucial gateways for the circulation of energy that sustains all physiological processes. By understanding and manipulating these junctures, practitioners can directly influence the flow of prana, aiming to restore balance and health within the body.

The concept of Prana in Ayurvedic philosophy extends beyond mere biological functions to encompass the essence of life itself. It is this energy that orchestrates cellular function, emotional well-being, and mental clarity. Marma points serve as critical hubs where prana can be accessed and regulated, making Marma Chikitsa a key therapeutic approach in the holistic healing arsenal of Ayurveda.

When these Marma points are stimulated, either through touch, pressure, or meditative techniques, the resultant effect on prana can lead to significant enhancements in health. This stimulation helps clear blockages and ensure a smooth flow of energy, thereby facilitating healing and restoring vitality. Marma Chikitsa thus stands as a testament to the esoteric medical wisdom of ancient Asia, offering not only physical relief but also profound spiritual elevation.

Marma and the 5 Koshas (Sheaths of Existence)

Marma Chikitsa extends beyond mere physical healing to influence the deeper layers of existence, as per Ayurvedic teachings, which are categorized into the Koshas.

More than just the origin of the body, it is the energetic construction of the body corporate, not necessarily the individual parts, which we will explore later, such as chakras, energy lines, and centers: the corporeal body.

The universe is composed of two fundamental elements: matter and energy. We say the matter elements are the universe with attributes and that energy elements are the universe without attributes.

The next statement is an algorithm:

- Matter is the vehicle of energy.
- Energy is consciousness, which manifests.
- When consciousness manifests, it finds a vehicle.
- When consciousness manifests in a human, the vehicle is the mind.
- When the mind manifests, it looks like a body.

Consciousness is fourfold. It has four different aspects:

- It has a mental aspect or "manas", which is the ability to recognize.
- It has an intellectual aspect, which is the "buddhi", the idea of discernment.
- It has identification or is-ness, "ahakara", which is the impulse of attraction and repulsion: I like, I do not like.
- It has a quality of being or "chitta", which is this sense of real, non-temporal, the idea of applying impulses and doing things.

Those four qualities make up the manifestation of consciousness. The ordinary mind is an organ just like your ears, tongue, nose, hands, feet and genitals. The energetic parts of the mind are these qualities of recognition, discernment, attraction and repulsion, attachment and a sense of being or "I am", of being able to do something.

When consciousness assumes physical forms, it exists in five bodies.

In yoga terminology these five bodies are called koshas or sheaths. The word kosha means envelope or sheath like the enclosure or wrapping for a knife or sword. It could also mean a sheath as in a layer like on an onion. Each layer in the onion, which is whole within itself, is distinctive and separate from every other layer. A sword goes into a sheath. The sword is the consciousness. When we talk about the Five Koshas, we are referring to the layered way the egos encapsulate. The three qualities of consciousness which are "sheathed" in the Koshas are Satvas, Rajas, and Tamas.

The five sheaths are from external to internal (outside to inside):
#5 The sheath of MATTER (Sans. Annamaya) (Physical Medicine) Pressure
#4 The sheath of VITAL AIR (Sans. Pranamaya) (Energy Medicine) Breath
#3 The sheath of MIND (Sans. Manomaya) (Education/ Psychology) Intellect
#2 The sheath of KNOWLEDGE (Sans.Vijnanamaya) (Awareness, Being) Application
#1 The sheath of BLISS (Sans. Anandamaya) (Spiritual, Ritual Medicine, Devotion and Surrender)

Traditionally, the Koshas present a five-tier model of the human being, ranging from the gross physical body to the more subtle realms of emotions, mind, knowledge, and bliss. These layers are interconnected, each influencing the well-being of the other. When Marma points are activated, the flow of energy impacts the Annamaya Kosha, or physical sheath, initiating healing that also penetrates the Pranamaya Kosha, the energy body that regulates life forces.

The energy body, or Annamaya Kosha, which governs the mental processes, experiences a balance in emotional energies, revealing the potential of Marma therapy to harmonize mental disturbances often expressed as physical ailments. Even more deeply, the Vijnanamaya Kosha, the sheath of wisdom, and the Anandamaya Kosha, the layer of bliss, are subtly nourished, promoting a profound sense of peace and spiritual awakening. Thus, Marma Chikitsa embodies a holistic therapeutic approach, pulling the threads of physical discomfort to uncover and heal subtle disturbances across all layers of human existence.

Link Between Marma and Prana Nadis (Subtle Energy Channels)

The profound linkage between Marma points and the Nadis, the subtle channels through which prana, or life energy, circulates, forms a cornerstone of Marma Chikitsa's esoteric anatomy. These Nadis serve not merely as conduits for vital energy but as pivotal axes around which physical and spiritual well-being revolves. By engaging these energy pathways, Marma Chikitsa facilitates a direct manipulation of prana, reshaping the body's energetic landscape toward equilibrium and health.
Central to this interaction is the principle that blockages within the Nadis can lead to both physical discomfort and spiritual dissonance. This understanding compels the Marma practitioner to adopt techniques that clear these energy blockages, thereby reinstating the unobstructed flow of life force, essential for healing. As prana flows freely through these channels, it not only detoxifies the physical body but also advances one's spiritual journey by enhancing subtle perception and deepening meditative experiences.
The therapy's effectiveness hinges on the precise stimulation of intersecting Nadis at Marma points. Through gentle pressure, resonance, or even meditative focus, these critical junctures are activated, fostering a cascade of healing energy that permeates the entire body. This

activation is conducive to revitalizing the mind and spirit, exemplifying the holistic approach of Marma Chikitsa, where the healing transcends the physical to embrace the spiritual essence of the individual.

Marma and the 7 Chakras: Energy Integration

In Marma Chikitsa, the convergence of Marmas with the chakras, the body's pivotal energetic centers, underscores a profound integration of physical therapies with energetic spiritual healing. Each of the seven main chakras, aligning from the base of the spine to the crown of the head, serves as a gateway to various aspects of human existence, influencing everything from our survival instincts to our connection to the divine.

The strategic manipulation of Marma points, located around these chakras, magnifies their therapeutic impact, orchestrating an enhanced flow of prana that transcends mere physical healing. By targeting these energetic hubs, practitioners can stimulate a deeper harmonization of bodily functions and emotional states, fostering wellbeing that resonates through the body's subtle energy system.

This holistic approach not only addresses ailments at their physical origin but also aligns the chakras, promoting spiritual balance and mental clarity. Therefore, Marma Chikitsa acts not only on the tangible body but also as a mediator of profound energy transformation, guiding the individual towards a state of enhanced vitality and higher consciousness.

Esoteric Meaning of Injury and Healing through Marma

In the esoteric tradition of Marma Chikitsa, injuries are not merely physical disturbances but disruptions in the energetic and spiritual layers of our being. These injuries, whether caused by physical harm, emotional stress, or spiritual disconnection, manifest as blockages in the flow of prana, the vital life energy. The healing process through Marma points is therefore understood as an intricate practice of re-aligning and rejuvenating this disrupted Pranic flow.

When a Marma point is stimulated, it acts as a portal through which healing energies can be directed to resolve both visible injuries and subtle energetic imbalances. This perspective highlights a more comprehensive approach to healing, where the recovery from physical ailments is closely tied to spiritual and emotional rejuvenation. The practitioner, by connecting with the cosmic energy through focused intention and touch, facilitates a deep healing that transcends the physical dimensions of the body.

Thus, Marma Chikitsa serves as a bridge between the tangible and intangible aspects of health, emphasizing that true healing occurs when harmony is restored not just within our physical body but across our entire existential spectrum. This holistic healing restores balance, ensuring the individual's return to a state of complete wellbeing.

Energetic Blockages and Their Spiritual Implications

In the intricate weave of Marma Chikitsa, energetic blockages are not mere physical impediments but signify deeper spiritual malaises. These blockages often result from unresolved traumas or karmic residues, manifesting as disruptions in the flow of prana, the life

force essential for health and vitality.
The spiritual implications of such blockages extend beyond physical discomfort, affecting our mental clarity and emotional stability. They are profound signs that the soul's journey is hindered, necessitating not only physical relief but also spiritual introspection and healing. Addressing these blockages through Marma Chikitsa involves a holistic remedy that purifies the Pranic pathways, thus reinstating spiritual alignment and promoting a deeper sense of well-being.
By targeting specific Marma points associated with these blockages, practitioners engage deeply with the patient's energy body, facilitating a release of these spiritual impediments. This release is often accompanied by profound emotional catharsis, heralding a restoration of both physical and spiritual order, and advancing the individual on their path to spiritual awakening and holistic health.

Emotional Release and Karma Healing Via Marma Points

Marma Chikitsa unveils profound pathways for emotional healing and karmic liberation, aligning ancient wisdom with the subtle dynamics of energy medicine. At its core, the practice targets Marma points, facilitating a profound emotional release that is often tied to karmic debts accumulated over multiple lifetimes. These specific points, when stimulated, act as gateways to unlock emotional baggage, facilitating a purgation of suppressed energies that burden the soul. This emotional catharsis is intimately connected to karma, the spiritual principle of cause and effect. Through targeted Marma treatments, practitioners can address the root causes of emotional turmoil, which may be rooted in past life experiences or inherited karmic patterns. The release at these critical junctures not only soothes the emotional body but also initiates a profound karmic healing, resetting energetic imbalances that perpetuate suffering.
Such therapeutic interventions serve not just to alleviate psychological distress but to foster a holistic renewal, weaving together the threads of spiritual growth and emotional resilience. By nurturing this intricate relationship between karma and the emotional self, Marma Chikitsa offers a transformative healing journey, leading to peace, clarity, and spiritual liberation.

Marma in Vedic Astrology and Spiritual Medicine

In the realm of Vedic astrology, Marma Chikitsa becomes an illuminating juncture where celestial mechanics intersect with terrestrial healing. Each Marma point is seen not just as a conduit for physical and spiritual energy, but also as an astral touchstone, reflecting the influences of planetary motions and alignments. This cosmic linkage suggests that the positions of planets at the time of one’s birth can dictate the vitality and susceptibility of specific Marma points.
Astrological charts, therefore, guide Marma therapists in customizing treatments that align with an individual's planetary influences, enhancing the therapeutic efficacy. The integration of spiritual medicine enables a holistic healing approach, addressing not only the physical but also the spiritual aspects of existence. The celestial alignment at the time of treatment can potentiate the activation of Marma points, making the healing process deeply transformative.
This profound synthesis of astrology with Marma therapy highlights a dimension where health is intricately connected to the universe’s rhythm, offering a path to harmony that transcends the physical and envelops the spiritual. This integration enables practitioners to administer more personalized and effective healing protocols, guided by the governance of cosmic forces.

Psychic Centers and Marma Point Resonance

Marma Chikitsa delves deeply into the psychic centers, where the mind's energies converge and resonate with Marma points throughout the human body. These centers, deeply embedded within the psyche, act as hubs for processing spiritual, mental, and emotional energies. When Marma points corresponding to these psychic centers are stimulated, it creates a resonance that unlocks profound psychic abilities and facilitates a deeper connection with the universal consciousness.

This resonance enhances the practitioner's ability to perceive and channel subtle energies for healing purposes. By fine-tuning the resonance between Marma points and psychic centers, a practitioner can amplify the healing energy transmitted, optimizing the therapeutic outcome. Such practices are not only healing in nature but are transformative, promoting significant growth in spiritual awareness and psychic development.

Through the systematic and deliberate stimulation of these critical points, Marma Chikitsa serves as a key to unlocking the hidden elements of the psyche, contributing to a more holistic and comprehensive understanding of both the self and the broader cosmos. The practice encourages the flowering of latent psychic potentials, fostering an environment where deep healing and spiritual evolution can occur.

Ajna and Sthapani Marma: Doors to Higher Perception

The Ajna and Sthapani Marma points are considered pivotal in Marma Chikitsa, acting as gateways to elevated states of consciousness and deeper perception. Located between the eyebrows, the Ajna chakra, often referred to as the third eye, serves as the command center for intuitive knowledge. Stimulating this Marma point facilitates a profound connection with one's inner wisdom and enhances the ability to perceive subtle energies and intuitive signals.

Conversely, the Sthapani Marma, closely associated with the Ajna chakra, impacts the frontal lobe of the brain, an area linked to higher cognitive functions, including decision-making and ethical reasoning. This Marma point is crucial for integrating spiritual insights into daily life, allowing individuals to navigate their existence with heightened awareness and purpose.

Together, these Marma points orchestrate a symphony of mental clarity and spiritual insight, providing practitioners and recipients access to layers of consciousness beyond ordinary perception. The stimulation of these points encourages transcendental experiences and insights, pivotal for holistic health and spiritual advancement.

Marma and Kundalini Energy Flow

In the profound science of Marma Chikitsa, the awakening and management of Kundalini energy hold a pivotal role. Marma points serve not only as physical junctions but also as spiritual gateways for the uncoiling and ascent of Kundalini energy, which resides dormant at the base of the spine. When activated correctly through precise Marma manipulations, this serpent-like energy travels upward through the Sushumna Nadi, energizing the seven chakras. This progression is crucial for holistic health, as each chakra aligns with specific psychological and physiological functions. The stimulation of Marma points catalyzes the Kundalini ascent, promoting the clearing and balancing of chakras, thus enhancing individual vitality and spiritual perception. An awakened Kundalini results in an expansion of consciousness, connecting the

individual with the divine.
The art of Marma Chikitsa, therefore, is not merely therapeutic but deeply transformative, facilitating an internal alchemy where physical healing is intertwined with spiritual enlightenment. Practitioners of Marma must approach Kundalini with respect and profound understanding to harness this energy safely and effectively.

Ritual Preparation for Marma Work: Mental and Emotional State

The ritualistic preparation for Marma Chikitsa is as vital as the practice itself, focusing intensely on the mental and emotional readiness of both the practitioner and the recipient. Before engaging in this sacred healing technique, one must attain a serene mental state, characterized by calmness and clarity. This preliminary step is crucial, as it sets the energetic tone for the session, ensuring the flow of prana remains uninterrupted and pure.
Emotional equanimity is equally essential. Practitioners often engage in meditation or chant mantras to stabilize their emotions and elevate their spiritual vibration. For recipients, the emotional state should be receptive and open, devoid of resistance or skepticism. This openness enables a more profound energetic exchange, thereby enhancing the healing potential of Marma interventions.
Thus, the ritual preparation transcends mere physical readiness, delving into the depths of psychological and spiritual attunement. It is a dance of energy where both participants synchronize their intent and emotions, crafting an atmosphere ripe for deep healing and spiritual awakening.

The Role of Silence, Intention, and Sankalpa in Healing

In the profound realms of Marma Chikitsa, silence is not merely the absence of sound but a vibrant space of potent healing potential. It provides a canvas upon which the intentions of healer and recipient are vividly painted, enabling a deep communion that transcends verbal communication. This silence enhances focus, allowing prana to flow uninhibitedly through the Marmas, driven by the purity of intent.
Intention acts as the directing force within this silent space, guiding the healing energies with precision and purpose. Every touch at a Marma point is imbued with this focused intention, orchestrated to awaken and realign life forces within the body. The practitioner's mindful intention is the essential ingredient that transforms routine touch into a curative gesture that reverberates through the body's energetic layers.
Sankalpa, or the healing resolution, further refines this process. It is a deeply held intention, a vow that reinforces the therapeutic journey. When combined with silence and focused intent, Sankalpa anchors the healing process, ensuring that the energies activated are consistent with the highest aspirations for health and well-being. Thus, these elements synergize, setting a profound course for healing that engages body, mind, and spirit in a harmonized pursuit of recovery and enlightenment.

Invocation and Mantras Used in Traditional Marma Practice

In the esoteric tradition of Marma Chikitsa, invocations and mantras play a critical role in channeling the healing energies of the universe into the practitioner's efforts. These sacred utterances are more than mere words; they are vibrations that align the healer's intentions with cosmic forces, enhancing the effectiveness of the treatments administered.

Each mantra is carefully selected based on its resonance with specific Marma points and the intended healing outcomes. The vibratory quality of these sacred chants helps to cleanse the aura, refine the energetic channels, and prepare the body for deeper therapeutic impacts.

Invocations, often recited at the beginning of a session, call upon divine energies and seek protection and guidance. They set a sacred space, marking the Marma practice as a holistic ritual that transcends physical manipulation.

Practitioners are trained to use these tools with deep respect and understanding, recognizing that their power is immense and sacred. This spiritual dimension is pivotal to Marma Chikitsa, as it enhances the healing journey, not just for the body, but also for the soul, facilitating a profound transformation that is both healing and enlightening.

Guru Initiation and Spiritual Qualification for Marma Healers

In the esoteric sphere of Marma Chikitsa, the initiation by a Guru stands as a pivotal rite, marking the transition into the deeper realms of spiritual and energetic healing. This initiation, known as 'diksha', is not merely a formality but a profound exchange of spiritual energy between the Guru and the disciple. It is believed that through this sacred ceremony, the practitioner is imbued with a refined sensitivity to energetic nuances, a gift essential for mastering Marma therapy.

The process of becoming spiritually qualified to practice Marma Chikitsa involves rigorous discipline and purification. Aspirants must delve deeply into the understanding of Pranic flow and the subtle dynamics of the body's energy centers. This spiritual and educational journey is underscored by a commitment to live in harmony with Ayurvedic principles, fostering purity in thoughts, diet, and lifestyle.

Moreover, the Guru ensures that the healer's intents align with the ethos of healing as service, steering them away from ego-driven motives. Only when a practitioner's heart and mind resonate with unconditional compassion and wisdom can the true essence of Marma Chikitsa be channeled through their touch. This holistic initiation cultivates healers who are not just skilled in technique but are embodiments of healing energy itself.

Attunement of the Practitioner's Hands

The attunement of the practitioner's hands in Marma Chikitsa is a delicate process of alignment and tuning to the vibrational energies essential for healing. This process is deeply rooted in the belief that the hands are not merely tools but extensions of the practitioner's own energy field. Through specific exercises and meditations, the hands are sensitized to detect slight variations in the energy flow within the Marma points, enabling precise interventions that catalyze profound healing.

This attunement involves rituals that purify and charge the healer's hands with prana, the life force. Practices such as mudras (hand gestures that lock and guide the flow of energy), and mantras (chanting) amplify the healing energy. Realignment through these spiritual exercises ensures that each touch by the practitioner becomes a conduit for transferring healing energies effectively to the recipient.

Furthermore, the emotional and spiritual purity of the practitioner plays a crucial role. It is believed that the cleaner the energetic resonance of the healer's hands, the more powerful and transformative the healing experience. Therefore, ongoing spiritual practices and ethical living are emphasized to maintain this attunement, making each Marma session not only a practice of healing but also an act of spiritual service.

Sacred Geometry and Marma Alignment

Sacred Geometry plays a pivotal role in aligning Marma points, which are considered gateways to body's vital energies. This ancient science emphasizes the interconnectivity of all life forms through geometric patterns, establishing a deep resonance with Marma practice, which helps restore and balance energy flow across the physical and spiritual planes.

The geometric shapes used in Marma Chikitsa, like circles and triangles, are believed to amplify healing energies. When placed around or over Marma points during treatments, these shapes channel cosmic energies that facilitate deeper healing. The specific alignments and placements are derived from extensive texts and are carefully tuned to match the body's energetic blueprint.

Further, practitioners often visualize these geometric patterns during the session, which enhances their focus and attunes the healing vibrations. This simultaneous application of visualized and physical sacred geometry helps to unlock blocked energies, promoting health, wellbeing, and spiritual awakening.

Incorporating these elements transforms Marma Chikitsa into a multidimensional healing toolkit, blending tangible touch with ethereal geometry to optimize the therapeutic potential.

Marma and Tantric Healing Traditions

Tantric healing within Marma Chikitsa incorporates profound spiritual and esoteric principles, blending physical touch with transcendent energetic practices. Rooted in the ancient Tantric scriptures, these methods engage not only the body but also the soul, fostering a deep and energetic purification and transformation. Within this tradition, Marma points are seen as portals for liberating trapped energies, enhancing spiritual awakening and physical well-being.

Practitioners of Tantric Marma utilize specific mantras and visualizations that correlate with different Marma points to stimulate and balance the body's vital energies. This practice is often accompanied using sacred sounds and geometrical patterns, which are believed to amplify the healing energies being channeled. Such rituals are thought to prepare the body's subtle energy fields for profound shifts, promoting healing and spiritual growth.

Moreover, Tantric Marma emphasizes the unity of dual energies within the body, aiming to harmonize male and female aspects, which are fundamental to personal and spiritual equilibrium. Through these intricate healing sessions, the practitioner guides the individual towards a state where health, energy, and spiritual enlightenment intersect, revealing paths to deeper self-understanding and cosmic connection.

Pranic Imprints and Aura-Clearing at Marma Points

The concept of Pranic imprints within Marma Chikitsa reveals the subtle layers at which energetic residues, or Samskaras, dwell within the human energy field. These imprints, held at Marma points, are residual energies from past experiences, emotions, and traumas that shape an individual's Pranic body, influencing health and consciousness.
Aura-clearing at these points is a profound practice designed to dissolve stored energies, thereby facilitating a purer state of being. By employing specific techniques such as directed Pranayama, strategic touch, and the use of sacred mantras, healers work to cleanse the aura, gradually lifting the veils of past impressions. This purification allows for a reinvigoration of vital energies, restoring balance and enhancing the bioenergetic field.
Effectively clearing these Pranic imprints catalyzes a deeper healing process, transforming the person's energy dynamics. Regular practice can lead to significant transformation, empowering individuals to experience greater clarity, vitality, and alignment with their higher self.

Use of Crystals and Yantras with Marma Points

Integrating crystals and yantras with Marma points unlocks a complex, resonant energy system. Crystals, with their discreet vibrational frequencies, align directly with the energetic needs of specific Marma sites. When placed appropriately, these stones empower the healing process by amplifying the Pranic movement and clearing blockages to restore energetic equilibrium.
Yantras contribute a sacred geometrical dimension to Marma therapy. These mystic diagrams are not just visual tools but dynamic, energetic instruments that organize and redirect energy flows. Positioned near or on the body during Marma sessions, yantras work in harmony with the physical touch and crystalline frequencies, establishing a lattice of healing vibrations.
The combination of crystals and yantras introduces a profound layer to Marma Chikitsa, transforming it into a holistic ritual. This synergy not only enhances energetic purification but also deepens the spiritual connection of the practitioner and recipient, guiding both towards a state of harmonious, vibrant health.

Colors and Marma Healing: Use of Light Frequency

In Marma Chikitsa, colors play a crucial role, each resonating with specific frequencies that interact with the body's energetic layers. This color therapy aspect utilizes the spectrum of light to enhance and direct the healing energy through Marma points. By applying distinct colored lights or fabrics during sessions, practitioners can invoke specific vibrations needed to balance and harmonize the body's prana, or life force.
The selection of colors is not arbitrary, correlating directly with the energetic needs identified at each Marma point. For instance, blue might be used to cool and calm an overheated system, whereas red could stimulate areas of sluggish energy. This tailored application of color frequencies supports a targeted healing response, addressing physical, emotional, or spiritual imbalances.
Further integrating the use of light frequency, practitioners often visualize the corresponding color energies during therapy, enhancing the therapeutic impact. This visualization technique, combined with the physical application of colors, fosters a profound energetic recalibration, vital for the healing process. Such practices exemplify how Marma Chikitsa transcends mere physical touch, entering realms of vibrational medicine that harmonize the entire being.

Ancient Alchemical Oils Used in Esoteric Marma Practice

In the realm of Marma Chikitsa, ancient alchemical oils serve as potent tools, imbued with therapeutic and esoteric properties. These special blends, crafted through sacred alchemical processes, are meticulously prepared to enhance the healing efficacy of Marma therapy. Derived from herbs, flowers, and minerals, these oils carry the vibrational signatures necessary for deep energetic shifts at Marma points.

When applying specific Marma points, these oils facilitate the unlocking and release of stagnant energy, promoting a flow that rejuvenates the body's vital systems. The alchemical transformation of these substances is believed to transmute earthly elements into divine forms, rendering the oils capable of not only physical healing but also spiritual awakening. Each oil is aligned with certain energetic qualities and planetary influences, chosen based on an individual's unique Pranic needs.

Moreover, the aromatic qualities of these oils play a crucial role in calming the mind and inducing a state conducive to healing. Their application becomes a ritual, setting the stage for profound transformations, both physically and spiritually. This traditional practice bridges ancient wisdom with contemporary spiritual disciplines, reaffirming the holistic approach of Marma Chikitsa.

The Science of Breath (Pranayama) and Marma Activation

Pranayama, the science of breath control, plays a pivotal role in the activation and regulation of Marma points, the vital energy junctions within the body. Through deliberate inhalation, retention, and exhalation, Pranayama enhances the flow of prana, or life force, directly influencing these potent sites.

Specific breathing techniques are tailored to activate different Marma points, depending on the desired healing outcome. For instance, 'Bhattarika', or the 'bellows breath', can energize the body, stimulating Marma points related to vitality and strength. Conversely, 'Sheetali', the cooling breath, is used to soothe Marma points associated with heat and inflammation.

Effective Marma activation through Pranayama not only regulates physical health but also balances emotional states. It prepares both the healer and the recipient for deeper spiritual work, harmonizing the energies across the body's subtle and physical layers.

This interplay of breath and energy points underscores Marma Chikitsa's holistic approach to healing, where breath is both a tool and a metaphor for the nurturing flow of life itself.

Yogic Siddhis and Marma Stimulation

The exploration of Yogic Siddhis—extraordinary powers gained through dedicated spiritual practice—intersects intriguingly with Marma Chikitsa. These siddhis, which include abilities such as telepathy, levitation, and heightened perception, are believed to be activated by stimulating specific Marma points, thereby enhancing the practitioner's energy flow and spiritual connectivity.

This stimulation is deeply tied to the advanced practices within yoga and tantra, where the focus is on transcending the physical to reach heightened states of awareness. Certain Marma points are specifically targeted to awaken these siddhis, acting as gateways to expanded consciousness and psychic abilities. By integrating Marma therapy with meditative focus and

disciplined energy work, practitioners can unlock these latent powers.
Such practices are not without their prerequisites; they require years of disciplined spiritual practice and ethical living. The holistic nature of Marma Chikitsa supports this journey, ensuring that the physical, emotional, and spiritual aspects are aligned, thereby facilitating a fertile ground for the blossoming of siddhis.

The Role of Dharma, Artha, Kama, Moksha in Healing

In the profound realms of Marma Chikitsa, the spiritual concepts of Dharma (duty), Artha (prosperity), Kama (pleasure), and Moksha (liberation) play crucial roles in promoting holistic healing. These four pursuits are traditionally seen as the objectives of human life in Vedic philosophy.
Dharma refers to righteous living and moral duties. When aligned with Dharma, Marma therapy focuses on healing as a service to one's spiritual growth, ensuring that every intervention is ethically grounded and supports the patient's journey towards spiritual integrity. Artha, pertaining to material success and security, influences the practical aspects of Marma therapy, where the provision and availability of treatments reflect the societal and personal resources, stabilizing the physical foundation necessary for spiritual and emotional healing.
Kama involves the enjoyment and fulfillment of desires, which in Marma healing, relate to balancing sensory inputs and nurturing emotional health. Finally, Moksha, the goal of liberation from the cycle of rebirth, is reflected in Marma practices that focus on releasing deeper energetic blockages, guiding both practitioner and patient toward spiritual freedom and enlightenment.

Interdimensional Healing Through Marma Points

Marma Chikitsa not only functions within the seen world but also extends into the realms of cosmic connectivity, where healing transcends physical boundaries, influencing the interdimensional aspects of the self. This profound aspect of Marma practice hinges on the understanding that human existence is layered across multiple dimensions that extend beyond our conventional perception.
Practitioners skilled in this esoteric aspect of Marma Chikitsa use specialized techniques to align these dimensional layers, facilitating a profound healing that resonates through the physical, astral, and causal bodies. This harmonization is believed to rectify imbalances that our earthly senses are unable to detect yet greatly impact our vitality and spiritual wellbeing.
Such healing is steeped in ancient wisdom, suggesting that Marma points are not only nexus points of physical nerves and tissues but also of time and space. Navigating this intricate matrix requires not just technical expertise but a deep, intuitive connection to universal energy flows.
Interdimensional healing highlights the vast, often untapped potential of Marma points in restoring health at the most fundamental levels of existence, marking a frontier in energy medicine where science meets the mystical.

Secret Marma Teachings of Kalari Masters

The Kalari masters, custodians of an ancient martial art form, also harbor secret teachings of Marma Chikitsa, a profound aspect of their training that transcends mere physicality. These esoteric teachings delve deeper into the spiritual dimensions of Marma, emphasizing not just the healing of bodily injuries but the elevation of the spirit and mind.

Traditionally, these secrets are passed down orally, from master to disciple, ensuring that the sanctity and purity of the knowledge are preserved. The Kalari masters teach that true mastery of Marma comes not from technical skill alone but through an understanding of the cosmic play of energy, where each Marma point is a confluence of spiritual and physical realities.

Among these teachings, particular emphasis is placed on synchronizing to activate and harness the energy flows at Marma points effectively. This synergy is vital during high-stakes performances, transforming ordinary movements into potent therapeutic gestures that aim at self-healing and the enhancement of vital energies.

Differences Between Physical and Esoteric Marma

Marma Chikitsa bridges the tangible and metaphysical, encompassing both physical and esoteric dimensions. Physically, Marma points are specific locations on the body where major veins, arteries, muscles, joints or bones intersect. Practitioners apply manual pressure or stimulate these points to enhance bodily health and alleviate pain, drawing from a deeply anatomical understanding.

Esoterically, these points transcend the mere physical components to act as portals to the subtler layers of one is being. Here, each Marma point is viewed as a confluence of consciousness and corporeal energy, tapping into psychic and spiritual realms. Esoteric practices focus on the energetic and vibrational aspects, utilizing Marma points to manipulate prana to facilitate deep spiritual healing and awakening.

Thus, while the physical application addresses immediate physiological issues, the esoteric approach aims to realign and purify the more elusive energetic imbalances, often tackling the root causes of physical discomforts at a spiritual level. This dual approach underscores the profound versatility and depth of Marma Chikitsa, melding the seen with the unseen.

Spiritual Protection During Marma Work

In the profound practice of Marma Chikitsa, spiritual protection is paramount, especially given the deep energetic interventions involved. As practitioners navigate the subtle realms manipulating prana, they must shield themselves and their patients from potential negative energies that could disrupt the healing process. This protective measure is not merely practical but deeply spiritual, rooted in the ancient wisdom of Vedic traditions.

The methodology involves various rituals and incantations that create a sacred space, sealing it from lower vibrational forces. The use of specific mantras chanted at the beginning and end of each session forms a vibrational barrier, harmonizing the energies within and repelling intrusive forces. Additionally, the layout of the healing space often incorporates symbols known for their protective properties, such as mandalas or yantras, strategically placed to enhance this safeguarding.

Ultimately, spiritual protection in Marma Chikitsa is about maintaining the purity and integrity of the healing space and the energetic transaction. It ensures that both healer and healee remain within a cocoon of heightened spiritual energy, fostering optimal healing and preventing any spiritual backflow or contamination that could impede the therapeutic journey.

How to Cultivate the Right Mindset for Marma Healing

Cultivating the right mindset for Marma Chikitsa is as pivotal as the technical skills required for its practice. This mindset begins with profound respect and an open, receptive state that acknowledges the sanctity of the energy being handled. Practitioners must cultivate a profound connection with the universal life force, Prana, enabling a tranquil yet focused state of mind that transcends ordinary consciousness.

The practitioner's intent should be clear and pure, directed towards the highest good of the recipient. This purity of intention forms the cornerstone of effective Marma therapy, ensuring that the energy manipulated is both beneficial and healing. It is vital that healers maintain a meditative poise throughout the session, an embodiment of the serenity and authority required to navigate these potent energetic dimensions.

Moreover, emotional resilience and humility are essential, allowing healers to serve as mere conduits for healing energy, detached from ego and personal gain. Cultivating such a mindset demands regular self-reflection and meditation, practices that not only refine one's healing capabilities but also deepen one's spiritual journey, aligning personal vibrations with the cosmic flows necessary for profound healing.

Summary

Marma Chikitsa, a vital component of Ayurvedic medicine, emphasizes the strategic manipulation of specific body points (Marmas) to regulate the flow of prana, or life force, which is essential for maintaining both physiological and spiritual health. This ancient practice encompasses not only physical healing but also spiritual and emotional rejuvenation across the body's five koshas, or sheaths, ranging from the physical to the blissful layer. Through techniques such as pressure application, meditative touch, and energy stimulation, these points serve as gateways to influence the deeper layers of existence, integrating with subtle energy channels (Nadis) and chakras to enhance overall wellbeing. Marma Chikitsa not only targets physical ailments but also addresses spiritual dissonances, acting on energetic blockages that manifest as physical or emotional discomfort. The practice interconnects with Vedic astrology and employs ritualistic preparations that enhance the healer's and recipient's emotional and spiritual states, which are essential for effective therapy. Silence, intention, and sacred mantras play pivotal roles, setting a profound healing course. Additionally, the involvement of crystals, yantras, and color therapy facilitates a more comprehensive healing approach, promoting energy balance and spiritual alignment. Marma Chikitsa's holistic approach is further exemplified in its capacity to facilitate emotional catharsis and karma healing, potentially engaging deeper spiritual transformations and accessing higher states of consciousness through the stimulation of specific Marmas such as Ajna (the third eye). Moreover, this therapy considers the spiritual principles of Dharma, Artha, Kama, and Moksha to promote holistic healing, linking personal health with spiritual evolution. Kaleidoscopically, Marma Chikitsa incorporates elements of breath control, sacred geometry, and alignments that resonate with the practitioner's intention, providing transformative health benefits. This ensures that the practice not only alleviates physical conditions but also promotes an integrated spiritual awakening.

References

[1] Subramanian, P. (2012). Ayurvedic Marma Therapy: Energy Points for Healing Body, Mind, and Consciousness. https://www.example.com/marma-therapy

[2] Frawley, D. (2000). Ayurveda and the Mind: The Healing of Consciousness. https://www.example.com/ayurveda-mind

[3] Lad, V. (1984). Ayurveda: A Comprehensive Guide to Traditional Indian Medicine for the West. https://www.example.com/ayurveda-lad

Case Study: The Integration of Marma Chikitsa in Managing Chronic Pain: A Holistic Approach

Martha, a 58-year-old woman, presented with a ten-year history of chronic lower back pain exacerbated by her job as a schoolteacher, which required prolonged hours of standing and occasionally lifting heavy objects. Traditional treatments, including physical therapy, pain medications, and occasional chiropractic adjustments, provided only temporary relief, leading her to explore alternative healing modalities.

Upon consulting with an Ayurvedic practitioner specializing in Marma Chikitsa, Martha underwent a thorough physical examination and detailed discussion of her health history, lifestyle, and emotional wellbeing. The practitioner identified several key Marma points along the spine and lower back that appeared to be blocked, disrupting the flow of Prana, or life energy, contributing to her chronic pain.

Treatment began with gentle stimulation of these Marma points through touch and pressure, accompanied by guided breathing exercises tailored to encourage the flow of energy through her body's subtle channels. The practitioner also incorporated meditative techniques to address Martha's emotional stressors, considering the Ayurvedic view that physical pain is often intertwined with emotional and spiritual health.

Over several weeks, Martha experienced a noticeable decrease in the intensity of her pain and an improvement in mobility. Sessions included the integration of specific dietary recommendations and herbal supplements to strengthen her body from within, aligning with the holistic aims of Marma Chikitsa. Additionally, the practitioner offered guidance on modifying her daily activities to maintain the balance of energy achieved through therapy.

The case of Martha illustrates the profound capacity of Marma Chikitsa not only to alleviate physical pain but also to foster a deeper healing that addresses the root causes of illness across the body's physical and subtle dimensions. This approach underscores the importance of viewing health through a holistic lens, where energy balance is fundamental to overall wellbeing.

Case Study: Revitalizing Well-being through the Esoteric Dimensions of Marma Chikitsa

Rajeev, a 45-year-old software developer, experienced a gradual decline in his mental clarity and physical vitality, attributed to the high demands and stress of his professional life. Traditional medical examinations revealed no specific physiological abnormalities, yet Rajeev felt consistently drained, mentally foggy, and emotionally unbalanced. This led him to explore alternative healing modalities, ultimately bringing him to a practitioner skilled in Marma Chikitsa.

The practitioner conducted a comprehensive assessment including a detailed discussion about Rajeev's lifestyle, emotional stressors, and daily routines. It was hypothesized that an imbalance in Rajeev's prana flow might be contributing to his symptoms. Marma Chikitsa, with its roots in Ayurvedic traditions, views health as a balanced flow of life energy through the body's Marma points—strategic energy junctures linked directly to the body's physiology and psychology.

Treatment commenced with gentle stimulation of specific Marma points traditionally associated with mental clarity and vital energy, such as the Sthapani (located at the center of the forehead) and the Hridaya (located at the center of the heart). These points were chosen to enhance cerebral circulation and strengthen heart energy, promoting both emotional and physical revitalization. Each session also included pranayama (breath control exercises) to enhance oxygenation and aid in the balancing of prana.

Rajeev was instructed in personal practices to maintain and enhance the benefits of the sessions, including dietary adjustments to promote clean and vital energy intake, as well as daily meditation and yoga to align his physical posture and mental state. Throughout his treatment, a noticeable improvement in his energy levels, concentration, and overall emotional resilience was observed.

This case study demonstrates how Marma Chikitsa, by targeting vital energy flow through specific points, can significantly enhance an individual's mental, physical, and emotional well-being. It highlights the profound depth of healing that can be achieved through understanding and manipulating the esoteric anatomy of the human body, based on ancient Ayurvedic wisdom.

Case Study: Harnessing Spiritual Awakening through Marma Chikitsa in a High-Stress Environment

Liam, a 37-year-old corporate executive, struggled with acute stress and anxiety due to the demanding nature of his job. Over time, his high-stress environment led to severe sleep disturbances and a diminished sense of well-being, prompting him to seek alternative treatments after conventional therapies had limited success. Liam's journey led him to a practitioner of Marma Chikitsa, aiming for not only physical relief but also a profound spiritual awakening as part of his healing process.

Initial assessments focused on understanding Liam's daily routines, stress levels, and overall health. The practitioner identified disruptions in the flow of prana around Liam's Ajna (the third eye) and Anahata (heart) Marma points, which according to Marma Chikitsa, significantly affected his mental and spiritual health. Considering these findings, the treatment targeted these points, aiming to unblock and rebalance Liam's life energy, which is essential in easing mental and emotional distress.

The sessions involved gentle stimulation of the Ajna and Anahata points through specific touch techniques supported by chanting and the burning of Ayurvedic herbs, known to amplify the healing energies. Additionally, the treatment was complemented by guided meditations designed to foster Liam's mental clarity and to connect him with his inner self, promoting emotional healing and spiritual insight.

Over the course of the treatment, Liam reported significant improvements in his cognitive functions and emotional stability. He experienced deeper, more restorative sleep and a renewed sense of vitality and peace. Follow-up sessions also included teachings on lifestyle adjustments and daily practices to support the sustained flow of prana, such as specific breathing exercises and dietary recommendations tailored to enhance his body's energy balance.

This case study elucidates the integrative approach of Marma Chikitsa, which addresses complex interconnections between the body's physical symptoms and spiritual health. By realigning the vital energy pathways, Marma Chikitsa not only alleviates physical ailments but also contributes to profound spiritual growth and emotional well-being, demonstrating its efficacy as a comprehensive healing modality in a high-stress modern environment.

Case Study: Navigating Post-Traumatic Stress and Physical Ailments with Marma Chikitsa

Anita, a 33-year-old former military officer, struggled with severe post-traumatic stress disorder (PTSD) and recurring migraines following an intense career in active combat zones. Her conditions were exacerbated by physical injuries sustained during service, including a partially healed leg fracture and chronic back pain. Despite various conventional treatments, including psychotherapy and pharmaceutical interventions, Anita's symptoms persisted, prompting her to explore alternative healing routes.

Anita's journey into alternative medicine led her to a seasoned practitioner of Marma Chikitsa. The initial sessions were devoted to a holistic evaluation, considering not only her physical injuries but also her emotional and psychic traumas. This comprehensive approach is a hallmark of Marma Chikitsa, recognizing the interconnectedness of physical and spiritual ailments. The practitioner pinpointed several blocked Marma points corresponding to Anita's symptoms, notably around the head for her migraines and along the spine and leg for her physical pains.

Treatment began with the gentle activation of these Marma points, aiming to restore the disrupted flow of prana that was believed to be contributing to her ailments. This was done through a combination of direct pressure, essential oils, and energy balancing techniques. The practitioner also integrated breathing exercises specifically designed to alleviate anxiety and stress, addressing the psychological aspects of PTSD.

Moreover, the practitioner recommended a series of lifestyle adjustments to support Anita's healing process. These included dietary changes to reduce inflammation, yoga practices to enhance physical alignment and strength, and meditation to support mental health and resilience. Over several months, Anita reported significant improvements in her symptoms. Her migraines became less frequent and less severe, her mobility improved, and, importantly, she experienced fewer PTSD episodes.

Anita's case underscores the effectiveness of Marma Chikitsa not only in treating physical symptoms but also in addressing deep-seated emotional scars. This holistic approach not only alleviates symptoms but also fosters a renewed sense of empowerment and balance, crucial for coping with complex conditions such as PTSD and chronic pain.

Case Study: Exploring the Depths of Emotional Healing with Marma Chikitsa: A Journey to Mental Clarity

Sophia, a 42-year-old artist and single mother, faced overwhelming emotional distress and anxiety that significantly impacted her creative output and personal well-being. Having tried various therapies with limited success, Sophia turned to Marma Chikitsa as a comprehensive approach to address her concerns holistically. Her frequent panic attacks and chronic insomnia prompted a need for a deeper, more sustaining healing modality than what she had encountered in conventional therapies.

Upon her first visit, the Marma practitioner conducted an extensive consultation to understand Sophia's lifestyle, emotional burdens, and physical health. It was discovered that the disruptions in her Prana flow, particularly around the heart (Anahata) and solar plexus (Manipura) Marma points, were contributing to her emotional and physical symptoms. These centers are heavily associated with emotional processing and personal power in Ayurvedic teachings, key areas that needed rebalancing in Sophia's case.

The treatment protocol initiated for Sophia involved targeted stimulation at these critical Marma points to release blocked energy and restore balance. Techniques included subtle and direct pressure, alongside the use of warm herbal oils specifically chosen for their calming properties. Each session also incorporated guided visualizations to enhance mindfulness and emotional release, fostering a deeper connection between her physical state and emotional health.

As therapy progressed, Sophia reported a significant reduction in her anxiety levels and improvements in sleep quality. The practitioner also recommended dietary adjustments to support her nervous and digestive systems, further promoting overall Pranic balance. Integrative breathing exercises (Pranayama) were introduced to maintain this balance daily and increase Sophia's ability to manage stress autonomously.

This case study underlines Marma Chikitsa's profound ability to heal emotionally driven conditions by addressing both the energy flow and the body. It highlights the importance of a holistic approach, considering not only the physical or visible symptoms but also the deeper emotional and energetic disruptions. Sophia's journey with Marma therapy exemplifies personal empowerment and revitalization, ultimately fostering both mental clarity and emotional resilience.

Case Study: Cultivating Spiritual Harmony: A Case of Integrating Marma Chikitsa with Yogic Practices for Enhanced Well-being

Kevin, a 40-year-old yoga instructor, found himself at a spiritual impasse despite his deep yogic practices. Over the years, he had developed sporadic digestive issues and a sense of emotional disconnection, which he suspected were affecting his spiritual growth and teaching capabilities. Traditional medical approaches had not yielded significant improvements, leading him to explore Marma Chikitsa, known for its integration of physical health with spiritual and energy healing.

During his first consultation, the Marma practitioner conducted a detailed evaluation of Kevin's health history, lifestyle, and emotional state. The initial assessment revealed potential blockages in the Anahata (heart) and Manipura (solar plexus) Marma points, crucial areas for emotional processing and energy distribution, respectively. These findings resonated with Kevin, as they mirrored the areas where he felt his yogic practices were stagnated.

The treatment plan consisted of bi-weekly sessions that focused on these key Marma points. Techniques included precise pressure application, the use of Ayurvedic oils chosen for their energetic properties, and incorporation of specific mantras that Kevin could resonate with during the sessions. These approaches were complemented by guided Pranayama exercises to deepen his breath's impact on Pranic flow.

As Kevin's therapy progressed, he noticed a marked improvement in his digestive symptoms, which was gradually restoring his vitality. More importantly, he experienced a profound reconnection with his emotional self, which he had not realized was so deeply rooted. The sessions became a space for significant spiritual reflection and healing, greatly enhancing his personal and professional life as a yoga instructor.

The insights gained from Kevin's case study demonstrate the powerful synergy between Marma Chikitsa and traditional yogic practices. By addressing the subtle imbalances in energy points associated with vital physiological functions and emotional well-being, Marma Chikitsa not only provided relief from physical ailments but also facilitated a deeper spiritual alignment and harmony. This holistic healing methodology reaffirmed the interconnectedness of body, mind, and spirit, offering a comprehensive approach to wellness that transcended conventional treatment boundaries.

Case Study: Transformation and Healing Through Marma Chikitsa After a Sports Injury

James, a 30-year-old professional basketball player, suffered a severe ankle sprain during a crucial game, leading to chronic pain and restricted mobility that adversely affected his performance and daily life. Conventional treatments such as physiotherapy and pain medication had offered only temporary relief. This ongoing issue led him to explore alternative therapies, culminating in his decision to try Marma Chikitsa, known for its holistic approach to healing and energy balance.

An experienced Marma practitioner conducted a comprehensive assessment of James's overall health, emphasizing the injuries and their implications on his energy flow, or Prana. The examination focused on identifying disruptions in the Marma points associated with his lower limbs and overall athletic performance. The practitioner identified blockages in the Gulpha (ankle) Marma point, crucial for mobility and stability, and the Kshipra (between the toes) Marma point, related to agile movements and quick reflexes.

Marma Chikitsa treatment for James involved the precise stimulation of these points to restore Prana flow and reduce pain. The practitioner used gentle pressure techniques combined with warm herbal oils that are known for their anti-inflammatory properties. Alongside these treatments, James was guided through specific Pranayama (breathing) techniques aimed at enhancing his internal healing processes and mental focus.

Throughout the course of his treatments, James noticed significant improvements not only in his ankle's functionality but also in his overall energy levels and mental clarity. These changes were vital for his return to professional sports. Additionally, the practitioner recommended lifestyle and dietary adjustments to support his physical robustness and to align his body's natural rhythm with his professional demands.

This case study sheds light on Marma Chikitsa's capability to address not just the physical dimensions of health issues, such as a sports injury, but also to impact the psychological and spiritual realms. By realigning James's energy pathways and encouraging the integration of body, mind, and spirit, Marma Chikitsa provided a comprehensive healing that traditional Western medicine could not fully offer.

Case Study: Enhancing Cognitive Function and Emotional Balance with Marma Chikitsa

Jennifer, a 52-year-old university professor, experienced increasing difficulties with memory retention and emotional fluctuations that significantly affected her professional responsibilities and personal life. Traditional neurologic evaluations and psychological assessments revealed mild cognitive impairment and anxiety without clear pathological origins, leading her to seek alternative therapeutic interventions.

During her initial consultation with a Marma Chikitsa practitioner, Jennifer described symptoms such as forgetfulness, difficulty in concentrating, mood swings, and unexplained bouts of sadness. After a comprehensive evaluation of her lifestyle, dietary habits, and emotional health, the practitioner identified potential disruptions in Jennifer's Pranic flow, particularly around the crown (Sahasrara) and heart (Anahata) Marma points, which are traditionally associated with cognitive functions and emotional regulation.

The treatment plan involved targeted stimulation of these specific Marma points, intending to clear blockages and enhance the flow of prana, thereby improving cognitive function and emotional stability. Each session included gentle pressure and the application of herbal oils known to support neurological and emotional health. Additionally, Jennifer practiced tailored pranayama (breathing techniques) designed to calm her mind and stabilize her mood.

Progressively, Jennifer noticed marked improvements in her memory and focus. Simultaneously, her emotional states became more balanced, with fewer instances of unexplained sadness or irritability. The practitioner also recommended dietary modifications incorporating Ayurvedic principles, focusing on foods that enhance cognitive function and stabilize emotional health.

The sessions fostered an integrative approach, combining physical touch with energetic and spiritual healing. Through ongoing Marma Chikitsa treatments, Jennifer rediscovered a sense of clarity and emotional equilibrium, attributes she had struggled to maintain. This case exemplifies the crucial role of energy balance in managing cognitive and emotional health and depicts how Marma Chikitsa can serve as a pivotal integrative therapy in addressing such complex neurological and emotional issues.

Case Study: Reviving Emotional and Physical Health through Esoteric Marma Healing

Emily, a 34-year-old graphic designer, presented with chronic fatigue syndrome and persistent emotional disturbances characterized by severe anxiety and depressive episodes. Her busy, deadline-driven environment exacerbated her symptoms, which conventional medical treatments—such as antidepressants and behavioral therapy—had failed to alleviate significantly. Desperate for relief and a more sustainable form of recovery, Emily turned to Marma Chikitsa after reading about its potential to balance body and mind energies.

The initial consultation with a seasoned Marma therapist began with an in-depth discussion about her medical history, emotional state, and lifestyle habits. The therapist conducted a subtle yet thorough analysis of Emily's energy points, pinpointing several blockages in her Anahata (heart) and Manipura (solar plexus) Marma points, which are often associated with emotional well-being and personal power, respectively. Her therapist suggested that these disruptions might be causing her physical and emotional symptoms.

Treatment commenced with precise, gentle pressure applied to these critical points using both direct touch and energy manipulation techniques. Emily received sessions twice a week where her therapist used aromatic oils specifically chosen for their properties to aid the flow of prana, or life energy. The scents helped to calm Emily's mind, making her more receptive to healing. Alongside Marma therapy, her practitioner recommended specific dietary changes and herbal supplements to better support her nervous system and overall energy levels.

As her therapy progressed, Emily experienced noticeable improvements in her anxiety levels and a significant boost in her energy. This positive change also led to improved sleep patterns and increased emotional resilience. Her therapist also integrated mindfulness practices and taught Emily meditation techniques to enhance the effects of the physical treatments and support her autonomy in managing stress.

This case exemplifies the effectiveness of Marma Chikitsa in treating conditions that span the physical and emotional spectrum, showcasing how ancient techniques can be adapted to relieve modern-day ailments. Emily's recovery journey highlights the importance of addressing both the energetic and physical disruptions to achieve overall balance and well-being.

Case Study: The Role of Marma Chikitsa in Combatting Chronic Insomnia and stress

Anita, a 47-year-old high school principal, was grappling with chronic insomnia and high stress levels, which began to adversely affect not only her professional performance but also her personal life. After trying various conventional treatments including sleep medication and cognitive behavioral therapy without significant improvement, Anita turned to Marma Chikitsa hoping for a more integrative and holistic remedy.

Her initial consultation involved a comprehensive personal health assessment by a seasoned Marma practitioner, who noted Anita's symptoms of prolonged sleep initiation latency, frequent nighttime awakenings, and non-restorative sleep, along with daytime consequences such as irritability, fatigue, and decreased concentration. The practitioner suggested that Anita's insomnia could be linked to Pranic imbalance primarily at the Talahridaya (palm heart) and Anja (third eye)

Marma points, which are closely associated with mental relaxation and sleep regulation.

Treatment commenced with gentle manipulations and specific pressure at these identified Marma points using soothing herbal oils selected for their calming properties. This was combined with Pranayama breathing techniques designed to reduce mental clutter and promote relaxation. The practitioner also introduced Anita to a series of guided meditations focused on releasing deep-seated tensions, which are often overlooked in conventional therapies.

Post-treatment sessions, Anita experienced noticeable improvements in her ability to fall asleep and the quality of her sleep. The sessions not only targeted her physical symptoms but also introduced her to lifestyle adjustments including dietary changes, evening routines, and the practice of nightly meditation to maintain and enhance the energetic balance achieved during treatment.

This case study highlights how Marma Chikitsa, when effectively integrated with behavioral modifications, provides a robust solution for managing chronic conditions such as insomnia. The holistic focus on energy pathways and their intersection with physical and mental health challenges demonstrates the modality's capacity to address underlying issues that contribute to sleep disturbances, highlighting its relevance in contemporary therapeutic practices.

Review Questions

1. A 35-year-old female patient visits an Ayurvedic practitioner due to recurring headaches and emotional disturbances. She describes her lifestyle as stressful due to high job demands and lacks adequate sleep. She often feels anxious and spiritually disconnected. Following an initial diagnosis, the practitioner decides to focus on Marma Chikitsa to help alleviate her symptoms. Which Marma point should the practitioner focus on to help improve her condition?
A) Anahata Chakra Marma point for heart and emotional balance
B) Ajna Marma point for mental clarity and relief from headaches
C) Manipura Chakra Marma point for digestive and metabolic enhancement
D) Vishuddha Chakra Marma point to improve communication skills
Answer: B
Explanation: The Ajna Marma point, located between the eyebrows, is associated with mental clarity, intuition, and relief of headaches. Stimulating this point can help in balancing the emotional state and enhancing spiritual connectivity, directly addressing the patient's complaints of emotional disturbances and recurrent headaches. This point is instrumental in promoting a sense of overall well-being by integrating spiritual and mental health, making it an ideal choice for this case.

2. During a session of Marma Chikitsa, the practitioner focuses on the Sthapani Marma, located between the eyebrows, alongside using specific mantras for a deeper spiritual impact. What are the expected outcomes of this integrative approach?
A) Decreased digestive function due to enhanced spiritual focus
B) Increased mental clarity and relief from frontal headaches
C) Strengthened lower back and alleviation of spinal discomfort
D) Enhanced lung capacity and easier breathing
Answer: B
Explanation: Stimulating the Sthapani Marma point (like the Ajna point discussed earlier) is

integral for improving higher cognitive functions and alleviating mental stress, including frontal headaches. The use of specific mantras heightens the spiritual impact, aligning the treatment more closely with the patient's psychosomatic framework. This enhances mental clarity and provides considerable relief from headache symptoms typically associated with stress and mental fatigue.

3. Given the patient's need for emotional and spiritual healing as well as her headache, which other Marma point would complement the stimulation of the Ajna Marma for an overall balanced therapy?
A) Kshipra Marma point for quick energy boost
B) Hridaya Marma point for emotional and cardiac balance
C) Guda Marma point to aid in digestive issues
D) Kakshadhara Marma point for shoulder and upper limb tension
Answer: B
Explanation: The Hridaya Marma point, situated over the heart, is closely linked to emotions and the cardiac system. Stimulating this Marma not only helps in stabilizing emotional disturbances but also enhances the heart's energy flow, which can be crucial for patients experiencing stress and emotional imbalance. Used in conjunction with the Ajna Marma, it can provide a holistic treatment focusing on both emotional balance and mental clarity.

CHAPTER FOUR: Tools, Oils, and Media Used in Marma Chikitsa

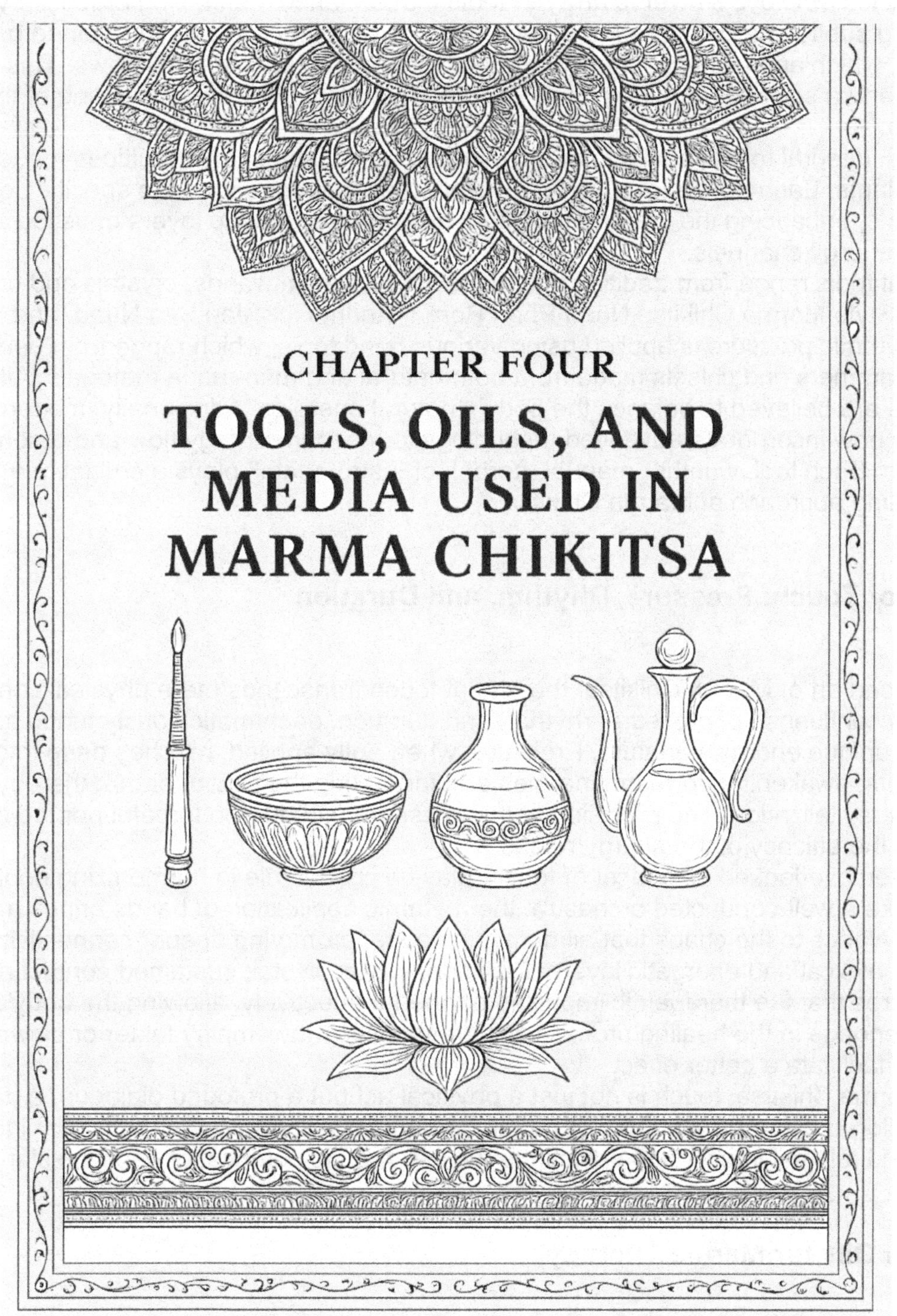

Overview of Tools: Manual, Herbal, Instrumental

Marma Chikitsa employs a diverse array of tools that enhance the healing process by manipulating subtle energy at Marma points. Manual tools are primarily the trained hands of the practitioner, which apply precise pressure to activate and balance energy flows. This touch is both an art and a science, requiring deep knowledge and intuitive understanding of the body's energy map.

Herbal tools, integral to this ancient practice, include oils, pastes, and poultices made from medicinal plants. Each herb is chosen for its properties that correspond to specific doshas and Marma points, enhancing the therapeutic effect by penetrating deep layers of tissue and influencing energy channels.

Instrumental tools range from traditional items, such as Kansa wands, crystals and copper rods. In the Thai Style Marma Chikitsa Nuad Phan Boran, Anantasuk, Jap Sen Nuad, and SriPai schools, rhythmic pressure is applied using various hand tools, which range from pen-like probes to hammers and chisels made from both natural and man-made materials. All these applications are believed to balance the body's natural energies. Additionally, modern implements now incorporate advanced technology to measure energy flow and resonance at Marma sites. Each tool, whether manual, herbal, or instrumental, plays a crucial role in the holistic healing approach of Marma Chikitsa.

The Role of Touch: Pressure, Rhythm, and Duration

In the nuanced art of Marma Chikitsa, the role of touch transcends mere physical contact; it embodies a confluence of pressure, rhythm, and duration, each meticulously tuned to the individual's unique energy signature. Pressure, when aptly applied, reaches deep into the Marma points, awakening dormant energies and facilitating the flow of prana, thereby catalyzing healing and revitalization. The precision of this pressure, neither too forceful nor too gentle, determines the efficacy of the energy release.

Rhythm, often overlooked as a facet of touch, plays a crucial role in harmonizing bodily systems. Like a well-conducted orchestra, the rhythmic application of hands brings a sense of order and balance to the chaos that ailment can cause, promoting deeper connectivity between the body's physical and energetic layers. Duration, too, is pivotal; sustained contact at Marma points ensures that the therapeutic impulses permeate effectively, allowing the body's innate wisdom to engage in the healing process. Different styles may employ faster or slower rhythmic pressure to facilitate a better effect.

Thus, in Marma Chikitsa, touch is not just a physical act but a profound dialogue, a dance of energies tailored to nurture and heal. Practitioners must wield these elements with intuitive precision and mindful intention to unlock the full therapeutic potential of each session.

Abhyanga Oils for Marma Therapy

Abhyanga oils serve as a pivotal medium in Marma Chikitsa, harmonizing and augmenting the therapeutic effects of touch. These specially formulated oils are infused with herbs that correspond to specific doshas and Marma points, enhancing their ability to penetrate deep tissues and vital energy pathways. The choice of oil is critical, as each holds properties that either soothe or stimulate the energy flow, aiding in the balance of bodily humors.

Traditionally, sesame oil is widely used for its warming and deeply penetrating qualities; however, coconut and mustard oils are also favored in certain treatments, depending on the patient's constitutional needs and local climatic conditions. These oils are often prepared using ancient recipes that include a variety of herbs, each selected for their Vata, Pitta, or Kapha pacifying qualities. This customization makes the oil a powerful tool in Marma therapy. Practitioners skillfully apply these oils in a rhythmic manner to enhance prana flow and aid in the detoxification process. The aromatic properties of these oils also play a role in psychological healing, making Abhyanga a holistic treatment modality. The use of these oils turns Marma therapy into a deeply soothing and rejuvenating experience.

Dosha-Specific Oil Formulations

In Marma Chikitsa, the formulation of dosha-specific oils is a refined art that aims to individualize and optimize healing by channeling nature's intelligence through Ayurvedic wisdom. Each oil is carefully crafted to address the unique imbalances of Vata, Pitta, or Kapha in an individual, maximizing the therapeutic potential of the Marma session. These formulations are not merely carriers of aromatic pleasure; they are potent alchemical mixtures that resonate deeply with the body's energy channels.

For instance, oils blended for Vata contain grounding herbs such as ashwagandha and bala, which confer warmth and stability, essential for calming Vata's cold and erratic nature. Pitta oils may feature cooling agents like sandalwood and rose, which are perfect for soothing Pitta's intense heat. Conversely, Kapha formulations are infused with invigorating substances, such as camphor and tulsi, to stimulate and energize Kapha's heavy and sluggish qualities.

This meticulous customization extends beyond mere symptom relief, fostering a deep, nourishing connection between the body's innate wisdom and the therapeutic intentions of Marma practice. Through these personalized oil blends, practitioners can direct healing with greater precision, targeting the energetic root causes of imbalance and disease.

Essential Oils and Their Corresponding Marma Effects

Essential oils, potent carriers of nature's deepest essences, play a crucial role in Marma Chikitsa, enhancing the therapeutic impact at vital energy points. These oils, extracted meticulously from plants, impart properties that are both healing and invigorating, acting on physical discomfort and emotional disturbances. Their unique molecular composition allows them to penetrate the skin swiftly and influence the subtle energy flows within the body.

Each essential oil aligns with specific Marma points to harness distinct energies. For instance, lavender, renowned for its calming qualities, is used to soothe Anahata (heart chakra) and alleviate stress-induced imbalances. Conversely, peppermint oil stimulates Manipura (solar plexus chakra), enhancing digestive fires and invigorating the spirit. The application of these oils in Marma therapy is not arbitrary but rather based on a profound understanding of the doshas and the energetic properties of each oil.

Thus, essential oils serve as powerful tools in Marma Chikitsa, facilitating dynamic shifts in energy and consciousness, steering the body towards balance and rejuvenation. Practitioners blend these oils with precision, creating a symbiotic relationship between aroma and therapy, each scent a whisper of nature's therapeutic dialogue with human physiology.

Herbal Pastes and Poultices

Herbal pastes and poultices stand as a cornerstone in Marma Chikitsa, offering targeted therapeutic benefits through natural concoctions. These pastes are meticulously crafted from finely ground herbs, chosen for their specific properties that align with the energy imbalances at Marma points. When these pastes are applied to the skin, the active ingredients penetrate deeply, initiating healing directly at the energetic epicenters.

The preparation of poultices involves mixing herbs with liquids, often medicated oils or warm water, to form a potent, malleable compound. This compound is then applied to the body, wrapped, and sometimes heated to enhance the absorption of the herbal properties. Such treatments are particularly beneficial for alleviating pain, reducing inflammation, and mobilizing the body's innate healing responses.

Integrating these herbal applications in Marma therapy elevates the energetic healing process, as the natural components work synergistically with the body's energy fields. Practitioners often tailor these formulations to meet individual needs, optimizing the therapeutic outcomes of each session to ensure profound and lasting health benefits.

Use of Heat and Fomentation in Marma Therapy

Heat and fomentation are indispensable tools in enhancing the efficacy of Marma Chikitsa, specifically in soothing pain and deepening the therapeutic influence at energy points. Applying warmth directly helps dilate blood vessels, which boosts circulation and facilitates the absorption of herbs and oils into the Marma points.

This application of heat opens channels, facilitates smoother flow of prana, and alleviates constricted energy pathways. Poultices or cloth bags filled with hot medicated herbs often serve this purpose, providing localized heat that penetrates deeply into tissues. Additionally, warm oil treatments enhance the soothing and penetrating capabilities of Marma therapy, facilitating a deeper release of blockages and restoration of vitality.

Practices like Kati Basti, where warm oil is applied to specific Marma points, harness the dual power of oil's herbal properties and heat's penetrative properties. Such techniques are tailored to individual needs, underscoring the personalized approach of Marma Chikitsa in harmonizing body, mind, and spirit.

Kati Basti Applications

Kati Basti stands out as an exceptional practice within Marma Chikitsa, concentrating on alleviating lower back pain and strengthening the spinal tissues. This technique involves creating a well-like structure on the lower back using dough made from black gram flour, which securely holds warm medicated oil in place directly over the painful area.

The selection of oil is paramount, often tailored to pacify specific doshas and address individual imbalances. The sustained heat and oil penetrate deeply, nourishing the dhatus (tissues) and soothing Vata dosha, known for its role in musculoskeletal pains. This process significantly enhances circulation and reduces muscle stiffness, offering profound pain relief and increased flexibility.

Incorporated wisely with therapeutic massages and other modalities of Marma Chikitsa, Kati Basti serves not only to relieve pain but also as a preventive measure against spine-related issues. Its holistic approach promotes not just physical healing but also emotional and spiritual well-being, catering to overall harmony and health.

Marma Massage Tools: Kansa Wands and Copper Rods

Kansa wands and copper rods make profound tools in Marma Chikitsa, contributing uniquely to the ancient wellness practice. Kansa, an alloy of copper, tin, and sometimes zinc, is famed for its dosha-balancing abilities. When expertly glided across Marma points, these wands enhance the body's natural healing responses by drawing out excess heat and toxins. The metal's subtle electrical conductivity resonates with the body's bioelectrical field, shifting energies to foster balance and rejuvenation.

Copper rods, similarly, are utilized for their conductive properties, offering a cooling sensation and reducing inflammation. They are particularly effective in targeting deeply buried Marma points, facilitating a more profound relaxation and energy release. This makes them invaluable in treating chronic pain and stiffness, as they transmit healing energies directly into the affected areas.

Integrating these tools with previously discussed herbal oils and poultices, practitioners can provide a comprehensive treatment that leverages the synergistic effects of various natural therapies. The precision in their use, aligned with the knowledge of Marma points, underscores the deep-rooted wisdom of Ayurvedic practices, ensuring a holistic approach to restoring health and vitality.

Energy Tools: Crystals and Yantras

In the realm of Marma Chikitsa, the use of energy tools such as crystals and yantras stands as a profound method to amplify healing. Crystals, with their intrinsic vibrational frequencies, optimize the energy flow through Marma points, acting as conduits for healing light and energy. Specific stones, such as rose quartz for emotional balance and amethyst for mental clarity, are strategically placed to resonate with corresponding Marma points, thereby enhancing the body's natural healing capabilities.

Yantras, geometric symbols deeply rooted in Vedic traditions, serve as focal points for meditation and energy alignment. When used in conjunction with Marma therapy, these sacred diagrams help in channeling cosmic energies, facilitating deeper spiritual and physical healing. Positioned near the patient or directly on Marma points, yantras work to clear blockages and restore the body's energetic equilibrium.

Integrating crystals and yantras in Marma Chikitsa not only accelerates the healing process but also deepens the patient's connection to their spiritual essence. This holistic approach ensures a restoration of vitality and promotes a profound sense of well-being.

Light and Color Therapy in Marma Practice

Light and color therapy, traditional components of holistic healing, have a distinctive role in Marma Chikitsa, interfacing directly with the body's energy centers to revitalize and heal. Utilizing specific wavelengths and hues, practitioners of Marma therapy can influence energy flow, facilitate detoxification, and enhance mood, each color addressing different energetic needs based on its vibrational frequency. For instance, blue light, known for its calming properties, might be used to soothe inflammation and reduce stress at critical Marma points. This practice often pairs with guided visualization to deepen the therapy's impact, directing light towards specific Marma points to activate and balance the energies. Moreover, integrating light therapy with complementary practices such as the use of herbal poultices or warm oils can amplify the therapeutic effects, creating a multi-sensory healing environment that targets both the physical and subtle energy bodies.

Overall, light and color therapy in Marma Chikitsa is not just about physical healing. It is a form of communication with the body's innate wisdom, a gentle reminder to the physiological systems to return to a state of harmony and optimal functioning. This method not only enhances the effectiveness of traditional Marma applications but also facilitates a holistic restoration of vitality and health.

Sound Tools: Binaural Beats, Gongs, and Chimes

Marma Chikitsa incorporates sound tools like binaural beats, gongs, and chimes, enabling profound shifts in energy and consciousness. Binaural beats involve playing two slightly different frequencies in each ear, producing auditory illusions that encourage specific brainwave states. This method can lead to deep relaxation and meditative states, enhancing the therapeutic effects of Marma therapy on the nervous system.

Gongs and chimes, with their resonant, penetrating sounds, play a crucial role in dispersing energy blockages. The vibrations produced by these instruments reverberate deeply within the body, reaching the Marma points to liberate trapped energy. These sound frequencies are not random but are carefully chosen to align with the body's natural rhythms, promoting healing from within.

Integrating these sound tools with other Marma modalities amplifies the healing process. Their application ranges from simple calming techniques to complex therapeutic sessions aimed at revitalizing and harmonizing the body's energies. Each session is tailored to patient-specific needs, making sound therapy a versatile and essential component of Marma Chikitsa.

Ghee and Medicinal Butters Usage

Ghee and medicinal butters play an indispensable role in Marma Chikitsa, contributing profound moisturizing and healing properties. Ghee, clarified butter, is highly revered in Ayurveda for its digestibility and for carrying the medicinal properties of herbs deeply into the tissues. When infused with Ayurvedic herbs, ghee becomes a potent medium that enhances the therapeutic effects of Marma therapy, targeting pain relief and tissue rejuvenation.

The application of herbal ghee in Marma therapy is tailored to individual needs, targeting specific doshas and enhancing the balance within the body's energy system. These formulations often include herbs like Ashwagandha for vitality, Turmeric for inflammation, and Brahmi for mental clarity. The penetrative nature of ghee ensures that these benefits reach the deeper layers of tissue, promoting healing from within.

These applications of lubricating medications are often made with "therapeutic prayers" for the well-being of the patient and are usually termed "oleation" protocols in the traditional literature. Moreover, medicinal butters like Shatadhauta Ghrita, prepared by washing ghee one hundred times, are used for their cooling and soothing properties. Applied directly to Marma points, these butters help calm the Pitta dosha and heal inflamed or irritated skin, making Marma Chikitsa a more comprehensive healing practice. The integration of ghee and medicinal butters underscores the holistic approach of Ayurveda, aiming not only at symptom relief but also at nurturing overall health and vitality.

Integration of Marma with Acupressure and Moxibustion

Marma Chikitsa's integration with acupressure and moxibustion bridges traditional healing wisdom across cultures, enhancing therapeutic approaches to pain and disease management. Acupressure, akin to Marma in its focus on energy points, complements the subtle energy manipulations by applying more structured, sustained pressure. This synergy maximizes energy flow and toxin release, broadening the scope of healing potential.

Moxibustion's use of heat to stimulate points parallels the heat applications in Marma, such as Kati Basti. Integrating moxibustion involves burning mugwort over specific Marma or acupressure points, which deeply warms the tissues and promotes circulation. This method helps eliminate cold and dampness from the body, which, in Eastern philosophies, is linked to pain and stiffness.

Together, these modalities extend Marma's efficacy, leveraging acupressure's precise pressure and moxibustion's penetrating warmth. The result is a potent therapeutic blend that addresses physical ailments and balances the subtle energy body, offering a holistic approach to rejuvenation and overall well-being.

Visualization and Guided Meditation Techniques

In the delicate art of Marma Chikitsa, visualization and guided meditation techniques play crucial roles. These practices empower the practitioner to direct healing energies through focused intention and mental imagery, complementing the physical aspects of Marma manipulation. By visualizing energy flow and healing lights enveloping the Marma points, patients can enhance their internal healing processes, facilitating a deeper connection between mind and body.

Guided meditation particularly serves as a bridge, linking the practitioner's therapeutic touch with the patient's cognitive states. Through soothing verbal cues and crafted imagery, practitioners guide individuals into profound states of relaxation. This mental tranquility is essential for opening energy pathways and allowing for the optimal reception of therapeutic interventions. It ensures that the session's benefits are not just superficial but deeply ingrained.

The synergy between visualization and the tangible tools and media used in Marma Chikitsa—like oils, crystals, and sound tools—creates a holistic healing environment. Each session is a carefully orchestrated experience, aiming not merely at physical relief but at nurturing serene mental landscapes, essential for lasting recovery and vitality restoration.

Preparation and Use of Ayurvedic Balms and Liniments

Ayurvedic balms and liniments play a pivotal role in Marma Chikitsa, as they are formulated to harness the healing powers of herbs and enhance the therapeutic effects of touch. These preparations are often enriched with potent, pain-relieving herbs such as turmeric and ginger, and penetrating oils like sesame or coconut, designed to target and alleviate discomfort at specific Marma points. The method of preparation involves a meticulous process of extracting herbal essences, ensuring the active components are preserved in their most potent form. Once crafted, the application of these balms and liniments is a ritual. A practitioner applies them in gentle, circular motions, focusing on Marma locations that correspond to the underlying imbalances. This method not only soothes physical pain but also aids in the subtle energy adjustments necessary for healing.

The integration of such treatments enhances the energetic exchanges during Marma therapy, creating deeper levels of relaxation and healing. Moreover, repetitive applications are recommended to maintain energy flows and sustain therapeutic benefits, helping restore vitality and alleviate chronic conditions, underlining the profound synergy between herbal therapy and energy healing in Marma Chikitsa.

Incorporating Marma Points in Panchakarma Procedures

Integrating Marma points within the framework of Panchakarma, a profound detoxification ritual in Ayurveda, enhances healing potential by aligning physical purification with subtle energy manipulation. Panchakarma—comprising five therapeutic actions—aims to thoroughly cleanse the body, rejuvenating it at a cellular level. By targeting specific Marma points during these procedures, therapists can amplify the detoxification effects, promoting deeper toxin release from both the physical and energetic bodies.

During Vamana (therapeutic emesis) or Virechana (purgation), for instance, stimulating corresponding Marma points can facilitate a more complete expulsion of doshic imbalances. Similarly, in Nasya (nasal administration of herbs), accessing Marma points around the nose and forehead enhances the absorption and efficacy of herbal medicines, clearing the mind and nourishing cerebral functions.

The strategic touch on Marma points during Snehana (oleation) and Swedana (sudation) also yields amplified results. This methodical stimulation not only deepens the therapeutic oils' penetration but also catalyzes the sweat-induced release of impurities. By incorporating Marma therapy in Panchakarma, practitioners offer a holistic revival, aligning the body's energies to foster profound healing and renewal.

Home Kits for Self-Marma Practice

The crafting of Home Kits for Self-Marma Practice enables individuals to experience the therapeutic benefits of Marma Chikitsa in the comfort of their own homes. These kits typically contain essential items such as herbal oils, Marma maps, and tools like wooden or copper wands. Each component is carefully selected to facilitate easy and safe self-administration of Marma therapy, catering especially to those with a basic understanding of the practice.

Instructions included in the kits emphasize the gentle activation of Marma points, suitable for daily routines. Users are guided on how to combine oils and apply precise pressure to enhance the flow of energy and alleviate common ailments. Videos or pamphlets often accompany these kits, providing visual and textual demonstrations that empower users to practice techniques such as rotational pressure and oil application confidently.

Moreover, the kits often include small booklets on dosha-specific practices, allowing for a personalized approach to health and well-being. The ability to adapt the intensity and frequency of treatments provides users with a flexible, tailored therapeutic experience, fostering self-reliance in managing health through ancient wisdom.

Ensuring Quality and Purity of Herbal Media Used

The integrity of Marma Chikitsa hinges significantly on the quality and purity of the herbal media utilized. Recognizing the profound impact of these materials on treatment efficacy, rigorous standards are essential for verifying and maintaining their purity. By sourcing herbs from reputable suppliers who adhere to traditional and sustainable cultivation methods, practitioners can safeguard against contaminants that might impair therapeutic outcomes.

Verification processes, which involve both modern laboratory testing and traditional assessments of sensory properties, ensure that each batch of herbs meets high standards of potency and purity. Certifications from trusted, standard-setting bodies further substantiate the quality, providing practitioners and patients with confidence in the herbal media used.

This meticulous oversight extends to storage and handling practices, where controlled environments prevent degradation of herbal properties. By committing to these high standards of quality assurance, Marma Chikitsa practitioners uphold the therapeutic potency of their treatments, ensuring that each application delivers optimal health benefits. These practices not only foster trust but also preserve the rich lineage of knowledge inherent to Marma therapy.

Selection of Oils: Criteria and Effects

The meticulous selection of oils in Marma Chikitsa is pivotal, governed by an understanding of their inherent properties and the specific needs of the patient. Criteria for choosing the right oil include its base consistency, herbal infusions, and the corresponding effects on the three doshas—Vata, Pitta, and Kapha. For instance, sesame oil is preferred for its penetrative qualities, ideal for pacifying Vata, while coconut oil is favored for its cooling properties, beneficial for Pitta-related imbalances.

The effects of these oils on Marma points are profound. They act as vehicles for directing healing energies into the body's subtle channels, amplifying the therapeutic impact of touch. This synergy between the oil's properties and Marma therapy enhances the flow of prana, promoting detoxification and rejuvenation.

Additionally, understanding seasonal and diurnal rhythms helps in selecting the ideal oil, aligning external treatments with internal circadian rhythms to maximize healing efficacy. Each selected oil thus plays a crucial role in the holistic health paradigm of Marma Chikitsa, tailored to individual healing journeys.

Sterilization and Maintenance of Tools Used in Marma Therapy

The sanctity of Marma Chikitsa is preserved through meticulous sterilization and maintenance of its therapeutic tools. Instruments like Kansa wands, copper rods, and even the simple wooden applicators require regular cleansing to prevent the buildup of biological contaminants that may compromise treatment quality and safety. Sterilization processes often involve both traditional methods, such as boiling in herbal decoctions and modern techniques like autoclaving, ensuring every instrument meets stringent hygiene standards.

Moreover, the maintenance of these tools extends beyond mere cleanliness. Regular inspections for signs of wear and tear are crucial, as damaged tools could potentially harm the delicate Marma points. Oiling and polishing with herbal compounds not only prevent material degradation but also enhance the tool's efficiency by maintaining their bio-energetic

compatibility with human tissue.
Lastly, practitioners are rigorously trained in the proper handling and storage of these instruments, ensuring that therapeutic integrity is maintained from one session to the next. By adhering to these protocols, Marma Chikitsa preserves its foundational elements of purity and effectiveness, fostering trust and deep healing amongst practitioners and patients alike.

Ethical Considerations in the Use of Tools and Media

Ethical considerations in Marma Chikitsa hold paramount importance, ensuring that the practice not only heals physically but also aligns with moral and spiritual values. Practitioners must exercise utmost responsibility in selecting and utilizing tools and media, keeping the patient's welfare at the forefront. Respect for personal boundaries and consent is fundamental, as Marma therapy often involves intimate bodily contact.
Beyond respecting physical boundaries, the energetic purity of the tools and substances used, such as oils and crystals, requires careful attention. Practitioners are responsible for maintaining the integrity of these tools through proper cleansing techniques, both physical and energetic, to prevent any adverse influence on the patient's energy body.
Furthermore, the ethical sourcing of materials, including herbs and oils, reflects the broader commitment of Marma Chikitsa to do no harm. This extends to environmental stewardship, where we source materials that are not only effective but also sustainably harvested, thereby supporting ecological health and community well-being. Thus, ethical considerations shape the practice, making it a holistic endeavor that honors both individual and collective integrity.

Training and Correct Use of Instruments and Appliances

Training in the correct use of instruments in Marma Chikitsa is a vital component of this ancient healing practice. It ensures that practitioners are not only adept in technique but also deeply attuned to the ethical deployment of these tools, respecting their potent interaction with the body's subtle energy points. Rigorous training programs, often spanning several months, cover the intricate use of Kansa wands, copper rods, and other specific applicators, such as the Thai Ayurveda use of "Tok Sen" tools, previously mentioned. These programs focus on pressure points, the angle of application, and the subtle nuances of energetic influence.
Furthermore, the curriculum includes extensive studies on physiological and energetic anatomy, ensuring that practitioners understand the profound impacts of their interventions. This knowledge is crucial when applying instruments to various Marma points, which can dramatically affect bodily systems and overall health. Continual assessment and feedback are integral to this training, enabling practitioners to refine their skills in real-world scenarios.
Lastly, adherence to traditional knowledge while integrating contemporary ergonomic practices maximizes both the efficacy and safety of instrument application. Dedicated sessions on maintenance and sterilization emphasize the profound respect required when handling these sacred tools, ensuring they are treated with care and reverence befitting their role in healing and wellness.

Application of New Media in Marma Practices: Innovations and Adaptations

The dynamism of Marma Chikitsa is evident in its evolving application of new media, embracing both tradition and innovation. Pioneering practitioners are increasingly integrating modern technologies to enhance the depth and efficacy of treatment. Electronic tools now help map Marma points with precision, providing digital overlays that guide therapeutic interventions and assure accuracy previously reliant on tactile skill alone.

Similarly, the adoption of virtual reality (VR) and augmented reality (AR) technologies provides immersive experiences that facilitate the training of new practitioners and enhance patient understanding of treatment processes. These technologies allow for a visual and interactive representation of Marma points, fostering a deeper connection and understanding between the practitioner and the therapy.

Further, advances in biofeedback mechanisms provide real-time insights into the physiological responses of patients during Marma therapy. This data-driven approach enables tailored treatments that respond dynamically to the individual's unique bio-energetic state, promoting more targeted and effective healing interventions.

Summary

The chapter on 'Tools, Oils, and Media Used in Marma Chikitsa' expertly details the various instruments, oils, and techniques pivotal in the practice of Marma Chikitsa, an ancient Ayurvedic healing technique that focuses on manipulating subtle energy through specific bodily points known as 'Marma points'. The diverse array of tools encompasses manual, herbal, and instrumental types. Manual tools require the skilled hands of the practitioner to apply pressure. In contrast, herbal tools include specialized oils and pastes that cater to distinct energetic needs dictated by the doshas (body constitutions). Instrumental tools range from traditional items, such as Kansa wands and copper rods, to advanced technological implements used for measuring energy flows. The chapter elucidates how careful manipulation of these tools aids in healing by facilitating the flow of prana (life force), thus promoting physical, emotional, and spiritual wellness. Special attention is given to the role of touch, rhythm, and duration in Marma therapy, all of which are crucial for achieving therapeutic effectiveness. Abhyanga oils are highlighted for their role in not only enhancing the healing touch but also in incorporating aromatherapeutic benefits. Each herbal oil, balm, and poultice is meticulously formulated from Ayurvedic recipes to maximize healing properties and align with individual patient needs. Techniques such as Kati Basti, which leverage heat and utilize sound tools like gongs or binaural beats, extend the sensory range of Marma Chikitsa, making it a holistic health modality. The innovative integration of modern technology with traditional methods enriches the practice, ensuring precise and effective treatments, while ethical considerations and training ensure the integrity and efficacy of the methods are maintained.

References

[1] Subtle Energy Body: The Complete Guide. https://www.books.google.com

[2] Traditional Ayurvedic Practices. https://www.ayurveda.com/resources/articles/traditional-ayurvedic-practices

[3] Effect of Ayurvedic oils on energy flow. https://www.journalofayurvedicstudies.com/article/effect-of-oils

[4] History of Marma Chikitsa. https://www.marmachikitsa.org/history

Case Study: Enhancing Therapeutic Efficacy through Integrated Marma Chikitsa and Modern Tools

In the bustling city of Mumbai, India, a wellness center has recently adopted a pioneering approach to traditional Marma Chikitsa by integrating it with contemporary medical tools. The case involved a 45-year-old male patient, Mr. Shah, who presented with chronic lower back pain and associated stress, which had resisted conventional treatments for months.

The practitioner, Dr. Anjali, an expert in Marma Chikitsa with a keen interest in integrating modern technology, decided to utilize a combination of traditional Kansa wands and an innovative biofeedback device. Kansa wands, known for their ability to harmonize the body's doshas, were used to stimulate specific Marma points across Mr. Shah's back and limbs. The biofeedback device, which measures physiological responses like skin conductance and heart rate variability, provided real-time data on the energetic shifts occurring during the session.

During the therapy sessions, Dr. Anjali applied herbal oils specifically crafted for Vata and Kapha doshas, previously diagnosed as imbalanced in Mr. Shah, to the Marma points before using the Kansa wands. These oils, infused with herbs such as ashwagandha and bala, were selected to bring warmth and stability to Mr. Shah's body, aiding in calming his Vata dosha, which is often associated with nervous and musculoskeletal disorders.

The integration of Marma Chikitsa with biofeedback allowed Dr. Anjali to achieve a deeper understanding of the patient's bio-energetic state. The feedback helped her adjust the pressure and duration of touch on Marma points in real-time, significantly enhancing the therapeutic efficacy. Over several sessions, Mr. Shah reported a noticeable reduction in pain and improved overall well-being.

This case illustrates the potential of integrating traditional Marma tools with modern technology to enhance healing and patient outcomes. It highlights the importance of a personalized approach in Marma Chikitsa, where understanding the subtle energy flows can be significantly enhanced by technological aid, paving the way for a new era in traditional practices.

Case Study: Revitalizing Marma Therapy with Customized Herbal and Oil Protocols

In the serene landscapes of Kerala, India, an Ayurvedic clinic has been exploring the profound impact of customized herbal formulations and specialized oils in Marma Chikitsa. The case centers around Mrs. Anitha, a 58-year-old woman experiencing severe arthritis and insomnia, conditions often exacerbated by her predominant Kapha dosha, which tends to cause sluggishness and fluid retention.

Dr. Lalitha, a seasoned Ayurvedic practitioner at the clinic, decided to tailor a unique Marma therapy regimen integrating vital herbal pastes and a dosha-specific oil selection. Recognizing the importance of individualized treatment, she formulated an herbal paste comprising potent anti-inflammatory herbs like turmeric and ginger and created a special blend of oils including eucalyptus and mustard oil, both known for their penetrating warmth and ability to reduce Kapha accumulation.

The Marma sessions began with the gentle application of the herbal paste on key Marma points known to influence joint health and sleep patterns. Dr. Lalitha then used the customized oils, meticulously applying them in a structured pattern to enhance absorption and effectiveness. By focusing on the Marma points corresponding to Vata regulation, she aimed to address the nerve impulses associated with pain and to promote better sleep.

Throughout the sessions, Mrs. Anitha reported a significant easing of her joint pains and a more relaxed state of mind, which contributed to better sleep. Dr. Lalitha adjusted the formulations across sessions based on Mrs. Anitha's feedback and progress, demonstrating the dynamic nature of this personalized therapy.

This case study underscores the importance of customization in Marma Chikitsa, showing that precise, personalized herbal and oil treatments can significantly enhance the effectiveness of traditional practices. It also highlights the broader applications of Marma therapy for chronic conditions, providing valuable insights into how traditional practices can be adapted and optimized for individual health needs.

Case Study: Holistic Healing through Marma Chikitsa: A Journey of Chronic Pain Management

In a quaint town nestled in the foothills of the Himalayas, an alternative therapy clinic has been pioneering a deeply integrated approach to Marma Chikitsa, tailored specifically for chronic pain management. The case revolves around a 62-year-old woman, Mrs. Mehta, who had been suffering from chronic fibromyalgia—a condition characterized by widespread pain and fatigue. Traditional medications provided her little relief, and she sought alternative treatments as a last resort.

The practitioner, Dr. Kumar, a seasoned expert in Marma Chikitsa with a profound interest in holistic healing methodologies, decided to employ a comprehensive treatment plan including manual and herbal tools. He began by mapping out the critical Marma points related to pain regulation and energy flow. Each session started with a gentle, rhythmic touch, applying appropriate pressure to these Marma points, aiming to release blocked prana, or life force, which, according to Ayurvedic belief, is often the cause of imbalance and pain.

Dr. Kumar enhanced the treatment by incorporating specially formulated Abhyanga oils. These were infused with herbs known for their Vata and Kapha-pacifying properties, such as turmeric for its anti-inflammatory qualities and Triphala for its detoxification properties. The oils were warmed slightly to facilitate deeper absorption and improve circulation around the targeted Marma points.

Additionally, Dr. Kumar incorporated sound tools, such as Tibetan singing bowls, at the beginning and end of each session. The vibrations from these bowls are considered beneficial in harmonizing the body's energy fields and enhancing the healing effects of Marma therapy. Mrs. Mehta participated in guided meditation sessions post-treatment to further support her mental and emotional well-being, vital components often overlooked in conventional treatments.

Through a series of twelve sessions, Mrs. Mehta experienced significant improvements not just in her physical symptoms but also in her overall energy levels and emotional state. Dr. Kumar's approach underscores the efficacy of Marma Chikitsa when combined with complementary tools and techniques, offering a robust framework for the holistic management of chronic conditions that respects the interconnectedness of body, mind, and spirit.

Case Study: Optimizing Marma Chikitsa with Advanced Heat and Fomentation Techniques

In the evolving field of Marma Chikitsa, an innovative clinic in Bangalore, India, has been incorporating advanced heat and fomentation techniques to enhance the therapeutic efficacy of traditional treatment methods. The case centers around Mr. Gupta, a 52-year-old businessman suffering from chronic shoulder pain and stiffness attributed to long hours of computer work and minimal physical activity.

Dr. Reddy, the attending Ayurvedic expert, noted that Mr. Gupta's condition was characterized by a significant Vata imbalance, as evidenced by localized dryness and restricted mobility. To address these issues, Dr. Reddy proposed a customized treatment plan utilizing specialized heat applications alongside traditional Marma point stimulation.

The treatment began with the gentle application of medicated oils infused with herbs like ginger, garlic, and sesame to effectively pacify the aggravated Vata dosha. Following the oil application, Dr. Reddy introduced a modern fomentation device specifically designed to provide consistent heat, thereby enhancing the oils' penetration and efficacy. The device targeted critical Marma points around the shoulder, facilitating a deeper release of blocked prana or vital energy.

Subsequent sessions incorporated poultices filled with heated medicinal herbs wrapped around Mr. Gupta's shoulder. These poultices were prepared fresh for each session, containing a blend of anti-inflammatory and pain-relieving herbs that synergistically worked to soften tissues and relax muscles, thus augmenting the Marma therapy's results.

Throughout his treatment journey, Mr. Gupta experienced a notable reduction in pain and an improvement in his range of motion. Dr. Reddy adjusted the intensity and duration of heat application based on Mr. Gupta's feedback and progress, showcasing the importance of personalized care in Marma Chikitsa.

This case illustrates how integrating traditional techniques with innovative heat delivery systems can significantly boost the healing process in Marma Chikitsa. The approach demonstrates the adaptability of ancient practices to modern therapeutic methods, ensuring a holistic treatment paradigm that respects the intricate balance of body energies.

Case Study: Implementing Multi-Sensory Marma Therapy for Enhanced Emotional Well-being

In the vibrant city of Chennai, a holistic wellness center specializing in Marma Chikitsa has pioneered the incorporation of multi-sensory stimulation into its treatments. The adaptability of Marma Chikitsa presents a unique opportunity to incorporate additional sensory modalities, thereby enhancing therapeutic outcomes. The case involves a 35-year-old female patient, Ms. Priya, struggling with anxiety and recurring depression, conditions that significantly affected her daily functionality and quality of life.

Dr. Nalini, an experienced Marma therapist and innovator in sensory therapies, designed a customized treatment regimen for Ms. Priya. Recognizing the interconnectedness of mind, body, and spirit in healing, she decided to combine traditional Marma therapy with sound, light, and aromatherapy, aiming to address both the patient's emotional and physical needs. Each session began with the application of dosha-specific oils, followed by the stimulation of Marma points through gentle, precise touches. Handcrafted essential oils with calming properties, such as lavender and chamomile, were diffused throughout the treatment area to create a soothing atmosphere.

To further enhance the experience, Dr. Nalini introduced a color therapy component. Soft blue and green lights bathed the room; colors known to promote tranquility and alleviate stress. This was accompanied by the sound of soft, rhythmic chimes and specially curated binaural beats playing in the background, targeting frequencies known to induce a meditative and relaxed state of mind.

Each session included guided visualization techniques, where Ms. Priya was encouraged to envision healing energies flowing through her body, focusing on rebalancing her energy fields and cleansing emotional blockages. Over several weeks, Ms. Priya reported substantial reductions in her anxiety levels and improvements in her overall mood and outlook on life.

This case demonstrates the potential of integrating multiple sensory therapies with traditional Marma Chikitsa to enhance emotional regulation and mental health. Dr. Nalini's approach showcases how tailoring treatments to the needs of the individual and engaging multiple senses can create a deeply therapeutic environment that supports comprehensive healing and emotional resilience.

Case Study: Reviving Traditional Practices with Technology-Enhanced Marma Therapy

In the quaint town of Coimbatore, India, a traditional Ayurvedic center recently incorporated cutting-edge technology into its Marma Chikitsa treatments, providing an enhanced therapeutic experience. The case study focuses on Mrs. Lata, a 67-year-old retired teacher suffering from chronic knee pain and mobility issues exacerbated by arthritis. Traditional methods had provided minimal relief, prompting the clinic to explore innovative approaches.

Dr. Vishnu, the center's lead practitioner with a background in both Ayurvedic and modern medical practices, introduced a newly developed Marma mat embedded with pressure sensors and heating elements. This mat was designed to stimulate Marma points accurately according to Ayurvedic scriptures while providing consistent heat to deepen the therapeutic impact.

Mrs. Lata's treatment began with the application of a customized herbal oil infused with anti-inflammatory herbs such as guggulu and nirgundi, known for their efficacy in treating joint pain. As Mrs. Lata lay on the mat, sensors detected pressure distribution and heat was gently applied, allowing for precise targeting of Marma points around her knees. Dr. Vishnu carefully monitored the real-time data displayed by the mat's connected device, adjusting the intensity and locations of stimulation to maximize therapeutic benefits.

Throughout the sessions, Mrs. Lata experienced significant improvements. The scientific precision of pressure and heat application ensured that the therapy was both safe and effectively tailored to her specific condition. The warming sensation of the mat not only soothed her pain but also improved the oil's penetration, enhancing the overall effect of the herbs.

This case exemplifies the potential of integrating traditional practices with innovative tools to revitalize ancient therapies, such as Marma Chikitsa. By combining the time-tested techniques with modern technology, practitioners can offer personalized, effective, and deeply healing experiences, setting a new standard in holistic treatment.

Case Study: Advanced Integration of Aromatherapy and Marma Chikitsa for Stress Reduction

At a well-known holistic health center in Pune, India, a novel approach to combining advanced aromatherapy with Marma Chikitsa has achieved remarkable success. The case involves Mr. Arjun, a 40-year-old IT consultant with chronic stress and anxiety symptoms exacerbated by a hectic work environment and poor sleep patterns. Understanding the deep-seated nature of his ailments, the center's lead practitioner, Dr. Seema, embarked on an innovative path integrating detailed essential oil therapy with traditional Marma techniques.

Dr. Seema, trained in both traditional Indian medicine and modern holistic techniques, initiated a comprehensive assessment of Mr. Arjun's doshic balance, identifying a significant Vata imbalance resulting in his nervous tension and restlessness. To address these issues, she employed a personalized blend of essential oils, including lavender for its calming properties, frankincense to enhance focus, and sandalwood for its grounding effects.

Additionally, Dr. Seema referred to the ancient texts of Marma Chikitsa to select strategic Marma points that correlate to stress relief and mental clarity. During the sessions, Mr. Arjun underwent a series of gentle stimulations at these Marma points using the essential oil blend, applied with rhythmic, mindful touches designed to penetrate deep into the tissue and soothe the nervous system. Each session also integrated the use of diffuse aromatic scents to facilitate a multi-sensory healing environment.

Through this dual approach, Dr. Seema created a highly customized therapeutic experience that leveraged the olfactory impact of essential oils with the energy-aligning capabilities of Marma therapy. Over a period of six weeks, Mr. Arjun reported notable improvements in his sleep quality, a significant reduction in anxiety levels, and an overall enhancement in his quality of life. He felt rejuvenated each time he stepped out of the session, carrying with him the nourishing fragrances and the calming energy from the therapy.

This case study illustrates the effectiveness of integrating aromatherapy with Marma Chikitsa in addressing mental and emotional well-being, demonstrating a progressive step towards holistic health practices where traditional and modern techniques coalesce to offer powerful healing solutions.

Case Study: Strategic Use of Herbal Pastes and Heat in Marma Chikitsa for Sports Injuries

In a sports rehabilitation center in Jaipur, India, a new integrative approach towards sports injuries combines Marma Chikitsa with specialized herbal pastes and heat treatments. The case revolves around a professional cricketer, Raj, aged 29, who sustained a significant hamstring injury during a national league game. Conventional physiotherapy provided limited relief, prompting the exploration of traditional Ayurvedic techniques to accelerate his recovery.

Dr. Gupta, an expert in both sports medicine and Marma Chikitsa, undertook Raj's treatment. Acknowledging the need for a tailored approach, Dr. Gupta decided to incorporate specific Marma points associated with muscle and tissue repair. He began by applying a custom-made herbal paste that included ingredients such as arnica, turmeric, and wintergreen. These herbs are known for their anti-inflammatory and pain-relieving properties, which are crucial for treating soft tissue injuries.

Following the application of the herbal paste, Dr. Gupta employed a traditional technique using poultices filled with heated medicinal herbs. The heat facilitated deeper penetration of the herbs into the tissue and increased blood flow to the injured area, which is essential for reducing swelling and promoting healing. Dr. Gupta carefully monitored the temperature to ensure maximum efficacy without causing discomfort or burns.

The Marma therapy sessions also involved gentle manipulations at specific energy points to further enhance circulation and support the body's innate healing mechanisms. By integrating heat therapy with the strategic application of herbal pastes, Dr. Gupta not only addressed the immediate symptoms of pain and inflammation but also promoted long-term healing and recovery. Over several weeks, Raj noticed a significant improvement in his mobility and a reduction in pain levels, attributing his faster recovery to the holistic treatment provided by Dr. Gupta.

This case underscores the effective integration of ancient Marma Chikitsa techniques with herbal and heat therapies to create a comprehensive treatment plan for sports injuries. It highlights the potential of traditional practices to complement modern sports medicine, providing athletes with a broader range of therapeutic options to enhance recovery and optimize performance.

Case Study: Integrative Marma Chikitsa for Comprehensive Stress Relief

In a bustling urban wellness clinic in Hyderabad, India, a unique case arose involving a 38-year-old IT professional named Mr. Karthik, who was battling severe stress, anxiety, and the onset of insomnia, exacerbated by a demanding work schedule and chronic back pain. The clinic, known for its holistic approach, proposed an integrative Marma Chikitsa regimen to address both his physical and emotional health comprehensively.

Dr. Priya, an experienced practitioner of Marma Chikitsa with a background in psychological counseling, undertook the case. Initial assessments indicated an imbalance in Mr. Karthik's Vata and Pitta doshas, manifesting as physical tension and mental unrest. To rectify these imbalances, Dr. Priya planned a treatment that incorporated tailored herbal oils, specific Marma points stimulation, sound therapy, and guided visualization techniques.

The treatment began with the application of a customized herbal oil blend, primarily designed to pacify Mr. Karthik's elevated Vata. This oil utilizes herbs such as Brahmi and Ashwagandha, renowned for their calming properties and effectiveness in supporting the nervous system. Following the oil application, Dr. Priya focused on stimulating key Marma points along Mr. Karthik's spine and near his head to release pent-up energy and enhance cerebral circulation, aiming to soothe his anxiety and ease his back pain.

Each session incorporated the use of Tibetan singing bowls, whose resonant sounds were employed to facilitate a deeper state of relaxation and meditation. Dr. Priya guided Mr. Karthik through visualization exercises, having him imagine a flow of healing energy cascading down his spine, washing away tension and restoring vitality. This multi-sensory approach not only targeted his physical ailments but also addressed his mental stressors, fostering a state of deep relaxation and mental clarity.

After twelve sessions spread over six weeks, Mr. Karthik reported significant reductions in back pain and anxiety, along with improved sleep quality. The comprehensive Marma Chikitsa approach adopted by Dr. Priya showcases the intricate interplay between traditional techniques and personalized care, providing effective relief from stress while promoting overall well-being and resilience in life.

Case Study: Innovative Application of Thermal Imaging in Marma Chikitsa for Chronic Digestive Disorders

In the serene environment of a specialized holistic clinic in Goa, a groundbreaking case arose involving the integration of advanced thermal imaging technology with traditional Marma Chikitsa to treat chronic digestive disorders. The patient, Mr. Rajan, a 49-year-old businessman, had been suffering from chronic irritable bowel syndrome (IBS) and related digestive issues, which traditional medications had failed to alleviate satisfactorily.

Mrs. Geeta, a highly skilled Marma Chikitsa practitioner with an interest in technological integration for enhanced healing outcomes, undertook his case. Her innovative approach involved using a thermal imaging camera to visualize the body's heat patterns before, during, and after the Marma therapy sessions. This technology enabled her to identify subtle physiological changes and determine the energetic status of specific Marma points related to digestive functioning.

During the sessions, Mrs. Geeta applied specially formulated herbal oils, known for their efficacy in balancing the Pitta dosha, which in Ayurveda is often linked with metabolism and digestive processes. She chose points like Nabhi (around the navel), which directly corresponds to digestive vitality in Marma therapy. The thermal imaging displayed shifts in thermal signatures, which helped assess the efficacy of the Marma applications in real-time and adjust the techniques accordingly.

Mrs. Geeta also customized the session duration and pressure applied, based on the thermal responses, which varied across different sessions. Over several weeks, Mr. Rajan reported a significant improvement in his digestive symptoms, reduced abdominal pain, and increased overall energy levels. The use of thermal imaging provided a non-invasive, insightful way to enhance the precision of Marma therapy and its adaptation to individual patient needs.

This case represents a significant advancement in Marma Chikitsa, demonstrating how the incorporation of modern diagnostic tools can revolutionize traditional practices. It highlights the potential of integrating contemporary scientific methods with age-old wisdom to create more effective, personalized therapeutic strategies, offering profound insights into both physiological and energetic changes during treatment.

Review Questions

1. A 42-year-old woman with chronic lower back pain seeks treatment after learning about Marma Chikitsa. Her Ayurvedic practitioner decides to use a Kati Basti treatment. Which essential component is used to create the well-like structure for the Kati Basti?

A) Kansa wand
B) Black gram flour dough
C) Coconut oil
D) Copper rod

Answer: B

Explanation: In the traditional practice of Marma Chikitsa, Kati Basti involves creating a well-like structure on the lower back using a dough made from black gram flour. This structure serves to hold warm medicated oil in place, targeting the lower back pain efficiently. The use of this specific type of dough is crucial as it ensures the containment of the oil, allowing optimal penetration of its medicinal properties into the tissues.

2. During a consultation for Marma Chikitsa, a practitioner assesses a patient with high Vata dosha. The practitioner decides to use a traditional oil in the treatment. Which oil is likely chosen due to its warming and deep-penetrating qualities, especially beneficial for pacifying Vata?

A) Sesame oil
B) Coconut oil
C) Mustard oil
D) Olive oil

Answer: A

Explanation: Sesame oil is traditionally favored in Marma Chikitsa for its warm and penetrative qualities, which are particularly effective in pacifying Vata dosha. This dosha is characterized by a cold and erratic nature; thus, warming sesame oil helps in stabilizing and soothing Vata-related imbalances.

3. A practitioner using Marma Chikitsa for an anxiety patient plan to incorporate essential oils to enhance treatment efficacy. Which essential oil is expected to be used for its renowned calming qualities and alignment with the Anahata (heart chakra)?
A) Peppermint oil
B) Lavender oil
C) Eucalyptus oil
D) Tea tree oil
Answer: B
Explanation: In Marma Chikitsa, lavender oil is highly valued for its calming and soothing properties, making it an excellent choice for treating stress and anxiety issues. It is particularly associated with Anahata, the heart chakra, where it aids in alleviating stress-induced imbalances, promoting relaxation and emotional balance.

4. Considering the profound role of rhythm in Marma Chikitsa's manual therapy, how does it affect the healing process when treating a patient with disrupted bodily systems due to chronic illness?
A) Increases cellular inflammation
B) Disrupts energetic balance
C) Harmonizes bodily systems
D) Blocks therapeutic impulses
Answer: C
Explanation: The rhythm in the manual touch during Marma Chikitsa plays a vital role, akin to a well-conducted orchestra, bringing order and balance to disrupted bodily systems caused by chronic ailments. This rhythmic application promotes connectivity between the body's physical and energetic layers, facilitating holistic healing and systemic harmonization.

5. A new practitioner of Marma Chikitsa enquires about the use of heat in treatments. What is the primary purpose of applying heat in the form of Swedana in Marma Therapy?
A) To cool down the body's exterior
B) To dilate blood vessels for improved circulation
C) To decrease the efficacy of herbal oils
D) To solidify the medicated pastes
Answer: B
Explanation: In Marma Chikitsa, the application of heat through methods like Swedana (fomentation) serves to dilate blood vessels. This dilation enhances circulation and promotes a more effective and deeper penetration of the therapeutic properties of herbs and oils into the Marma points, thus optimizing the healing process.

CHAPTER FIVE: Step-by-Step Application Techniques for Beginners

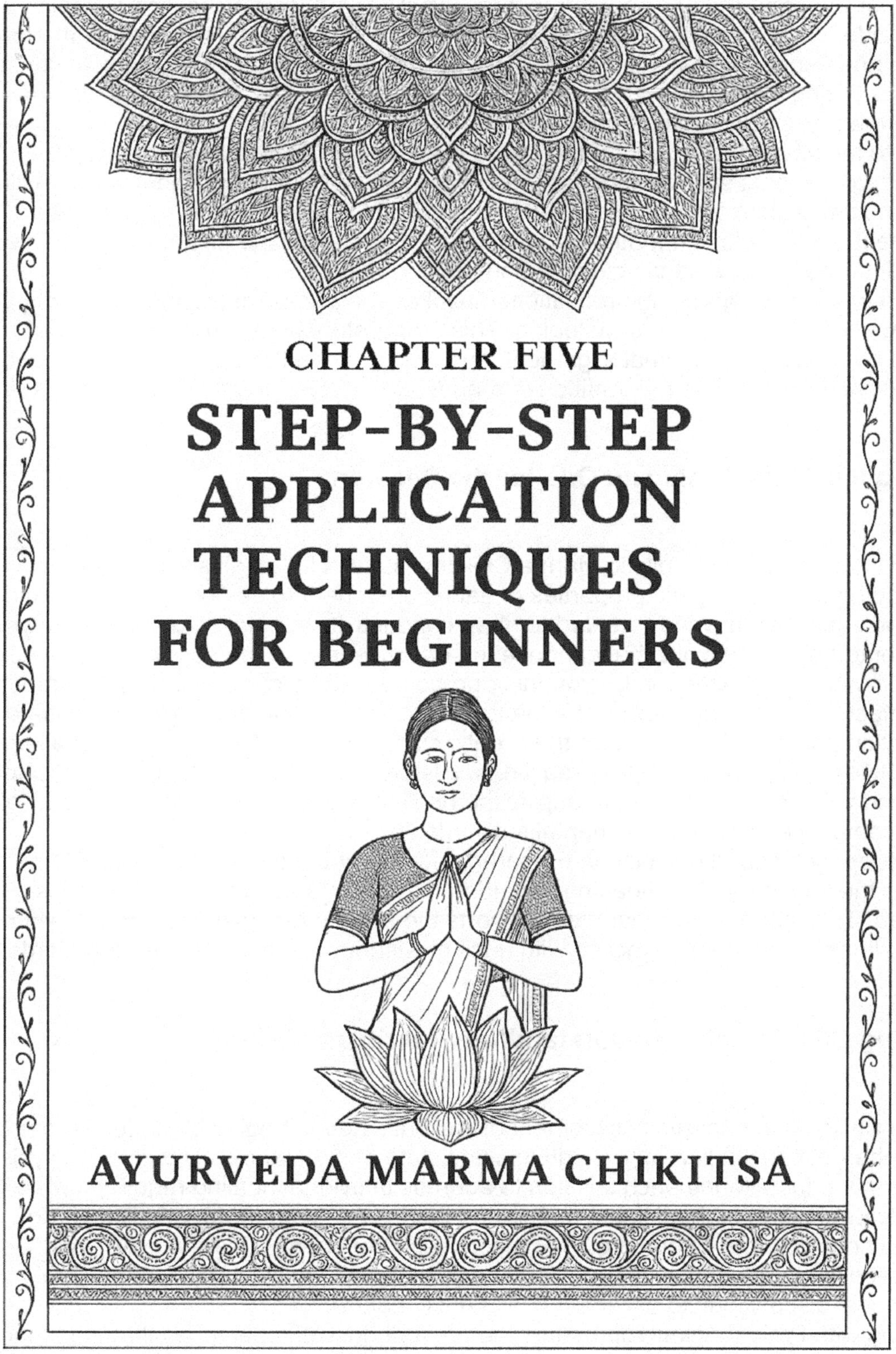

Preparing the Healing Space: Setting the Stage for Healing

The establishment of a tranquil and sacred healing space is crucial in Marma Chikitsa, as it sets the stage for the profound energy work that follows. Preparation begins with choosing a location that is shielded from external noises and disturbances, fostering an environment that promotes relaxation and openness to healing energies. The ambient setting should evoke a sense of calmness, utilizing elements such as dim lighting, soothing colors, and natural materials that align with the Earth's grounding energies.

Attention to the vibrational quality of the space is essential. This can be enhanced by incorporating elements such as incense, soothing music, or natural sounds, which facilitate a deeper meditative state for both practitioner and client. Cleanliness and a systematic arrangement of the tools and materials, which have been sterilized as per the guidelines discussed, further invite a sense of order and readiness.

In creating this sacred space, the practitioner invokes the ancestral wisdom of Marma Chikitsa, setting intentions for healing and wellbeing. This preparatory step is not merely about physical readiness but also about spiritual alignment, ensuring that the therapeutic session conducted is as effective and elevated as the tradition demands.

Selecting the Right Tools and Oils for the Session

Choosing the right tools and oils in Marma Chikitsa is pivotal. It begins with a deep understanding of the energetic properties of each component to establish a therapeutic synergy. Copper rods and Kansa wands, valued for their conductivity in balancing bodily energies, are complemented by specific oils that enhance the effectiveness of the session. For instance, sesame oil might be chosen for its grounding properties, while coconut oil is preferred for its cooling effect, which is essential in treatments aimed at pacifying an aggravated Pitta dosha.

The selection process also considers the client's current state of health, including allergies and skin sensitivities, to prevent adverse reactions. It is crucial to use only high-quality, cold-pressed oils, imbued with organic herbs that amplify the healing properties and adhere to ethical sourcing commitments for environmental stewardship.

Ultimately, every tool and oil must be prepared and presented in its most pristine form, as outlined in the sterilization subheading, ensuring that the integrity of the Marma session is maintained. This thoughtful preparation supports the profound healing potential of Marma Chikitsa, aligning therapeutic practice with ancient wisdom and modern care standards.

Assessing Client Needs: Understanding Prakriti and Vikriti

In Marma Chikitsa, the holistic assessment of a client's needs begins by understanding their Prakriti (inherent constitution) and Vikriti (current state of imbalance). This dual analysis forms the cornerstone for tailoring each session to address individual healing requirements effectively.

Prakriti, determined at birth, dictates the natural balance of Vata, Pitta, and Kapha doshas in the body. This constitutional blueprint guides the selection of specific Marma points and techniques to harmonize innate tendencies. The practitioner observes physical traits, behavioral patterns, and emotional dispositions to ascertain this intrinsic nature.

Contrasting with Prakriti, Vikriti represents the present doshic imbalances that manifest as diseases or health disturbances. An accurate assessment of Vikriti involves a detailed exploration of symptoms, recent health changes, and lifestyle behaviors. Addressing Vikriti is imperative for restoring doshic equilibrium and achieving lasting healing.

Thus, a meticulous evaluation of both Prakriti and Vikriti allows Marma therapists to devise a personalized treatment plan that not only addresses current ailments but also aligns with the client's fundamental nature, promoting overall wellness and preventing future health issues.

Guidelines for Hygiene and Sterilization in Marma Practice

Maintaining impeccable hygiene and adhering to proper sterilization protocols is crucial in Marma Chikitsa to ensure safe and effective healing practices. These guidelines safeguard both practitioners and clients from infections and guarantee the integrity of the healing environment.

Firstly, all Marma tools, including Kansa wands and copper rods, must be sterilized before and after each session. Autoclaving, an effective sterilization method, is recommended to eradicate all microbial life that could potentially compromise the therapeutic process. Similarly, practitioners are to use disposable gloves and maintain personal hygiene by routinely sanitizing their hands and forearms.

The healing space itself deserves attention; regular cleaning regimes using natural, non-toxic disinfectants help maintain an energetically and physically pure environment. Proper disposal systems for used materials, such as cotton pads or paper towels, should be in place to prevent contamination.

Lastly, adherence to these hygiene and sterilization standards reflects the practitioner's commitment to client safety and respect for the ancient art of Marma Chikitsa, preserving its credibility and effectiveness in contemporary practice.

Basic Hand Positions and Touch Techniques

Mastering basic hand positions and touch techniques is foundational in Marma Chikitsa. These initial gestures are not mere physical contacts but deeply meditative interactions that channel healing energies through the practitioner's palms to the client's Marma points. The hands are softened and sensitized through preliminary exercises that heighten tactile perception, enabling the practitioner to detect subtle imbalances in the client's energy flow.

The most widely used touch techniques involve gentle pressing, circular movements, and light tapping. Each technique has a specific purpose: pressing to stimulate energy flow, circular motions to distribute this energy, and tapping to awaken dormant energy. The precise execution of these techniques ensures that they resonate with the inherent vibrational frequencies of the Marma points, facilitating effective healing.

Through conscious touch, the practitioner conveys compassion and healing intention, creating a therapeutic connection that transcends the physical. Training in these techniques prioritizes not only skillful application but also the cultivation of an empathetic and energetically conducive touch that honors the ancient wisdom and therapeutic potential of Marma Chikitsa.

Initial Client Consultation: Exploring Health History and Goals

The initial client consultation forms a cornerstone of Marma Chikitsa, laying the groundwork for a tailored therapeutic experience. This consultative phase is crucial, as it delves into the client's

detailed health history and wellness goals. A comprehensive understanding of past medical conditions, surgeries, chronic issues, and familial health patterns is gathered. Such in-depth knowledge enables practitioners to identify potential vulnerabilities and strengths in the client's health constitution.
Additionally, discussing the client's current lifestyle, including diet, exercise habits, and stress levels, provides insights into various factors that could influence their energy (Prana) flow and overall well-being. This holistic view facilitates the creation of a personalized healing strategy that aligns with the individual's unique needs and aspirations for health and vitality.
Setting clear and achievable health goals during this consultation is paramount. It ensures that both practitioner and client have a common understanding and commitment to the healing journey, fostering an environment of trust and focused intent, which is vital for the success of the Marma therapy.

Mapping Marma Points: Anatomical Locations and Significance

In the realm of Marma Chikitsa, understanding the precise anatomical locations and the profound significance of Marma points is crucial for effective therapy. These strategic points act as junctions where consciousness and physiology intersect, influencing not only the physical body but also the emotional and spiritual layers of one is being.
Each Marma point located on the body corresponds to a specific organ or system. For instance, the 'Ani' Marma found on the shoulder is crucial for maintaining respiratory health and emotional release. Effective stimulation of these points can enhance vitality, promote balance, and initiate deep healing responses, which is why accurate mapping is essential.
The practitioner's ability to localise these points accurately derives from a deep anatomical knowledge complemented by an intuitive understanding of energy pathways. Thus, the mapping process is both a scientific procedure and an artistic exploration, demanding precision and sensitivity. This intricate knowledge empowers the practitioner to tailor treatments that resonate deeply with the client's unique physiological and energetic constitution.

Sequence of Application: Order and Flow of Marma Point Stimulation

Developing a coherent sequence of Marma point stimulation is not just a technique but an art that requires understanding of the body's energetic map and the client's unique Prakriti and Vikriti. The practitioner begins with grounding points to stabilize the client's energy. This is crucial for preparing the body to receive more profound healing without overwhelming the system.
Following the grounding, the sequence proceeds to more specific points related to the identified imbalances. This could involve moving from lower to higher points on the body to facilitate the upward flow of energy, promoting detoxification and revitalization. Each point is stimulated in a manner that respects the natural flow of Prana, ensuring that the energy distribution harmonizes the doshas instead of aggravating them.
The session concludes with points that encourage reintegration and balance, allowing the client's energy to settle into a new state of equilibrium. This careful orchestration of point application maximizes therapeutic efficacy and supports profound healing transitions.

Pressure Techniques: Degrees of Application

In Marma Chikitsa, the application of pressure is not uniform but varies significantly depending on the Marma point, the client's condition, and the desired therapeutic outcome. The nuances of pressure application are integral for achieving specific healing responses. Typically, the pressure can range from gentle to moderate and even firm, each catering to different layers of the body's tissues and energetic pathways.

Initially, light pressure helps in acclimating the client's body and energy system, facilitating a receptive state for deeper work. As the session progresses, pressure intensifies to engage more profound Marma points that influence core physiological processes. However, it is crucial to monitor the client's feedback and adjust pressure accordingly to avoid discomfort or overstimulation, which can counteract the healing process.

Understanding when to modulate the degree of pressure ensures that the Marma therapy session is both effective and harmonious, aligning deeply with the principles of Ayurveda that emphasize balance and gentle healing. This tailored approach respects the individual's unique physical and energy constitution, promoting optimal health and vitality restoration.

Duration of Marma Point Stimulation

The duration of stimulating each Marma point is a critical facet of Marma Chikitsa that must be carefully calibrated. Unlike more overt healing modalities, where prolonged exposure to a therapy is typically required, Marma therapy emphasizes precision over duration. Each point's engagement time significantly influences the therapeutic impact, balancing subtle energy flows without overwhelming the client's system.

Typically, the duration of stimulation for each Marma point varies from a few seconds to several minutes, depending on the client's condition and the desired healing outcome. Beginners are advised to start with shorter durations, gradually extending as they gain sensitivity and understanding of the energetic responses elicited by different points. This careful timing ensures that the energy is neither under-stimulated, which would render the therapy ineffective, nor over-stimulated, which could lead to energy imbalances or discomfort.

Practitioners must observe the client's reactions closely and adjust the duration accordingly. For instance, if a client feels discomfort or excessive sensitivity at a specific point, it indicates a need to shorten the engagement time. This responsive approach helps tailor a session to the unique energetic needs of everyone, enhancing the overall efficacy and safety of the treatment.

Combining Breath Work with Marma Stimulation

Integrating breath work with Marma stimulation enriches the healing process by synchronizing the client's energy flow with physical touch. This technique leverages the natural rhythm of breath to deepen the therapeutic impact of Marma point activation, promoting a harmonious balance between the body's vital energies. As breath work encourages relaxation and activation of the parasympathetic nervous system, it sets an ideal physiological state for receiving Marma therapy.

During a session, practitioners guide clients through specific breathing patterns—such as deep abdominal breathing or controlled exhales—tailored to enhance the responsiveness of Marma points. Conscious breathing helps distribute Prana smoothly throughout the body, intensifying the healing experience. It also aids in releasing blockages more effectively, as the client's focused breathing aligns with the precise application of pressure on Marma points. Furthermore, practitioners observe the client's breath to gauge their comfort and emotional state, adjusting techniques to maintain a serene healing environment. This integration not only facilitates more profound physical healing but also supports mental tranquility and emotional release, ensuring a holistic Marma practice that nurtures all facets of human wellness.

Integration of Aromatic Oils and Their Impact on Marma Points

The integration of aromatic oils in Marma Chikitsa enhances the healing potency of Marma point stimulation. Each oil possesses unique properties that can either soothe or stimulate the energy flow at various Marma points. For example, lavender oil promotes relaxation and is often used on points that aid in reducing anxiety and stress.

When applied, these oils penetrate the skin, influencing the subtle energies that govern physiological functions. A practitioner might select peppermint oil to invigorate the senses and clear the mind when working on Marma points related to cognitive functions. The synergy between the selected oils and Marma points can significantly amplify the therapeutic effects, making the session profoundly impactful.

Moreover, the aromatic scents act on the olfactory senses, which are directly linked to the brain's limbic system. This connection facilitates an emotional release, crucial for healing. Thus, understanding the appropriate oil and its dosage is vital for the practitioner, ensuring the session's success while maintaining the integrity of the holistic practice

Cautions and Contraindications: When to Avoid Certain Marma Points

While Marma Chikitsa offers profound healing benefits, awareness of its cautions is pivotal to ensure safety. Certain conditions necessitate avoiding specific Marma points to prevent exacerbating health issues. For instance, it is recommended to skirt the Marma application around abdominal points during pregnancy as this could risk uterine contractions and endanger the fetus. Similarly, in cases of acute infections or malignant tumors, stimulating relevant Marma points may inadvertently promote the dissemination of toxins or increase metabolic activity at the site, thereby complicating the medical condition.

Cardiovascular issues also present contraindications; points correlating to heart energy should be approached with extreme caution or avoided altogether with conditions like severe hypertension or recent heart attacks, due to the potential for triggering cardiac distress. Recognizing these sensitive scenarios is essential for safeguarding client well-being.

Moreover, it is crucial to consider the client's pain thresholds and current medications that might alter sensory perceptions or the body's response to Marma therapy. Practitioners must persistently communicate with the client to monitor any discomfort and adjust their techniques, accordingly, ensuring a therapeutic session that respects both the art of Marma Chikitsa and the client's physiological limits.

Post-Session Care: Guidelines for Clients

Following a Marma Chikitsa session, the healing journey continues with meticulous post-session care. Clients are advised to remain in a state of relaxation, allowing the body's energies to stabilize after the stimulation of Marma points. It is recommended to drink warm water to help flush out any released toxins and hydrate the tissues, enhancing the therapeutic effects.
Clients should avoid strenuous activities for at least 24 hours after the session, allowing the body ample time to integrate the benefits of the therapy. A gentle walk or light stretching can be beneficial, but heavy lifting or vigorous exercise might disrupt the energetic adjustments made during the session.
Diet plays a crucial role in consolidating the gains from a Marma therapy session. A light, easily digestible meal soon after the session is ideal. Clients should avoid overly spicy or heavy foods that could overburden the digestive system during this sensitive time.
Finally, establishing a serene environment at home or the workplace post-therapy can significantly aid in maintaining the calmness and balance achieved through Marma Chikitsa. Soft lighting, minimal noise, and a comfortable setting can help extend the session's soothing effects, fostering deep and lasting healing.

Recording and Monitoring Healing Progress

In Marma Chikitsa, recording and monitoring the healing progress of each client is a foundational aspect of the practice. This systematic tracking not only reveals the effectiveness of the treatments but also guides future sessions to address the client's needs better.
Practitioners typically use a detailed log to note each session's specifics, including the Marma points stimulated, the oils used, and the client's responsiveness to different pressures and durations.
Documenting the client's initial state before commencing Marma therapy provides a baseline against which to measure improvements or changes. This could include physical symptoms, emotional states, and energy levels. As sessions progress, updates to this record reflect shifts in these areas, offering tangible evidence of Marma Chikitsa's impact.
Moreover, ongoing monitoring enables the practitioner to adjust techniques according to the evolving needs of the client. Regular review of the documented progress ensures a highly personalized approach, maximizing the therapeutic benefits while maintaining an optimal balance of the body's energies. This diligent recording fosters a deep understanding and fine-tuning of the healing journey.

Frequency of Sessions: Creating a Treatment Schedule

The frequency of Marma Chikitsa sessions is crucial in optimizing the healing trajectory for each client. Initially, more frequent sessions may be necessary to establish momentum in energy flow and symptom relief. Typically, sessions might start weekly, allowing the practitioner to closely observe and react to the client's evolving response to treatment.
As improvement becomes apparent, the interval between sessions can be extended. This adjustment is based on sustained positive changes in the client's physical and emotional states. For chronic conditions, a longer duration of consistent treatments may be required to achieve significant healing outcomes. The practitioner, by diligently monitoring progress, determines the

optimal session frequency reflective of the client's current health dynamics.
Ultimately, the goal is to taper the sessions as the client gains autonomy in managing their well-being. Educating clients on self-maintenance techniques enables them to support the continuity of healing benefits. Regular reviews ensure the treatment remains aligned with the client's health status, refining the schedule to the most therapeutic frequency.

Adapting Techniques for Different Age Groups and Health Conditions

Marma Chikitsa, though universally beneficial, requires careful technique adaptation for various age groups and specific health conditions to ensure maximum effectiveness and safety. For elderly clients, gentler pressure is often necessary, considering their potentially fragile skin and bones. Additionally, a focus on Marma points that enhance joint mobility, and balance can significantly uplift their quality of life.
Children, on the other hand, have a more dynamic energy flow and faster response to Marma stimulation. Treatments are generally shorter, and the touch is lighter than with adults. Special attention is given to nurturing growth and developmental Marma points that support their rapidly changing bodies and temperaments.
Adapting Marma techniques for chronic health conditions involves an in-depth understanding of the interplay between the Marma points and the diseased state. For instance, Marma therapy for someone with chronic inflammation might include techniques that aim to cool and calm the body's energy pathways.
Thus, expertly adjusting Marma techniques based on age and health nuances not only personalizes healing but also enhances the efficacy of the practice, promoting health and vitality across all life stages.

Introduction to Advanced Marma Techniques

Venturing into advanced Marma techniques marks a pivotal progression in a practitioner's journey. These sophisticated methods target deeper layers of the body's energy system, aiming to unlock profound healing potential. Advanced techniques not only require a refined understanding of Marma points but also mastery in manipulating subtle energies. Practitioners learn to synchronize deeper breathing rhythms with precise touch, significantly enhancing the energy flow.
The application of these techniques requires an adept ability to integrate multiple Marma points simultaneously, promoting holistic healing that extends beyond localized pain relief. This could involve dynamic sequences that connect bodily regions, facilitating the wider distribution and harmonization of energy. Such sessions often target chronic ailments, aiming for long-term relief and systemic health improvements.
Moreover, ethical considerations become increasingly complex at this level. Practitioners must navigate not just physical but also emotional and spiritual dimensions, ensuring a safe and respectful engagement with the client's entire being. Advanced practice thus becomes an eloquent dance of intuition, skill, and profound respect for the subtle energies of life.

Client Feedback: Listening and Adjusting Techniques Accordingly

The practice of Marma Chikitsa transcends mere technique; it embodies a dialogue between practitioner and client. Listening to client feedback is phenomenally crucial as it furnishes insights into their subjective experience of the session. Eliciting honest responses helps practitioners assess the suitability of applied pressures, the comfort with chosen Marma points, and the overall effects perceived by the client.

This direct feedback facilitates the critical adjustment of techniques. It serves not just to enhance the comfort level in subsequent sessions but also to refine the therapeutic approach to better match individual sensitivities and needs. Whether it is altering the pressure applied, modifying the sequence of Marma point stimulation, or incorporating different aromatic oils, each adjustment is designed to enhance the therapy's efficacy.

Ultimately, embracing client feedback embeds a spirit of continual improvement within the practice. It encourages a bespoke healing journey for each client, ensuring that Marma Chikitsa not only alleviates physical or emotional ailments but also enriches the overall well-being of the individual.

Ensuring Client Comfort and Safety During Sessions

Ensuring client comfort and safety during Marma Chikitsa sessions is paramount. A comforting environment facilitates an immersive healing experience, while safety measures guard against potential risks associated with the application technique. Comfort is initially cultivated by creating a soothing ambiance, utilizing elements like soft lighting, gentle music, and an optimal room temperature that aligns with the client's preferences and physiological needs.

Safety measures are meticulous, starting with the practitioner's thorough awareness of the client's medical history and potential allergens, which impacts the choice of oils and the intensity of application. All equipment and surfaces are sterilized, and high hygiene standards are maintained to prevent the spread of infections. During the session, the practitioner continually engages with the client, gathering feedback on comfort levels and adjusting pressure or technique as needed.

Moreover, practitioners ensure that each client feels respected and secure throughout the process. Clear communication about each step of the procedure, along with maintaining a professional yet empathetic demeanor, is fundamental to fostering a safe and reassuring therapeutic environment.

Utilizing Marma Therapy as a Preventive Tool

Marma Therapy, traditionally rooted in Ayurvedic medicine, serves not only as a remedy but also as a proactive health measure. By strategically stimulating Marma points, this therapy enhances the body's natural resilience, potentially averting the onset of disease by maintaining energy balance and strengthening the immune system. Regular Marma sessions help in the early detection of energy imbalances that could escalate into physical symptoms, thus acting preemptively.

The preventative aspect of Marma Therapy is particularly valuable in today's fast-paced world, where stress triggers numerous health issues. Through calming the nervous system and optimizing energy flow, Marma sessions equip the body to handle stress more effectively. This

not only prevents stress-related ailments but also improves overall vitality and mental clarity, keeping the body and mind in a state of harmony and alert health.
Educating clients on incorporating Marma Therapy into their wellness routine can instill a habit of health consciousness and self-care. Emphasizing its utility in prevention encourages consistent practice, which can potentially reduce the need for healthcare interventions and promote a long-term, holistic approach to health.

Ethical Considerations in Marma Practice

Ethical integrity is fundamental in Marma Chikitsa, guiding practitioners to uphold responsibilities that transcend the technical execution of their skills. The sensitivity of engaging energetically with clients demands strict confidentiality, ensuring their personal and health-related information is protected fiercely. This confidentiality builds trust, a cornerstone in therapeutic relationships, which in turn enhances the healing experience.
Furthermore, practitioners are obligated to practice non-judgment. Each client's emotional and physical states are to be met with unconditional positive regard. This ethical stance prevents any bias or prejudice that could affect the treatment process and supports an inclusive practice welcoming to all individuals. Practitioners must continually self-reflect, recognizing their own limits in skill and knowledge, and refer clients to additional healthcare providers when a client's needs exceed what Marma Chikitsa can effectively address.
Lastly, informed consent is crucial. Practitioners should provide clients with clear explanations of the therapies proposed, including any potential risks. This transparency enables clients to make informed decisions about their health interventions, fostering autonomy in their healing journey. Ethical practice thus ensures that safety, respect, and informed choice are always at the forefront.

Building a Professional Marma Practice: Tips for Beginners

Establishing a new Marma practice requires thoughtful preparation and a strategic approach. Initially, beginners should focus on creating a welcoming environment that speaks to the holistic nature of Marma therapy. This includes choosing a tranquil location, setting up a serene workspace with all necessary equipment, and ensuring privacy and comfort for every client.
Marketing is crucial; new practitioners must effectively communicate the benefits of Marma Chikitsa. Utilizing social media platforms, local wellness events, and collaborations with other healthcare providers can increase visibility. Additionally, maintaining a professional online presence with educational content about Marma therapy can attract those curious about alternative healing methods.
Finally, continual education and certification in Marma Chikitsa enhance credibility and expertise. Attending workshops and seminars not only broadens one's knowledge but also connects with a network of practitioners. This community can be invaluable for support and referrals as one navigates the early stages of establishing a practice.

Continued Learning and Mastery: Pathways for Beginner Practitioners

Aspiring Marma Chikitsa practitioners must recognize that initial training marks just the beginning of their educational journey. Stepping beyond foundational skills, continuous learning is essential for deepening one's understanding and refining techniques. It is advisable to regularly engage in advanced workshops and seminars that introduce more complex aspects of Marma therapy, while also providing the latest research and developments in the field. Subscription to relevant journals, participating in practitioner forums, and being part of Ayurvedic healing communities can also enhance one's learning curve. These platforms offer valuable insights and peer discussions that challenge and extend a practitioner's capacity.

Mentorship is another pivotal aspect, where experienced Marma therapists can provide practical guidance and advice. This relationship fosters a more nuanced appreciation of Marma applications, instilling confidence through firsthand shared experiences.

Thus, the commitment to continued education ensures that practitioners not only maintain their competency but also excel, adapting innovatively to meet diverse client needs and staying relevant in the evolving landscape of holistic health.

Summary

The chapter 'Step-by-Step Application Techniques for Beginners' is a comprehensive guide to Marma Chikitsa, an ancient Ayurvedic practice. It begins with setting up a healing space characterized by tranquility and organized with elements promoting relaxation and receptivity to healing. The selection of tools and oils, critical for effective therapy, is thoroughly discussed, emphasizing the use of materials like copper rods and specific oils like sesame or coconut, based on their properties and the client's dosha imbalance. Understanding the client's Prakriti (inherent constitution) and Vikriti (current imbalance) is crucial in customizing the therapy session to individual needs. This is achieved through detailed initial consultations that consider the client's health history and goals. Proper hygiene and sterilization practices are prescribed to maintain the safety and integrity of the therapeutic environment. Mastery of hand positions and touch techniques is essential for the effective stimulation of Marma points, which are specific locations on the body that influence health and energy flow. The chapter also explains the mapping of these points in terms of their anatomical significance, followed by the appropriate sequence of Marma point stimulation, emphasizing the symbiotic relationship between pressure application and the desired therapeutic outcomes. Furthermore, integration of breath work with Marma stimulation is highlighted as enhancing the healing process. The use of aromatic oils is also introduced as an additional layer to Marma therapy, enhancing the sensory experience and therapeutic impact. Cautions are provided to avoid complications in vulnerable conditions. Post-session care tips and progressive tracking of the client's healing journey underline the importance of continued care. The chapter serves not only as an instructional guide for performing Marma Chikitsa but also reflects on how practitioners should align their practice with ethical standards, consider contraindications, and adapt techniques based on the specific needs of clients, ranging from children to the elderly. It concludes with strategies for building a professional practice and emphasizes the necessity of continued learning and mastery in Marma Chikitsa.

References

[1] Subramania, K., et al. 'Fundamentals of Marma Therapy: Implications in Modern Medicine', International Journal of Engineering Science, 2020. https://www.ijer.com/v1/issue3/p5.pdf

[2] Mishra, A., 'Ayurvedic Marma Therapy: Case Studies and Clinical Applications', AYU Journal, 2019. https://www.ayujournal.org/text.asp?2019/35/4/117/129917

Case Study: Enhancing Therapeutic Outcomes through Optimized Marma Chikitsa Practices

Sanjana, a seasoned Marma Chikitsa practitioner, has seen numerous success stories over her 15-year career. However, she recently encountered a challenging case with her client, Rohan, a 42-year-old software engineer suffering from chronic back pain and insomnia. Understanding the depth of Marma Chikitsa's healing potential, especially with her extensive training in assessing Prakriti and Vikriti, Sanjana was determined to tailor a session that addressed both Rohan's physical and emotional distress.

The initial consultation revealed Rohan's Vata-Pitta constitution, with an evident aggravation in Vata leading to his insomnia and irregular digestion. For the therapeutic session, Sanjana emphasized grounding techniques utilizing sesame oil for its warming and soothing properties, recommended particularly for Rohan's Vata imbalance. Rohan was advised to continue with a Vata-pacifying diet post-session, to complement the Marma therapy and provide more sustained relief.

During the session, Sanjana employed a sequence of hand positions and touch techniques that focused on the Marma points correlating to spinal health and stress alleviation. Special attention was given to soft circular motions and gentle pressure on specific points that aligned with Rohan's energetic needs, intuitively guided by her in-depth understanding of the energy channels influenced by both age and his current health condition. She combined this with aromatic oils, such as lavender, to aid in relaxation.

The session did produce noticeable improvements in Rohan's sleep patterns and back pain within a few weeks. Reflecting on the outcome, Sanjana realized that a critical component of her success stemmed from meticulous documentation during the session, which enabled her to refine her approach based on observed results and feedback, thereby adapting techniques for subsequent sessions to optimize healing.

To enhance community knowledge, Sanjana plans to conduct a detailed seminar focusing on the integration of breathwork with Marma point stimulation, highlighting her experiences and outcomes from cases like Rohan's, and advocating for continuous learning and mastery among fellow practitioners.

Case Study: Integrative Approach to Marma Therapy for Age-Related Ailments

An experienced Marma Chikitsa therapist, Dr. Anil Desai, faces a compelling challenge with his new client, Mrs. Lakshmi Patel, a 68-year-old retired schoolteacher who experiences severe arthritis pain in her knees and frequent episodes of anxiety. Managing the complexities associated with aging, Dr. Desai plans a holistic session that aims not only to alleviate symptoms but also to explore the preventive aspects of Marma Chikitsa, thereby enhancing Mrs. Patel's overall quality of life.

Dr. Desai begins with a thorough initial consultation, where he discovers Mrs. Patel's Kapha-Vata constitution, with a significant Vata imbalance manifesting as joint pain and anxiety. Given the delicate nature of administering therapy to an elderly patient, Dr. Desai decides on a conservative approach based on the chapters discussing the adaptation of techniques for different age groups and health conditions. He emphasizes mild pressure techniques and limits the duration of stimulation on each Marma point to avert any discomfort or overwhelming of her energy pathways.

The treatment plan includes utilizing ginger-infused oil, known for its anti-inflammatory and warming properties, which are beneficial against joint pain. Recognizing her anxiety, Dr. Desai also integrates calming aromatic oils like sandalwood to facilitate emotional relief. The session is conducted in a serene environment, enhancing therapeutic effects through a combination of soft background music and dim lighting, which soothes Mrs. Patel's overall senses and promotes a parasympathetic response.

Following the session, Dr. Desai outlines a detailed care plan for Mrs. Patel to ensure ongoing benefits. He incorporates gentle, daily exercises tailored to her condition and age, along with dietary suggestions to balance her doshas. Acknowledging her psychological well-being, he proposes regular mindfulness practices to mitigate anxiety and improve mental health.

This case demonstrates the power of integrating comprehensive Marma Chikitsa applications with bespoke adjustments catered to an elderly client. Dr. Desai schedules follow-up sessions to monitor progress and make necessary adjustments, emphasizing the importance of recording and frequent consultation to optimize Marma therapy outcomes continually.

Case Study: Strategic Use of Marma Chikitsa in Sports Rehabilitation

Amit, a 30-year-old professional basketball player, sustained a knee injury during a game, resulting in acute pain and reduced mobility. His physiotherapist, Deepa, who also specializes in Marma Chikitsa, recognized an opportunity to integrate these techniques to facilitate Amit's healing process while addressing the physical and energetic impacts of the injury.

The initial examination focused on assessing Amit's Prakriti, which revealed a predominant Pitta-Kapha constitution. This was critical, as the inflammatory nature of his injury (Pitta) compounded by his Kapha build, suggested a susceptibility to fluid retention and swelling. Considering his active lifestyle and the demands of his profession, Deepa decided to employ a specific combination of Marma points that would not only address the injury but also support Amit's overall energy flow, crucial for his athletic performance.

During the treatment sessions, Deepa utilized cooling coconut oil to counteract the heat of Pitta and selected Marma points, such as Janu (knee) and Gulpha (ankle), to enhance joint health and mobility. She meticulously applied gentle but firm pressure techniques to stimulate these points, promoting circulation and reducing inflammation. The sessions were augmented with light tapping around the affected areas to encourage energetic awakening and healing.

To deepen the therapeutic experience, Deepa incorporated guided breathwork designed to align with the rhythmic application of pressure, thereby enhancing Amit's body awareness and relaxation. This integration proved essential in managing pain and facilitating a faster recovery. She also advised Amit on lifestyle adjustments and dietary changes to sustain the benefits of Marma therapy, emphasizing the consumption of anti-inflammatory foods to reduce Pitta aggravation.

Amit's recovery was meticulously documented by Deepa, who noted each session's progress, and any adjustments made, which informed the subsequent treatments. The recorded data demonstrated significant improvements in his mobility and a decrease in pain levels, underscoring the efficacy of Marma Chikitsa in sports rehabilitation settings.

Case Study: Implementing Marma Chikitsa for Chronic Digestive Disorders: A Comprehensive Treatment Approach

Leela, a 34-year-old graphic designer, presented with persistent digestive issues including irritable bowel syndrome (IBS) and related anxiety, which had impaired her quality of life over the past five years. She sought out Marma Chikitsa, having exhausted conventional treatments with limited success. Her practitioner, Dr. Mehta, a seasoned Marma therapist, was tasked with creating a treatment plan that not only addressed Leela's digestive complaints but also targeted the underlying stress contributing to her condition.

The initial evaluation was meticulous, focusing on the assessment of Leela's Prakriti and Vikriti. Dr. Mehta determined that Leela's primary dosha was Pitta, with a significant Vata imbalance manifesting as anxiety and irregular digestive patterns. This detailed diagnostic approach allowed Dr. Mehta to tailor a multi-faceted treatment plan specifically for Leela.

Sessions commenced with the careful selection of Marma points known to enhance digestive health and reduce anxiety. Points such as Nabhi (navel) and Hridaya (heart) were targeted to balance the digestive fire (Agni) and calm the mind. Dr. Mehta utilized sesame oil to calm Vata and coconut oil to soothe Pitta, applying them with precision to different Marma points to harmonize Leela's doshic imbalances. The tactile applications involved gentle circular motions to stimulate the energy flow, followed by mild pressure to maintain the stimulation without causing discomfort.

Furthermore, Dr. Mehta incorporated breathing exercises into the sessions to aid relaxation and enhance the effectiveness of the Marma therapy. This combination significantly alleviated Leela's symptoms by the end of the treatment series. Enhancing the treatment, dietary recommendations were provided, focusing on cooling, easy-to-digest foods that pacify Pitta, and lifestyle changes were suggested to incorporate mild exercise and stress reduction techniques.

The treatment concluded with Dr. Mehta advising Leela on self-care practices that included specific Marma points she could stimulate at home to manage acute stress and digestive flare-ups. This comprehensive approach not only addressed her immediate health concerns but also equipped Leela with the tools to manage her symptoms in the long term, showcasing the profound capabilities of Marma Chikitsa in treating complex health issues comprehensively.

Case Study: Revitalizing Mental Health: A Holistic Marma Chikitsa Approach

In a significant exploration of Marma Chikitsa's capabilities beyond physical ailments, Ananya, a 28-year-old software developer, sought help for her escalating issues related to stress and burnout, which had begun manifesting as severe migraines and insomnia. Deepali, a Marma therapist with a profound understanding of the interconnections between mental and physical health, received Ananya for an initial detailed assessment.

The assessment delved deeply into Ananya's daily routines, stress levels, and background, alongside a traditional evaluation of Prakriti and Vikriti. Ananya's constitution was identified as primarily Vata, with current imbalances also pointing towards Vata aggravation, characterized by her restlessness, anxiety, and digestive irregularities. This insight was crucial, guiding Deepali's selection of Marma points and techniques tailored to not only soothe Ananya's immediate symptoms but also to restore long-term balance.

Deepali's treatment plan incorporated both direct Marma stimulation and supplementary techniques like aromatherapy and breath work, aimed at calming Ananya's overactive Vata. Specific Marma points like 'Brahmarandra' at the crown were targeted to alleviate headaches, while 'Anahata' over the chest area was focused on to soothe anxiety. Deepali used gentle circular motions with moderate pressure, employing sesame oil known for its grounding properties. Furthermore, lavender and chamomile oils were diffused during the sessions to aid relaxation and sleep.

Each session incorporated guided breath techniques, synchronized with the stimulation of Marma points to enhance the therapeutic effect. This integration not only facilitated a deeper state of relaxation during treatments but also empowered Ananya to manage stress independently through breathing exercises.

As treatments progressed, Deepali observed notable improvements in Ananya's migraine frequency and sleep quality. This case illustrates the profound impact of an integrated Marma Chikitsa approach on mental health. Her continued improvement reinforced the need for holistic treatment plans in dealing with stress-related disorders, validating the ancient wisdom of Marma therapy in addressing modern-day health challenges.

Case Study: Navigating Complex Pediatric Cases with Marma Chikitsa

Rita, a skilled Marma Chikitsa practitioner specializing in pediatric care, faced a unique challenge with her young client, 8-year-old Arjun. Arjun had been diagnosed with attention deficit hyperactivity disorder (ADHD) and exhibited symptoms such as hyperactivity, difficulty maintaining focus, and temperamental issues. His parents, keen on exploring holistic treatment avenues, sought Rita's expertise to complement Arjun's ongoing behavioral therapies.

During the initial consultation, Rita conducted a thorough examination to understand Arjun's Prakriti. According to her assessment, Arjun displayed a predominant Vata constitution with noticeable imbalances contributing to his restlessness and attention fluctuations. In addressing a child's condition, especially one as delicate as ADHD, Rita recognized the importance of a gentle approach as discussed in the chapters about adapting techniques for different health conditions and age groups.

The treatment plan Rita devised involved carefully selected Marma points that are known to promote calmness and mental clarity. She incorporated the use of milder, soothing oils, such as coconut oil, known for its cooling properties, which is ideal for pacifying the aggravated Vata dosha in Arjun. Rita applied soft, gentle touches on the scalp and feet, areas directly linked to grounding Vata and enhancing cognitive functions.

Each session began with Rita guiding Arjun through simple breathing exercises, which were crucial in settling his initial hyperactivity and preparing him for the Marma treatment. The tactile stimulation, combined with controlled breathing, helped subtly balance his Prana, thereby promoting a state of calm and focus. Rita observed a gradual but noticeable improvement in Arjun's ability to concentrate and a reduction in his hyperactive episodes over several sessions.

Reflecting on this case, Rita emphasized the necessity of patience and persistence in treating pediatric cases with Marma Chikitsa. She meticulously documented the details of each session, noting the changes and adjusting her approach according to Arjun's responsiveness. Her case study makes a significant contribution to the pediatric applications of Marma Chikitsa, offering insights into the strategic use of specific Marma points and techniques that cater to young clients with neurological and behavioral challenges.

Case Study: Holistic Management of Chronic Fatigue Syndrome through Marma Chikitsa

Mira, a 38-year-old content writer, had been struggling with Chronic Fatigue Syndrome (CFS) for nearly three years. The persistent tiredness had not only affected her professional life but had also significantly diminished her social interactions. Despite trying various conventional treatments, Mira found only temporary relief. This led her to explore alternative therapies, and she eventually decided to try Marma Chikitsa, having heard of its holistic benefits.

Dr. Kumar, an experienced Marma therapist, conducted an extensive initial consultation to understand Mira's health history, lifestyle, and previous treatments. He also assessed her Prakriti and found her to exhibit a predominant Kapha imbalance, which was manifesting as lethargy and mental fog, typical symptoms of CFS. Dr. Kumar formulated a personalized Marma therapy plan that not only targeted her physical symptoms but also aimed at revitalizing her mental and emotional health.

In the sessions, Dr. Kumar focused on vital Marma points that stimulate energy flow and enhance vitality. Points like Surya (solar plexus) and Hridaya (heart) were emphasized to boost Mira's core energy. To address the mental fog, points on the head, such as Brahmarandra and Adhipati, were stimulated. Dr. Kumar used a combination of moderate pressure and specific oils like eucalyptus, known for its invigorating properties, to activate these points. Each session also included guided breathwork, synchronizing the breath with the rhythm of Marma point stimulation to enhance oxygen flow. and aiding in mental clarity.

Throughout the treatment, special attention was given to integrating lifestyle adjustments. Mira was advised on dietary changes to reduce Kapha aggravation and encourage light, energy-boosting foods. Gentle yoga and meditation were recommended to maintain the balance achieved in the sessions.

Dr. Kumar meticulously documented each session's effects, adapting the approach based on Mira's feedback and progress. Over several weeks, Mira reported a significant improvement in energy levels and a reduction in her symptoms. This case highlights the efficacy of Marma Chikitsa in managing complex, chronic conditions like CFS, demonstrating its potential to revitalize both physical and mental health through targeted, personalized treatment plans.

Case Study: Advanced Marma Techniques for Managing Severe Migraines and Stress

Aaliyah, a 35-year-old executive in a high-stress tech firm, had been grappling with severe migraines and chronic stress, affecting her productivity and overall quality of life. Despite various medical treatments, the relief was short-lived, prompting her to explore alternative therapies like Marma Chikitsa. Upon consultation, her Marma therapist, Nikhil, identified her dominant Dosha as Pitta with a secondary Vata imbalance, which was aggravating her symptoms of migraines and stress.

Nikhil decided to initiate treatment with a focus on advanced Marma techniques, as Aaliyah's condition required interventions that went beyond basic touch and pressure applications. Nikhil crafted a session sequence tailored to address the heightened Pitta and soothe the nervous system. He incorporated specific points such as '*Sthapani*' (forehead point for calming the mind and alleviating headaches) and 'Manya' (neck points to relieve tension). Utilizing a cooling oil blend of coconut infused with peppermint helped counteract the Pitta's heat, essential for soothing Aaliyah's migraines.

The treatment protocol was complemented by integrating breath work with Marma stimulation, enhancing therapeutic impact. Nikhil guided Aaliyah through controlled breathing exercises synchronized with each point's stimulation to deepen relaxation and maximize the healing process. This approach not only helped in managing her immediate pain but also facilitated a deeper state of relaxation during the sessions.

In addition to the therapy, Nikhil advised Aaliyah on lifestyle adjustments, including dietary changes to reduce Pitta aggravating foods and incorporating daily meditation to manage stress effectively. These recommendations were aimed at sustaining the benefits of the Marma therapy and preventing the recurrence of symptoms.

Reflecting on the treatment success, Nikhil emphasized the effectiveness of combining advanced Marma techniques with holistic lifestyle changes in managing complex health issues like migraines and stress, illustrating the profound capabilities of Marma therapy when adapted to the unique needs of clients. This case enhanced the knowledge base about the strategic application of Marma points that are crucial in chronic conditions, accelerating recovery and promoting long-term wellness.

Case Study: Comprehensive Marma Therapy for Autoimmune Disorder Management

Emma, a 47-year-old teacher, was diagnosed with rheumatoid arthritis, an autoimmune disorder characterized by prolonged inflammation and joint pain. Traditional medications provided limited relief and considerable side effects, leading Emma to explore alternative therapies like Marma Chikitsa. She hoped that it would offer a gentle yet effective solution to manage her condition holistically.

Dr. Singh, a Marma therapist with experience in autoimmune disorders, conducted an exhaustive initial evaluation to understand Emma's health history, dietary habits, emotional state, and, more importantly, her Prakriti (constitutional type) and Vikriti (current imbalances). This detailed assessment was crucial as it informed the personalized therapeutic approach that would balance her aggravated doshas and potentially ease her symptoms.

During the therapy, Dr. Singh focused on key Marma points known to reduce inflammation and boost immunity. Points like Kshipra (located near the base of the thumb) and Gulpha (near the ankle), which are traditionally associated with alleviating joint pain, were given special attention. The stimulation of these points was carefully integrated with the use of specially selected oils; turmeric oil for its anti-inflammatory properties and ginger oil to improve circulation and reduce stiffness, applied with gentle, soothing motions to avoid discomfort at the tender joints.

Furthermore, Dr. Singh incorporated guided breathwork techniques to enhance the efficacy of the Marma sessions. This combination is aimed not only at physical relief but also at emotional and psychological well-being, as stress reduction plays a significant role in managing autoimmune disorders. Emma was also advised on dietary changes that align with Ayurvedic principles to support her overall treatment plan.

Over several weeks, Emma experienced noticeable improvement in joint mobility and a reduction in pain levels. Dr. Singh documented each session meticulously, adjusting techniques and oils based on Emma's feedback and progress. This adaptive approach underlines the importance of personalized care in Marma Therapy, showcasing its potential in managing chronic conditions effectively. The positive outcome not only improved Emma's quality of life but also reaffirmed the value of integrating traditional wisdom with modern therapeutic practices.

Case Study: Optimal Utilization of Marma Therapy Techniques in Workplace Stress Reduction

Anita, a 40-year-old corporate executive at a high-demand tech firm, had been experiencing escalating levels of stress due to her strenuous workload. This persistent stress manifested physically as neck stiffness, headaches, and occasional bouts of anxiety. Given her interest in holistic therapies, Anita decided to explore Marma Chikitsa after reading about its efficacy in alleviating stress-related symptoms. Her therapist, Dr. Roy, a seasoned practitioner of Marma Chikitsa with extensive experience in corporate wellness programs, had a detailed initial consultation with Anita to evaluate her Prakriti (constitutional type) and Vikriti (current imbalances). This comprehensive assessment revealed a pronounced Vata-Pitta disturbance marked by her systemic stress and anxiety symptoms.

Dr. Roy strategized a session plan integrating Marma points known for relaxation and stress alleviation. He focused on 'Talahridaya' (palm center linked to heart energy), 'Manya' (neck base for relieving tension), and 'Sthapani' (forehead center associated with emotional and mental stress). Utilizing a blend of soothing oil infused with sandalwood for its calming properties, Dr. Roy applied gentle yet precise pressure on these critical points to balance Anita's disrupted Doshas and energy flow.

In addition to Marma point stimulation, the treatment included guided breathwork, encouraging Anita to follow deep, rhythmic breathing to complement the physical intervention. This dual approach aimed to maximize relaxation and restoration of Anita's energy balance. Dr. Roy also advised her to integrate short Marma-based self-care routines into her daily work schedule to manage stress proactively.

Reflecting on Anita's sessions, Dr. Roy noted significant improvement in her symptoms within a few weeks. He emphasized the effectiveness of combining traditional Marma therapy with modern lifestyle adaptations to meet the needs of busy professionals. This case highlighted the practical application of Marma Chikitsa in a corporate environment and its potential to enhance workplace wellness significantly, reflecting the adaptability and relevance of ancient practices in contemporary settings.

Review Questions

1. During a Marma Chikitsa session, a practitioner named Anu sets up her healing space. She chooses a quiet room, dims the lights, plays soft nature sounds, and arranges her tools systematically before inviting her client, Ravi. Ravi is a middle-aged man suffering from chronic stress and insomnia. Based on Anu's preparations, which element is missing and crucial for aligning with Earth's grounding energies during the session?

A) Enhanced lighting for brightness
B) Placement of synthetic materials
C) Incorporation of natural materials
D) Increased room temperature

Answer: C

Explanation: Incorporation of natural materials is crucial for aligning with Earth's grounding energies in the healing space. All other options are counterproductive to creating a tranquil and sanctified environment emphasized in the practice of Marma Chikitsa. Natural materials resonate with calming energies, helping to foster a more conducive environment for healing and alleviating conditions such as stress and insomnia.

2. Ravi is nervous about his first Marma Chikitsa session. Anu decides to use specific oils to help pacify his aggravated Pitta dosha, which is characterized by heat and inflammation according to Ayurveda. Which oil should Anu choose for its cooling effects?

A) Sesame oil
B) Coconut oil
C) Olive oil
D) Almond oil

Answer: B

Explanation: Coconut oil is preferred for its cooling effects, essential in treatments aimed at pacifying aggravated Pitta dosha. Sesame oil, by contrast, is known for its grounding properties but is warming, which might not be as effective for Pitta imbalances. Olive and almond oils are not specifically mentioned for their dosha-specific effects in Marma Chikitsa.

3. Anu begins her holistic assessment of Ravi by determining his Prakriti and Vikriti to tailor the Marma Chikitsa session. She notices his dry skin, quick speech, and variable digestion, all symptoms indicating a Vata imbalance. Which approach should Anu take to effectively address Ravi's current state following the principles of Marma Chikitsa?

A) Vigorous stimulation of Marma points
B) Gentle stimulation with warming oils
C) Use of cooling oils and rapid movements
D) Ignoring Prakriti due to the dominance of Vikriti symptoms

Answer: B

Explanation: To address a Vata imbalance characterized by dry skin, rapid speech, and irregular digestion, Anu should opt for gentle stimulation with warming oils. Vata is cold and dry, so warming oils can help balance these qualities. Vigorous stimulation may aggravate Vata further, while cooling oils are more suitable for a Pitta imbalance. Ignoring Prakriti is not recommended as it can provide critical insight into the inherent constitution of the client.

4. Anu is meticulous about hygiene and sterilization in her Marma practice. She sterilizes her Kansa wands and copper rods using autoclaving before each session. Moreover, her routine includes wearing disposable gloves. Why is autoclaving an optimal choice for sterilization in this scenario?

A) It is a natural herbal method of cleansing
B) It uses intense heat to eradicate all microbial life
C) It enhances the electrical conductivity of the tools
D) It is the least expensive method available

Answer: B

Explanation: Autoclaving is optimal for sterilization because it uses intense heat (steam under pressure) to eradicate all microbial life. This ensures that the tools used in Marma Chikitsa are free from contaminants that could potentially compromise the therapeutic process. It does not directly enhance electrical conductivity nor is it characterized by its cost but rather its effectiveness in achieving a high level of sterilization.

CHAPTER SIX: Case Studies and Clinical Applications of Marma Chikitsa

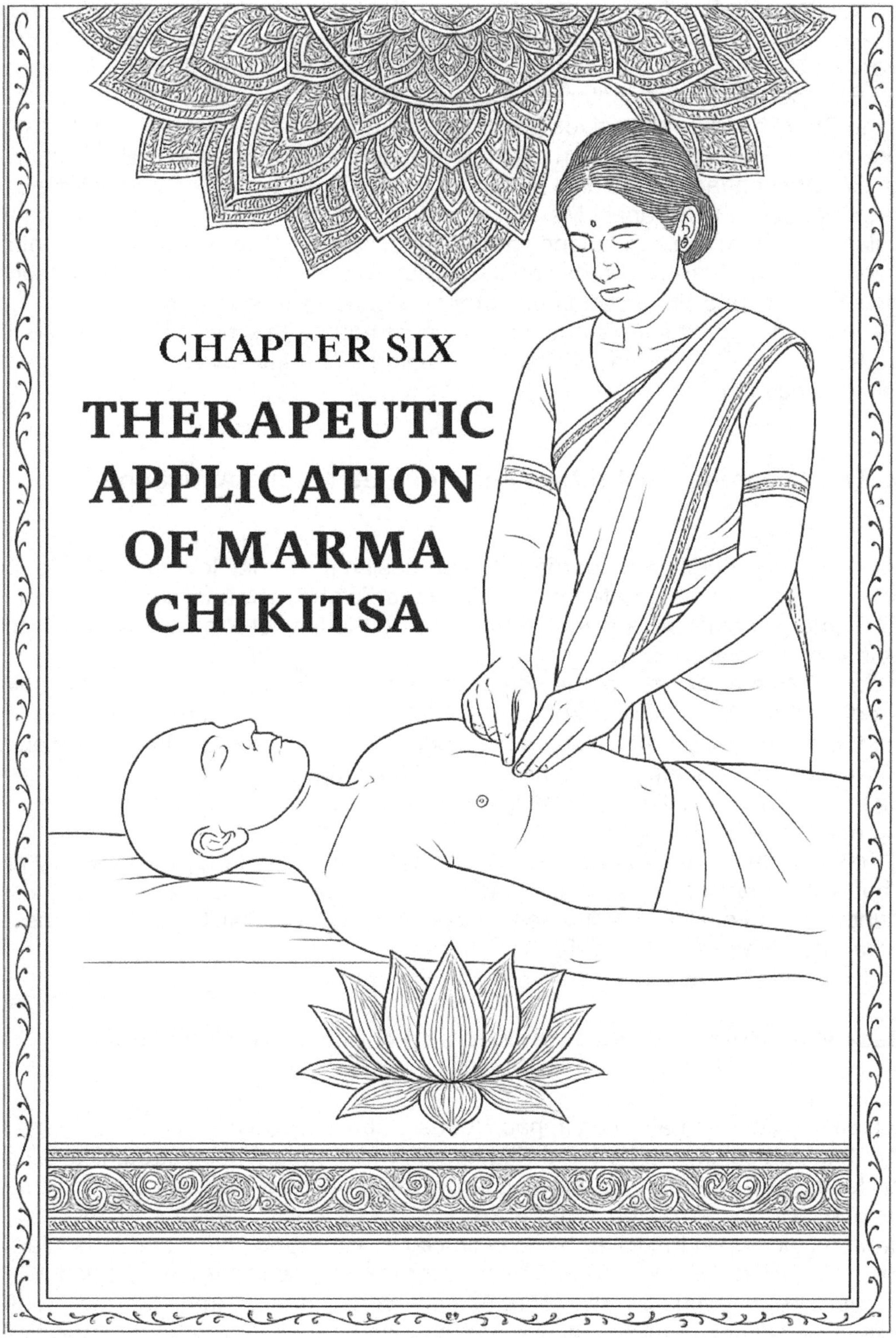

Chronic Headache Relief Through Shankha and Sthapani Marma

Chronic headaches, a prevalent ailment affecting millions globally, often resist conventional treatments, leading sufferers towards holistic alternatives like Marma Chikitsa. The ancient science of Ayurveda identifies specific energy points, or 'Marmas,' which, when stimulated, can alleviate various ailments. In the treatment of chronic headaches, the Shankha (temporal region) and Sthapani (forehead center) Marmas are pivotal.

Activating the Shankha Marma involves gentle pressure and rotational movements, targeting the temporal area to relieve the tension accumulating in the head muscles. This technique not only helps alleviate headaches but also enhances sensory function, promoting overall calmness. Conversely, the Sthapani Marma, located at the mid-forehead, is known as the 'third eye.' Stimulation here focuses on balancing the Ajna Chakra, which is pivotal for mental clarity and emotional stability, thereby addressing the psychosomatic components of headaches.

Case studies demonstrate significant improvement in patients suffering from chronic headaches, with reduced frequency and intensity after regular Marma therapy. These findings underscore the potential of Marma Chikitsa in providing a non-invasive, rejuvenating solution for chronic pain management.

Insomnia Treatment via Talahridaya and Adhipati Marma Activation

Marma Chikitsa offers a profound approach to addressing insomnia, leveraging the ancient wisdom of Ayurveda through targeted activation of the Talahridaya and Adhipati Marma points. These critical energy points are known for harmonizing the flow of Pranic energy, which is essential for sleep regulation and mental peace.

The Talahridaya Marma, situated at the center of the palm, plays a crucial role in calming the mind and reducing anxiety, which are often leading contributors to insomnia. By applying gentle pressure to this Marma point, practitioners help induce a state of deep relaxation, thereby paving the way for restful sleep. Meanwhile, the Adhipati Marma, positioned at the crown of the head, aligns the body's circadian rhythms that control sleep-wake cycles, further facilitating a natural and healthy sleep pattern.

Together, these Marma points form a synergistic treatment that not only alleviates symptoms of insomnia but also enhances overall well-being. In clinical applications, patients report significant improvements in sleep quality and duration, showcasing Marma Chikitsa's effectiveness in restoring vitality and reversing sleep disturbances.

Lower Back Pain Resolved Through Kati and Nitamba Marma Points

Lower back pain, a common affliction impacting the global population, often finds relief through Marma Chikitsa, particularly via Kati and Nitamba Marma points. These strategically located energy points, integral to Ayurvedic therapy, target the root causes of pain and facilitate the healing process.

The Kati Marma, located in the lower back, is crucial in alleviating spinal and muscular discomfort. By applying specific pressure techniques, therapists influence energy flow, promoting pain relief and muscle relaxation. Simultaneously, the Nitamba Marma, located near the buttocks, is stimulated to further alleviate tension and enhance circulatory dynamics. Together, these points synergistically work to restore balance and reduce inflammation.

Clinical case studies highlight the efficacy of this approach in chronic lower back pain scenarios. Patients report significant improvements in mobility and a decrease in pain levels after undergoing targeted Marma therapy. This testament to the potential of Marma Chikitsa underscores its value as a non-invasive alternative in pain management.

Knee Osteoarthritis Improvement Using Janu and Indrabasti Marmas

Knee osteoarthritis, characterized by chronic pain and joint degeneration, often impedes daily activities. However, the ancient art of Marma Chikitsa offers a unique approach to mitigating these symptoms by stimulating the Janu and Indrabasti Marma points. These specific points are strategically located around the knee, believed to be pivotal in regulating energy flow and alleviating pain.

The Janu Marma, situated at the knee joint, directly influences the flow of Vata, the Ayurvedic principle associated with movement and pain. By applying gentle pressure techniques to this Marma, practitioners aim to reduce stiffness and enhance mobility. The Indrabasti Marma, meanwhile, lying just above the knee, serves to fortify the surrounding tissues and stabilize the knee structure. Stimulation in this area supports overall joint health and reduces inflammation.

Practical case studies have shown that patients experiencing knee osteoarthritis report significant improvements in pain levels and joint function after undergoing therapy focused on these Marmas. This treatment, emphasizing holistic well-being, exemplifies the potential of Marma Chikitsa in restoring vitality and reversing degenerative ailments.

Frozen Shoulder Treated with Amsa and Kakshadhara Marma

Frozen shoulder, a condition characterized by stiffness and pain in the shoulder joint, finds promising relief through specific Marma points known as Amsa and Kakshadhara. These points are central in Ayurvedic therapy for mobilizing stagnant energy that contributes to joint immobility and discomfort.

The Amsa Marma, located at the shoulder, is integral in alleviating pain and enhancing joint function. Therapy involving this Marma point utilizes targeted pressure and manipulative techniques to restore movement and reduce pain. Conversely, the Kakshadhara Marma, situated along the scapular region, complements the treatment by addressing underlying tension and aiding in the flow of prana, or life energy, through the affected area.

Clinical case studies showcase remarkable outcomes where patients experiencing frozen shoulder report improved range of motion and reduced pain after undergoing treatments involving these Marma points. This approach not only highlights the efficacy of Marma Chikitsa but also underscores its value as a non-invasive alternative in managing complex musculoskeletal conditions.

PCOS Symptoms Relieved with Guda and Basti Marma Therapy

Polycystic Ovary Syndrome (PCOS) challenges countless women with symptoms ranging from irregular menstrual cycles to insulin resistance. Embracing the holistic vistas of Ayurveda, Marma Chikitsa has emerged as a beacon of hope for managing these multifaceted symptoms through the stimulation of the Guda and Basti Marma points.

The Guda Marma, crucially positioned near the anus, is instrumental in regulating the Apana Vayu, which in Ayurvedic terms is vital for maintaining reproductive health and alleviating menstrual irregularities. Gentle manipulations of this Marma help in harmonizing hormonal imbalances, a common plight in PCOS sufferers. Meanwhile, the Basti Marma, located in the sacral area, primarily focuses on enhancing the functionality of the urinary and reproductive systems. This stimulation is believed to enhance the body's detoxification processes, thereby supporting hormonal balance and potentially reducing the occurrence of ovarian cysts.

Clinical observations underscore significant improvements in symptoms, with many women reporting regular menstrual cycles and reduced PCOS-related discomfort after undergoing this therapy. This natural and non-invasive approach underscores the healing potential embedded within ancient Ayurvedic practices, offering a sustainable alternative for women battling PCOS.

Sciatica Relief Through Kurchashira and Gulpha Marma Work

Sciatica, characterized by pain that radiates along the path of the sciatic nerve, finds innovative relief through the ancient technique of Marma Chikitsa, specifically targeting the Kurchashira and Gulpha Marmas. These vital energy points are strategically located to influence the nerve pathways that are often implicated in the development of sciatica.

The Kurchashira Marma, located on the calf, plays a pivotal role in modulating the painful sensations transmitted along the sciatic nerve. Practitioners apply precise pressure to this point to pacify the aggravated Vata dosha, which is often responsible for the nerve discomfort and pain. Similarly, the Gulpha Marma, located near the ankle, supports joint health and helps reduce stiffness and inflammation along the sciatic pathway.

Clinical practice has shown promising results, with many patients experiencing significant reductions in pain intensity and frequency. This non-invasive treatment leverages the body's own healing mechanisms, enhancing mobility and promoting long-term relief from sciatica.

Asthma Symptom Management with Urah and Apastambha Marma

Asthma, a prevalent respiratory condition, often restricts individuals through chronic inflammation and airway constriction. Marma Chikitsa, through the targeted stimulation of Urah and Apastambha Marma points, offers an ancillary modality for managing asthma symptoms, emphasizing a holistic recovery path beyond conventional treatments.

The Urah Marma points, located near the chest, play a crucial role in enhancing respiratory function and reducing chest tightness. Activation of these Marma points encourages better Pranic flow, which helps alleviate stress on the respiratory system. Meanwhile, the Apastambha Marma, located near the lower back, plays a crucial role in stabilizing energy flows that impact overall vitality, including lung capacity and respiration.

Case studies present a promising outlook where patients with chronic asthma have noted a marked improvement in breathing ease and a reduction in asthmatic attacks. This treatment approach not only supports lung health but also contributes to balancing the body's innate energy fields, showcasing Marma Chikitsa's potential in enhancing overall quality of life.

Constipation Alleviation via Nabhi and Parsruti Marma Stimulation

Constipation, a common yet distressing condition, often disrupts daily well-being and health. Marma Chikitsa offers a compelling solution by focusing on the Nabhi and Parsvati Marma points, which, according to Ayurveda, are believed to influence digestive processes significantly. The Nabhi Marma, located around the navel, is central to the body's digestive fire, known as Agni. Stimulating this Marma is thought to enhance gastrointestinal motility and balance the body's Vata Dosha, the energy that governs movement, including digestion and elimination. Techniques involve gentle circular massage and pressure application, aimed at kickstarting the digestive mechanisms and addressing the sluggish bowel movements.

Conversely, the Parsruti Marma, found near the lower abdomen, supports the Nabhi in energizing the digestive tract. Together, these Marmas create a synergistic effect that stimulates bowel movements and promotes a natural, gentle relief from constipation. Clinical case studies demonstrate that patients experience improved bowel regularity and a decrease in associated symptoms, such as abdominal discomfort, following this therapy.

Facial Paralysis Recovery Through Hanusandhi and Nasa Marma Points

Facial paralysis, often characterized by an inability to control the muscles on one side of the face, can be profoundly distressing. In the realm of Ayurvedic medicine, Marma Chikitsa presents a nuanced approach to this condition through the strategic stimulation of Hanusandhi and Nasa Marma points, located around the jaw and nose, respectively.

The Hanusandhi Marma is crucial due to its location at the jaw hinge, where it interfaces with facial nerve pathways. Treatment involving this Marma involves gentle pressure and rotational movements, aiming to restore neural control and alleviate muscle stiffness. Concurrently, the Nasa Marma serves to enhance these effects by targeting the nasal area, pivotal in reflex connections with facial muscles. Through sequential and combined stimulation of these points, Marma Chikitsa enables a reduction in symptom severity and encourages a faster recovery process.

Clinical observations have been promising, with patients reporting improvements in facial symmetry and muscle control. This non-invasive therapy underscores Marma Chikitsa's potential in addressing neurological disorders and enhancing quality of life through ancient practices.

Bell's Palsy Marma Intervention Protocol

Bell's palsy, characterized by sudden facial paralysis, may find hope in the ancient Ayurvedic practice of Marma Chikitsa. This unique approach addresses the underlying imbalances by precisely stimulating specific Marma points, thereby fostering nerve revitalization and muscle recovery.

Focus is placed on the Hanusandhi and Nasa Marma points, instrumental in neural pathways relevant to facial movements. The Hanusandhi, located at the jaw hinge, directly impacts nerve control, influencing facial symmetry and expression. Nasa Marmas, near the nasal passages, further enhance therapeutic effects by stabilizing Pranic flow, essential for nerve function. This dual-point regimen is designed to restore nerve conductivity and normal muscle function.

Clinical cases illustrate substantial success, with many patients experiencing accelerated recovery periods and significant reduction in paralysis symptoms. This protocol not only illuminates the therapeutic potential of Marma Chikitsa in neuromuscular rehabilitation but also underscores its role in integrative health strategies for neurological disorders.

Anxiety Reduction Using Hridaya and Talahridaya Points

Anxiety, often manifesting as a pervasive sense of unease and nervousness, can disrupt daily life and diminish overall wellness. Marma Chikitsa's approach to alleviating anxiety focuses on the strategic activation of the Hridaya and Talahridaya Marma points, known for their ability to regulate emotional and cardiac rhythms.

In the realm of Ayurvedic energy healing, the Hridaya Marma, situated at the center of the chest, is regarded as a vital point for accessing the heart's subtle energy. Stimulating this point influences the heart chakra, fostering emotional release and stability. Similarly, the Talahridaya Marma, located at the center of the palm, complements this by promoting a grounding effect, which is pivotal in managing acute stress and anxiety episodes.

Clinical observations indicate that patients undergoing therapy with these Marma points experience noticeable reductions in anxiety symptoms. This non-invasive technique facilitates a deeper connection with one's body, enhancing personal resilience and emotional equilibrium.

Depression Case Study with Marma and Breath Integration

Depression, marked by pervasive sadness and a lack of interest in life, often challenges conventional treatment approaches. In this case study, Marma Chikitsa integrates with breathwork to target the mental and emotional disbalances inherent in depression. The stimulation of specific Marma points, combined with controlled breathing techniques, works synergistically to restore mental clarity and emotional stability.

Key to this therapy are the Hridaya and Manas Marma points, located at the heart and head, respectively, which are believed to have a direct influence on emotional and mental wellness. Activation of these points, combined with deep, rhythmic breathing exercises, facilitates a flow of prana that uplifts the spirit and alleviates depressive symptoms. This method harnesses the body's inherent energy to restore emotional equilibrium and naturally enhance mood.

Positive outcomes from this integrated approach include improved emotional regulation and reductions in depressive symptoms, as observed in patient testimonials. Through Marma Chikitsa and breath integration, individuals can reclaim joy and a zest for life, illustrating the profound impact of this method on mental health.

Hormonal Imbalance Balanced by Guda and Apasthambha Marma

Hormonal imbalances, affecting countless individuals, disrupt normal bodily functions. Marma Chikitsa, an ancient Ayurvedic healing practice, demonstrates significant promise in restoring endocrine health, particularly through the Guda and Apasthambha Marma points.

The Guda Marma, located in the rectal area, is closely linked with the body's elimination processes and adrenal function. Treatment of this Marma involves applying careful pressure techniques to stimulate organ detoxification and adrenal health, which are crucial for balanced hormone production. Activities targeting this Marma impact the body's overall energetic flow and

facilitate recovery of adrenal fatigue, a common issue in hormonal disorders.
On the other hand, the Apasthambha Marma, located near the base of the spine, is associated with reproductive and spinal health. By energizing this site, therapists aim to recalibrate the reproductive hormones. These two points, together, strategically foster a harmonious hormonal environment, providing evidence of tangible benefits seen in enhanced energy levels and normalized hormone profiles among clients.

Sinusitis Relieved by Applying Marma to Nasa and Avarta

Sinusitis, characterized by inflammation and congestion of the sinuses, disrupts comfort and respiratory function. Ayurvedic energy healing, through Marma Chikitsa, offers substantial remediation by focusing on Nasa and Avarta Marma points, strategically positioned at the bridge of the nose and around the eyes. These points are vital in Ayurvedic diagnostics, as they are intrinsically connected to the sinus passages and associated mucus membranes.
Treatment involves gentle, circular pressure at these Marma sites, synchronized subtly with the patient's breathing to maximize prana distribution through the affected areas, facilitating decongestion and reducing inflammation. This approach not only aims to alleviate physical symptoms but also to restore the energetic balance, crucial for overall nasal health. The therapy harnesses the natural body's energies and is complemented by aromatic oils that are inhaled during the session to enhance the healing process.
Clinical successes include reported relief from chronic sinus congestion and a marked improvement in breathing efficiency. Patients often experience these benefits after just a few sessions, underscoring Marma Chikitsa's effectiveness in treating sinusitis naturally.

Liver Detox Support Using Phana and Kurcha Marmas

In the realm of Ayurvedic therapy, liver health is paramount, as it significantly impacts overall vitality and the body's natural detoxification processes. Marma Chikitsa, through targeted stimulation of Phana and Kurcha Marma points, offers a profound method for enhancing liver function and supporting detoxification pathways. The Phana Marma, located near the temples, is intricately connected to the head's Pranic flow, which indirectly influences liver health through neural and hormonal balance. Kurcha Marmas, positioned at the base of the fifth toes, directly correlate with the body's eliminative systems, promoting the removal of toxins that burden the liver.
This dual-point activation promotes a detoxifying effect, reducing hepatic stagnation and promoting the regeneration of liver cells, which is crucial for individuals suffering from toxin overload or chronic liver conditions. Regular treatment can lead to noticeable improvements in liver enzyme levels and a reduction in symptoms associated with toxic buildup, such as fatigue and jaundice.
Clinical observations reveal that patients undergoing this Marma therapy report enhanced energy levels and a greater sense of well-being. The non-invasive nature of Marma Chikitsa, combined with its efficacy in stimulating vital energy pathways, makes it a valuable component of holistic liver health management.

Parkinson's Support Through Dhamani Marma Therapy

Parkinson's Disease, characterized by tremors, rigidity, and slow movement, finds promising interventions in Marma Chikitsa, particularly through Dhamani Marma therapy. This subheading explores the application of Marma Chikitsa in alleviating Parkinson's symptoms by targeting the Dhamani Marma, located along the energy channels that govern neurological and motor functions.

The therapy involves precise stimulation of the Dhamani points to enhance Pranic flow, thereby improving motor control and reducing tremors. The activation of these Marmas is believed to regulate the Vata Dosha, which in Ayurveda is considered responsible for neurological movements.

Patients undergoing Dhamani Marma therapy have reported improvements in their motor skills and a decrease in rigidity. This non-invasive approach not only addresses physical symptoms but also contributes to emotional and psychological well-being, offering a holistic remedy for those battling this debilitating condition.

Through continuous clinical observations and patient feedback, Marma therapy has proven to be a vital component of Parkinson's management, highlighting the effectiveness of traditional Ayurvedic practices in modern therapeutic contexts.

Chronic Fatigue Syndrome Reversed Through Full-Body Marma Activation

Chronic Fatigue Syndrome (CFS), characterized by profound tiredness that remains unrelieved by rest, often confounds standard medical treatments. Marma Chikitsa, through full-body activation, offers an innovative and revitalizing approach to healing. The therapy involves stimulating holistic Marma points to energize and balance the body's vital energies or prana.

This treatment uniquely targets multiple interconnected Marma points to orchestrate a comprehensive resurgence of vitality. Key points, such as the Brahmarandhra and Surya Marma, located at the crown and the solar plexus, respectively, are emphasized to elevate the core energy flow and enhance metabolic processes, which are crucial in combating fatigue.

Patients undergoing this treatment experience a rebalancing of their vital energies that manifests in reduced fatigue and improved overall stamina.

Clinical cases illustrate significant improvements in patients' energy levels, mood, and sleep patterns. This case study highlights the transformative potential of Marma Chikitsa, demonstrating its efficacy in enhancing the quality of life for individuals suffering from CFS.

Stroke Rehabilitation with Marma-Based Neuroregulation

Stroke rehabilitation, which focuses on restoring functions lost due to neurological damage, taps into the ancient wisdom of Marma Chikitsa. By activating specific Marma points, this therapeutic approach aims to enhance neuroplasticity—the brain's ability to reorganize itself by forming new neural connections.

Practitioners target the Brahmarandhra and Bindu Marma points located at the crown and back of the head, respectively. Stimulating these zones is believed to potentiate healing energies, facilitating improvements in cognitive and motor skills affected by the stroke. The touch technique, gentle yet profound, is synchronized with subtle breathwork, supporting a holistic recovery pace adjusted to individual needs.

The result is not only physical but significant emotional and psychological rejuvenation. Patients report enhanced clarity and reduced anxiety, which are essential for recovery. Continual therapy sessions often yield incremental benefits, underscoring Marma Chikitsa's potential in stroke rehabilitation through meticulous and nurturing energy modulation.

Autonomic Dysfunction Treated Through Sthapani and Apanga Points

Autonomic Dysfunction, a complex condition marked by irregularities in the autonomic nervous system, orchestrates involuntary bodily functions such as heart rate and digestion. Ayurvedic practices, such as Marma Chikitsa, offer non-invasive solutions through the targeted activation of specific points, primarily Sthapani and Apanga, located on the forehead and near the eyes, respectively.

Marma therapy at these sites focuses on restoring balance within the autonomic functions. Sthapani, being centrally located, is integral for calming the mind and harmonizing the neural activities that command the body's baseline operations. Apanga points, slightly lateral, support this by alleviating stress around the ocular area, which often impacts autonomic stability. Together, they create an environment that fosters neurophysiological equilibrium.

Patients receiving this treatment report significant reductions in symptoms such as erratic heartbeats and digestive troubles. The gentle stimulations encourage vital energy flows, reestablishing the natural rhythms essential for health. This approach exemplifies Marma Chikitsa's ability to address complex bodily dysfunctions through precise, holistic touch.

PTSD Management with Hridaya and Urvi Marma Protocol

Post-Traumatic Stress Disorder (PTSD) profoundly impacts the emotional and physiological aspects of individuals, often manifesting in persistent anxiety, nightmares, and intrusive thoughts. Marma Chikitsa, a traditional Ayurvedic healing technique, offers a unique approach to alleviating these symptoms through the activation of Hridaya and Urvi Marma points.

The Hridaya Marma, located at the heart center, is pivotal for emotional regulation and heart function. Marma therapy focusing on this point seeks to soothe the heart's energy, facilitating emotional release and stability. Conjointly, the Urvi Marma, positioned on the thighs, targets the energetic pathways that influence fear and anxiety responses. Stimulating Urvi works in tandem with Hridaya to enhance resilience and ground emotions.

Clinical cases of PTSD treated with this protocol report reduced anxiety levels and improved sleep patterns. Patients experience a notable decrease in hyperarousal symptoms and an increased sense of calm, evidencing the integrative potency of Marma Chikitsa in healing trauma without invasive intervention.

Post-Surgical Recovery Enhanced with Gentle Marma Touch

Post-surgical recovery can be daunting, with pain and limited mobility often prolonging the healing process. Marma Chikitsa offers a unique approach to expedite recovery through gentle Marma touch, which stimulates specific energy points to foster healing and reduce discomfort. By focusing on vital Marma points, this method enhances the body's natural recuperative processes. The gentle touch technique not only eases pain but also minimizes inflammation,

which is crucial in the post-operative period. Key Marma points like Anahata (heart) and Janu (knees) are often targeted, depending on the surgical site, to promote energy flow and assist in tissue regeneration.
Patients who have undergone Marma therapy post-surgery report a noticeable reduction in pain and quicker return to daily activities. This holistic approach, therefore, not only addresses the physical aspects of healing but also supports emotional well-being, making it a comprehensive adjunct therapy in post-surgical care.

Hypothyroidism Managed by Kanth and Adhipati Points

Hypothyroidism, a prevalent endocrine disorder, often presents challenges in conventional treatment plans, particularly in achieving optimal thyroid function without side effects. Marma Chikitsa introduces a potent, non-invasive method to manage this condition through the stimulation of Kanth and Adhipati Marma points. Located at the throat and crown, respectively, these points are central to thyroid regulation and hormonal balance.
The Kanth Marma, directly influencing the thyroid gland, is gently stimulated to enhance metabolic processes and energy production. This specific point's activation helps in normalizing the sluggish thyroid operations that characterize hypothyroidism. Concurrently, the Adhipati Marma, situated at the top of the head, is targeted to regulate the pituitary gland, the master gland controlling hormonal secretions, including thyroid hormones.
Patients undergoing this dual-point Marma therapy report improvements in energy levels, reduction in symptoms like fatigue and weight gain, and a notable stabilization in emotional states. This treatment exemplifies how traditional practices can harmoniously integrate into modern therapeutic landscapes for effective disease management.

Joint Instability Case Study Resolved with Snayu Marma Work

Joint instability, a debilitating condition that undermines skeletal stability and mobility, presents significant challenges in conventional treatment. The ancient Ayurvedic technique of Marma Chikitsa offers a promising alternative through the activation of Snayu Marma points, specifically targeting the connective tissues that support joint health.
In a compelling case study, a patient suffering from chronic knee instability experienced profound improvement following a regimen of Snayu Marma therapy. This technique involved precise, gentle stimulation of Snayu points around the affected knee, effectively enhancing ligament strength and joint function. The therapy was complemented by bespoke herbal treatments and tailored dietary guidelines to support tissue regeneration and reduce inflammation.
Remarkably, the patient reported not only a significant reduction in joint pain but also an increased range of motion and stability. This case underscores Marma Chikitsa's potential in addressing complex musculoskeletal issues through holistic, non-invasive interventions, illustrating its role in modern therapeutic practices.

Summary

The chapter 'Case Studies and Clinical Applications of Marma Chikitsa' explores various therapeutic applications of Marma Chikitsa, an ancient Ayurvedic healing practice. It begins by addressing chronic headaches through the activation of Shankha and Sthapani Marma points located in the temporal region and forehead, respectively. This technique is said to relieve pain and enhance mental clarity by balancing the Ajna Chakra. Next, the chapter discusses insomnia management via the Talahridaya and Adhipati Marma points, which are pivotal for sleep regulation and emotional stability.

The treatment of lower back pain is also explored, utilizing the Kati and Nitamba Marma points to alleviate muscle tension and enhance circulatory dynamics, offering significant improvements in mobility and pain reduction. Knee osteoarthritis is addressed through the Janu and Indrabasti Marma points around the knee, improving joint function and reducing pain. Additionally, the chapter covers the management of frozen shoulder through the Amsa and Kakshadhara Marma points, leading to improved range of motion and reduced discomfort.

PCOS symptoms are managed through the Guda and Basti Marma points, aiding in hormonal balance and reproductive health, while sciatica relief is provided through the Kurchashira and Gulpha Marma points, reducing pain and improving mobility. Marma Chikitsa is also described as beneficial for managing asthma, relieving sinusitis, supporting liver detoxification, and promoting stroke rehabilitation through various strategically located Marma points. Furthermore, the text discusses the treatment of autonomic dysfunction, PTSD, post-surgical recovery, and hypothyroidism, emphasizing Marma Chikitsa's role in restoring balance and enhancing the body's natural healing abilities. The chapter not only illustrates how Marma Chikitsa addresses a wide range of physical conditions but also highlights its impact on emotional and psychological well-being, offering a holistic approach to healing and overall health.

References

[1] Charaka Samhita. https://www.ncbi.nlm.nih.gov/pmc/articles/PMC3215410/

[2] Clinical Applications of Ayurvedic and Chinese Herbs: Monographs for the Western Herbal Practitioner. https://books.google.com/

[3] Fundamentals of Complementary and Alternative Medicine. https://www.elsevier.com/books/fundamentals-of-complementary-and-alternative-medicine/micozzi/978-1-4377-0925-4/

Case Study: Optimizing Mental Wellness with Marma Chikitsa: A Case Study on Depression and Anxiety

Marma Chikitsa, a traditional form of Ayurvedic therapy, focuses on activating specific energy points known as 'Marma' points to heal and revitalize the body and mind. This case study explores the application of Marma Chikitsa in treating mental health issues, particularly depression and anxiety, which are prevalent in modern society. The patients involved in this study, Mark and Sarah, presented with persistent symptoms of depression and anxiety that interfered significantly with their daily functioning.

Mark, a 35-year-old IT professional, experienced chronic anxiety characterized by palpitations, frequent panic attacks, and social withdrawal. Sarah, a 42-year-old teacher, suffered from long-standing depression with symptoms including sustained low mood, lack of interest in activities, and fatigue. Both patients sought alternative treatments after conventional therapies provided limited relief.

The treatment plan incorporated stimulating the Hridaya (heart) and Manas (mind) Marma points, recognized for their influence on emotional regulation and mental clarity. The therapist employed gentle pressure techniques to activate these points, which are thought to regulate the flow of prana (vital life force), thereby harmonizing the body's intrinsic energetic balance.

Over a series of sessions, Mark observed a notable reduction in his anxiety levels, with fewer panic attacks and an improved ability to engage in social situations. Sarah experienced alleviation of depressive symptoms, reporting enhanced mood, increased energy, and renewed interest in her hobbies and social interactions.

This case study illustrates how Marma Chikitsa can be a potent non-pharmacological intervention in mental health care. The targeted activation of Marma points, based on individual needs, potentially offers a customized therapeutic approach that addresses the roots of psychological distress. Furthermore, this practice highlights the importance of integrating traditional healing techniques with modern psychological understanding to provide holistic care that encompasses physical, emotional, and mental health.

Case Study: Revitalizing Chronic Fatigue with Comprehensive Marma Therapy: An In-depth Analysis

Marma Chikitsa, an ancient Ayurvedic therapy, focuses on vital energy points that vitalize and heal the body. This detailed case study examines its efficacy in treating Chronic Fatigue Syndrome (CFS), a complex disorder characterized by extreme fatigue that does not improve with rest and cannot be explained by any underlying medical condition. The subject of this study is Emily, a 29-year-old graphic designer, who has been battling persistent fatigue, muscle pain, and cognitive impairments, affecting her quality of life and work productivity for over three years. Traditional medical treatments had minimal impact, leading her to seek alternative therapies.

Emily's treatment plan was uniquely tailored, utilizing a holistic approach targeting multiple Marma points known to enhance energy flow and alleviate fatigue. Key points included Brahmarandhra and Surya Marma at the crown and solar plexus, respectively, to regulate vital energy pathways and boost overall vitality. The therapist applied gentle yet precise pressure to stimulate these points, intending to restore Emily's energetic balance and improve her body's self-healing capacity.

The therapy sessions were conducted twice a week for four months. After the initial few sessions, Emily reported noticeable improvements in her energy levels and mental clarity. Gradually, the muscle pains diminished, and her sleep quality improved significantly, which contributed to further enhancements in her daily functioning. The continuous application of Marma therapy, coupled with dietary adjustments and mild physical exercises as recommended by her therapist, led to substantial improvement in her symptoms.

This case study not only supports the effectiveness of Marma Chikitsa in managing symptoms of chronic fatigue but also illustrates the potential of this ancient practice to be integrated into modern therapeutic strategies for comprehensive and non-invasive treatment solutions. The personalized care and understanding of the body's energy system inherent in Marma Chikitsa can offer a significant benefit to those who struggle with the complexities of CFS, providing a path to recovery and enhanced life quality.

Case Study: Enhancing Cardiovascular Health with Marma Chikitsa: A Comprehensive Case Study

Marma Chikitsa has been traditionally used in Ayurvedic medicine to balance the body's vital energies through the stimulation of specific Marma points. This case study delves into its application for enhancing cardiovascular health, focusing on a patient, John, a 58-year-old male with a history of hypertension and borderline high cholesterol, conditions typical in those with elevated risk for cardiovascular diseases. Traditional Western medicine had only been partially effective in managing his symptoms, prompting him to explore alternative treatments.

John's therapy began with an in-depth consultation to understand his lifestyle, diet, and previous health history, ensuring a tailored treatment plan. The Marma therapist identified key points such as Hridaya (heart), Anahata (chest area), and Apalapa (under the arms), which are traditionally associated with heart health and circulation. Gentle stimulation of these points was intended to improve Pranic flow around the cardiovascular system, thus reducing John's risk factors for hypertension and balancing his cholesterol levels.

Over a series of bi-weekly sessions spanning three months, John's therapist applied light pressure and circular massage techniques to these points, which are believed to detoxify the body energetically and enhance heart function. Alongside Marma Chikitsa, John was advised on dietary changes, including reducing sodium intake and incorporating more plant-based foods, as well as a moderate exercise regimen.

John reported a gradual but noticeable improvement in his energy levels and a reduction in blood pressure readings within the first month. By the end of the therapy cycle, his cholesterol levels had normalized, and his doctor noted an overall improvement in cardiovascular function. This case not only highlights the potential of Marma Chikitsa as a complement to conventional cardiac care but also underscores the importance of a holistic approach to health, combining physical, energetic, and lifestyle interventions to maximize well-being.

Case Study: Transformative Relief for Migraine Sufferers Through Marma Chikitsa

Marma Chikitsa, renowned for its profound impact on balancing bodily energies in Ayurvedic medicine, was employed in the transformative care of Ava, a 45-year-old software developer suffering from debilitating migraines for over a decade. Despite trying various medications, her condition frequently resulted in lost workdays and diminished quality of life. Ava's migraines were typically characterized by intense throbbing pain on one side of her head, accompanied by nausea and extreme sensitivity to light and sound.

The treatment strategy devised for Ava focused on the Sthapani (forehead center), Adhipati (crown), and Anja (between the eyebrows) Marma points, critical for their influence on neurological function and mental stress relief. The holistic approach included gentle stimulation of these points to realign her body's energies, particularly aiming to regulate the Pitta (fire and water) dosha, commonly associated with heat and inflammation linked to headaches.

Sessions were conducted weekly over a three-month period. Initially, Ava's therapist used light fingertip pressure to delicately activate each Marma point, following a precise protocol aimed at calming the excess Pitta. Additionally, essential oils with cooling properties, like sandalwood and camphor, were incorporated to enhance the efficacy of the treatments. Gradually, as the sessions continued, Ava reported a significant reduction in migraine frequency and intensity, which she described as life changing.

This case study not only underscores the potential of Marma Chikitsa to treat chronic conditions such as migraines but also highlights the importance of a tailored therapeutic approach. It provides valuable insights into how traditional techniques can be adapted into contemporary therapeutic practices, offering holistic alternatives to pharmaceutical interventions. The success of Ava's treatment reaffirms the necessity and effectiveness of addressing the energetic imbalances within the body, which are often overlooked in conventional medicine.

Case Study: Advanced Recovery in Paraplegic Patients Through Marma Chikitsa

Marma Chikitsa, an esteemed branch of Ayurvedic medicine, focuses on the body's vital energy points to stimulate healing and balance bodily functions. This extended case study delves deep into its applications in treating nerve damage in paraplegic patients, particularly examining the case of James, a 30-year-old man who suffered severe spinal injuries in a car accident, resulting in lower limb paralysis.

James's treatment began with a comprehensive evaluation of his physical health and residual limb sensations, during which specific Marma points linked to spinal and neurological health, such as Gulpha (ankle), Janu (knee), and Kati (lower back)—were identified for therapy. These points are believed in Ayurveda to regulate energy flows that can stimulate nerve function and potentially restore mobility.

The therapy sessions were meticulously designed, involving gentle but firm pressure on the identified Marma points to activate the body's innate healing responses. This stimulation was combined with traditional Ayurvedic oils known for their efficacy in nerve regeneration, which were applied during the sessions to enhance the treatment's effectiveness.

Over the ongoing treatment period, there was a noticeable improvement in James's condition. Initial changes involved increased sensation in areas that had been numb since his accident. As the sessions progressed, James reported a reduction in neuropathic pain, which is a significant indicator of nerve healing. Moreover, there was a slight improvement in muscle tone and strength in his lower body, which he had not experienced since the accident.

This case study not only highlights the potential of Marma Chikitsa in managing and potentially reversing nerve damage in paraplegic patients but also raises important considerations about the integration of traditional therapeutic practices with modern medical treatments. It underscores the need for a holistic approach in treating spinal injuries, considering not just the physical symptoms but also the energetic and neurological wellness of the patient. Through James's case, we observe how ancient practices can offer new avenues for rehabilitation and recovery in spinal injury cases, contributing deeply to the field of integrative medicine.

Case Study: Reviving Respiratory Health: A Case Study on Chronic Bronchitis and Marma Chikitsa

Chronic bronchitis, marked by persistent cough and difficulty in breathing, significantly impairs quality of life. This case study focuses on the use of Marma Chikitsa, an Ayurvedic therapy technique, to manage and potentially alleviate symptoms of chronic bronchitis in a 55-year-old male patient, Michael. Traditional treatments, including inhalers and steroids, provided Michael only short-term relief, prompting him to seek alternative therapies.

The treatment strategy incorporated stimulating key Marma points associated with respiratory health, specifically the Kurpara (arm), Uru (thigh), and Anahata (heart). These points are traditionally believed to influence prana distribution which is vital for lung and airway function. Sessions were handled by an experienced Marma therapist who applied gentle but firm pressure on these points to possibly remove energy blockages impacting the respiratory channels.

Treatment was scheduled twice a week for a period of three months. During each session, the therapist focused on the rhythmic application of pressure to stimulate the flow of prana, aiming to reduce inflammation and ease breathing. Essential oils like eucalyptus and peppermint, known for their respiratory benefits, were also used during the therapy to complement the energy work by helping decongest the airways.

As the weeks progressed, Michael reported a noticeable decrease in his cough frequency and an improvement in his breathing. His reliance on inhalers decreased, and there was a marked improvement in his overall energy levels and mood. The therapist also recommended dietary adjustments and herbal preparations to support respiratory health and reduce mucus production.

This case highlights how Marma Chikitsa can be effectively incorporated into holistic health strategies, addressing the underlying energy imbalances associated with respiratory ailments like chronic bronchitis. It also demonstrates the potential of integrating traditional Ayurvedic practices with lifestyle and dietary changes to enhance overall efficacy and improve patient outcomes.

Case Study: Enhanced Mobility and Reduced Pain in Arthritis Patients Through Marma Chikitsa

Marma Chikitsa, rooted in the ancient Ayurvedic tradition, taps into the power of the body's vital energy points (Marma points) to treat various ailments, including arthritis, a condition marked by painful inflammation and stiffness in the joints. This extensive case study focuses on the treatment of arthritis using Marma therapy to offer profound insights into its efficacy and mechanism. Let us examine the experience of Linda, a 67-year-old retired schoolteacher, who suffered from osteoarthritis in her knees and hands for several years, which greatly hampered her mobility and daily activities.

Linda's treatments involved stimulating specific Marma points, primarily the Janu (knees) and Kshipra (hands), which are believed to be crucial in managing joint health and providing pain relief. Her therapist utilized a combination of gentle pressure, essential oils, and movement therapies aimed at these points to reduce pain and inflammation. Each session began with a thorough evaluation of her joint flexibility and pain levels to tailor the stimulation to her specific needs.

Over several bi-weekly sessions, Linda experienced a notable reduction in her joint pain, which allowed increased mobility and improved quality of life. The therapy sessions also incorporated advice on dietary changes to support joint health, emphasizing anti-inflammatory foods and hydration to enhance treatment outcomes.

The success of Linda's case sheds light on the potential Marma Chikitsa holds as a holistic alternative or complement to conventional treatments for arthritis. The therapy's focus on not just the physical symptoms but also on the energetic and emotional layers facilitates a comprehensive healing environment. This case study illustrates the intricate connection between Marma points and bodily functions and provides a foundation for further exploration and integration of Marma therapy into general healthcare practices.

Case Study: Holistic Management of Rheumatoid Arthritis Through Marma Chikitsa

Marma Chikitsa, rooted in the ancient Ayurvedic tradition of healing, utilizes the body's vital energy points to treat various ailments. This case study explores its application in managing Rheumatoid Arthritis (RA), a chronic inflammatory disorder affecting numerous joints, including those in the hands and feet. The patient, Susan, is a 52-year-old female with a ten-year history of RA, characterized by joint pain, stiffness, and swelling, leading to decreased mobility and quality of life. Traditional pharmacological treatments had offered some relief but were accompanied by side effects such as gastrointestinal distress and increased risk of infections.

Susan's treatment plan incorporated Marma therapy, focusing on specific points believed to reduce inflammation and pain. These points included Kshipra (located at the base of the fingers), Janu (knees), and Gulpha (ankles). The selected Marma points are considered pertinent in managing joint health, vital for RA patients. The therapist applied gentle, circular pressure to stimulate these Marmas to potentially rebalance the body's vital energies or Prana, aiming to alleviate pain and improve joint mobility.

Over the three-month treatment cycle, with sessions occurring twice a week, Susan noted a significant decrease in joint stiffness each morning and reduced swelling in her fingers and knees. The therapy involved not only Marma point stimulation but also dietary recommendations to decrease inflammation and lifestyle modifications focusing on gentle exercises like yoga to enhance joint flexibility and strength.

Throughout the course, Susan's reliance on nonsteroidal anti-inflammatory drugs decreased substantially. The holistic approach embraced by Marma Chikitsa, integrating physical touch, dietary changes, and therapeutic exercises, proved vital in managing her RA symptoms effectively. This case study not only highlights the relevance of ancient healing practices in contemporary health scenarios but also showcases the importance of a comprehensive, tailored therapeutic approach in managing chronic conditions like Rheumatoid Arthritis.

Case Study: Targeted Marma Therapy for Enhanced Recovery Post-Stroke

The case study presented here examines the therapeutic effects of Marma Chikitsa on a 68-year-old retiree, Thomas, who suffered a mild ischemic stroke. While conventional rehabilitation methods such as physical therapy and medications were initially helpful, Thomas continued to experience residual weakness on his left side and difficulty with speech. Seeking complementary therapies, he turned to Marma Chikitsa, intrigued by its holistic approach and potential to enhance neurological function.

The treatment plan prioritized Marma points known to influence brain health and motor skills, notably the Brahmarandhra and Bindu points at the cranial apex, and the Gandhara and Simanta, which are located at the throat and heart, respectively. Each session involved precise, gentle pressure and rotational movements on these points to stimulate nerve pathways and promote better energy flow throughout the central nervous system.

Initial sessions focused on establishing a baseline of Thomas's energy distribution and identifying areas of significant energy disruption or blockage. The therapist used a combination of direct touch and aromatic oils known to aid neural health, such as frankincense and sandalwood, to enhance the sensory experience and therapeutic efficacy. As treatments progressed, noticeable improvements were observed in Thomas's speech fluency and motor coordination. His recovery not only included gains in physical abilities but also improvements in cognitive functions like memory and focus, which are often impacted by stroke.

After several months of consistent Marma therapy, alongside his ongoing conventional rehabilitation, Thomas reported feeling more energetic and mentally alert. His family noted a significant reduction in the post-stroke fatigue that initially plagued his daily activities. The integration of Marma Chikitsa into his recovery plan demonstrated a promising adjunct to traditional stroke rehabilitation by capitalizing on the holistic healing principles of Ayurveda to facilitate recovery not just on a physical level but also improving the emotional and psychological well-being of the patient.

Case Study: Integrative Approach to Managing Type 2 Diabetes with Marma Chikitsa

This comprehensive case study explores the use of Marma Chikitsa, an ancient Ayurvedic therapy, in the management of Type 2 Diabetes, a widespread chronic condition characterized by high blood sugar levels and insulin resistance. The focus is on a 53-year-old patient, Robert, who has been battling Type 2 Diabetes for over 8 years. Traditional medications had provided some regulation of his glucose levels, but with side effects like gastrointestinal distress and fatigue, prompting Robert to seek alternative therapies.

Robert's treatment incorporated Marma Chikitsa to specifically target energy points believed to influence metabolic processes and pancreas function, namely the Surya (solar plexus) and Talahridaya (palm center) Marma points. The therapy sessions, conducted weekly, combined gentle pressure with rotational movements at these points to stimulate and balance the body's energy pathways, potentially enhancing insulin sensitivity and glucose metabolism.

The practitioner also integrated dietary consultations into the therapy, emphasizing low-glycemic, nutrient-rich foods which are critical in managing blood sugar levels. Robert was encouraged to engage in daily mild to moderate exercise, like walking and yoga, which are known to improve insulin sensitivity and support the overall effectiveness of Marma therapy.

Over a period of six months, Robert observed notable improvements — his average fasting blood sugar levels reduced, and his dependence on medication decreased significantly. Additionally, Robert reported increased energy levels and an overall improvement in his vitality and mood, attributing these changes to the holistic approach of Marma Chikitsa combined with lifestyle modifications.

This case study exemplifies the potential of an integrative approach to diabetes care, where traditional therapies like Marma Chikitsa complement medical treatment. It highlights the importance of a holistic strategy in chronic disease management, addressing not only the physical but also the energetic imbalances in the body.

Review Questions

1. A 35-year-old female patient with a history of chronic headaches seeks alternative treatment after failing to achieve relief with conventional medicine. She has been treated with medication therapy without significant improvement. An Ayurvedic practitioner suggests activating the Shankha and Sthapani Marma points. What would be the expected outcome of stimulating these specific Marma points?
A) Increase in headache frequency
B) Significant reduction in headache severity and frequency
C) Worsening of her sensory functions
D) Triggering of additional pain in other body parts
Answer: B
Explanation: The stimulation of Shankha and Sthapani Marma points is intended to relieve headache pain. Shankha, located in the temporal area, helps ease muscle tension and enhance sensory functions. Sthapani, or the 'third eye' Marma in the forehead, aids in balancing the mental and emotional states, addressing the psychosomatic aspects of headaches. Regular therapy could lead to a significant reduction in the frequency and intensity of headaches, as observed in various case studies.

2. A chronic insomniac, resistant to traditional sleep aids, is introduced to Marma Chikitsa therapy focusing on Talahridaya and Adhipati points. What effect does stimulation of these points have on the individual's sleep patterns?
A) Disruption of the circadian rhythm
B) Localized pain relief without affecting sleep
C) Enhancement of mental clarity but no effect on sleep
D) Improved sleep quality and regulation of sleep cycles
Answer: D
Explanation: Activating the Talahridaya and Adhipati Marma points has a direct influence on calming the mind and stabilizing the sleep-wake cycles. Talahridaya, located in the palm center, is known for alleviating anxiety, facilitating deep relaxation, and promoting restfulness. Adhipati, positioned at the crown, helps in aligning the body's natural circadian rhythms. These interventions can significantly improve sleep quality and restore natural sleep patterns, offering a non-invasive solution to insomnia.

3. A patient suffering from lower back pain due to prolonged hours at a desk is treated using Marma Chikitsa, targeting the Kati and Nitamba points. What benefits are typically observed from the stimulation of these Marma points?
A) Increased discomfort due to muscle tension
B) Temporary relief followed by worsening of symptoms
C) Notable pain reduction and increased mobility
D) No change in pain but increased stress levels
Answer: C
Explanation: The activation of Kati and Nitamba Marma points is specifically beneficial for ameliorating lower back pain and enhancing mobility. Kati Marma, found in the lower back, facilitates spinal and muscular relief, aiding in the alleviation of discomfort and promoting relaxation. Nitamba Marma, located near the buttocks, works to reduce tension and improve circulatory dynamics. Together, these points help restore balance, reduce inflammation, and significantly improve mobility and pain levels.

4. Following a Marma Chikitsa session focusing on Janu and Indrabasti points for knee osteoarthritis, a patient reports changes in their condition. What outcomes might be expected from this Marma therapy?
A) Increased stiffness and pain in the knee
B) Decreased inflammation and enhanced joint mobility
C) No change in joint health but increased energy levels
D) Development of secondary muscular issues
Answer: B
Explanation: Janu and Indrabasti Marma points are strategically located to impact knee health directly. Stimulation of the Janu point, which coordinates with the knee joint, helps mitigate stiffness and improve flexion and movement, which are essential for osteoarthritis patients. Indrabasti, situated above the knee, supports overall knee stability and reduces inflammation. This specific Marma therapy is thereby effective in decreasing pain and inflammation while enhancing mobility and joint function, providing considerable relief from osteoarthritis symptoms.

5. A person undergoing treatment for chronic frozen shoulder is advised to undergo Marma Chikitsa, including stimulation of Amsa and Kakshadhara points. Which benefits are expected to manifest from this therapy?
A) The immediate full range of shoulder motion is restored
B) Gradual improvement in range of motion and pain reduction
C) Shoulder stiffness increases, but lessened pain
D) No noticeable change in shoulder condition
Answer: B
Explanation: Amsa and Kakshadhara Marma points are key in addressing stiffness and pain in the shoulder area. The Amsa point, located in the shoulder region, is effective in relieving pain and promoting improved joint function. Kakshadhara, found along the scapula, complements Amsa by alleviating underlying tension and facilitating energy flow. Marma therapy on these points collectively facilitates a gradual restoration of mobility and a significant reduction in pain, leading to progressive improvement in frozen shoulder conditions.

CHAPTER SEVEN: Marma Chikitsa in Chronic Disease Management

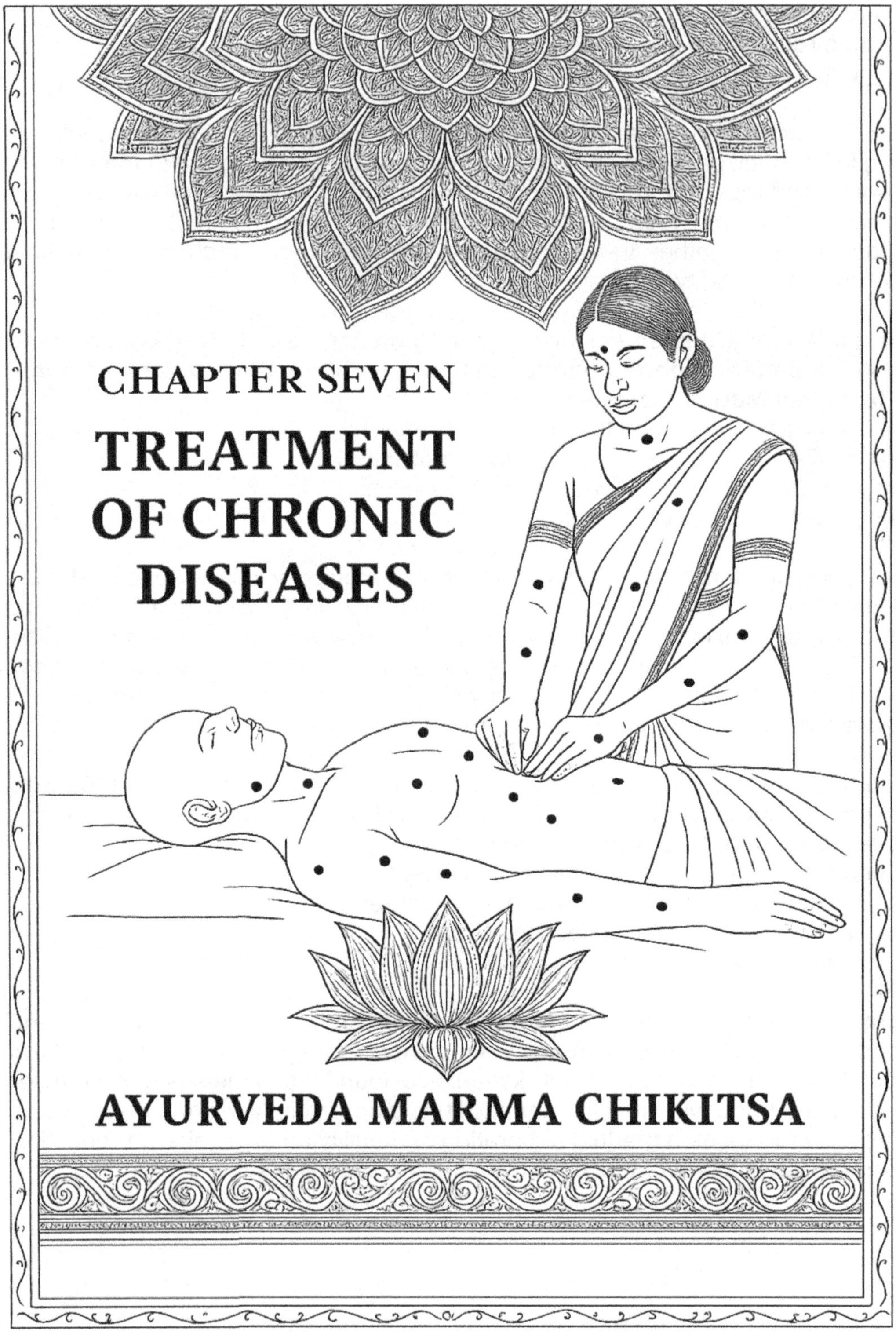

Overview of Chronic Illness Through an Ayurvedic Lens

Ayurveda, the ancient science of life, provides a unique perspective on chronic illness, stressing the balance of the body's energies (doshas) and the flow of life force (prana). Chronic diseases, according to Ayurveda, often manifest from prolonged dosha imbalances, primarily due to lifestyle inconsistencies, dietary errors, and psychological stressors.

Marma Chikitsa, an integral part of Ayurveda, focuses on Marma points, strategic body locations where flesh, veins, arteries, tendons, bones, and joints converge. These points are seen as portals through which the body's energy can be influenced. By manipulating these vital points, Marma Chikitsa seeks to restore equilibrium to the doshas and enhance the distribution of prana, thereby addressing the root causes of chronic conditions.

This form of treatment views each patient holistically, considering their unique constitution and the interplay of their physical, mental, and emotional health. It is a personalized approach that not only aims to alleviate symptoms but also to rejuvenate the body and prevent further progression of ailments, distinguishing it significantly from conventional Western methods that often focus solely on symptomatic relief.

Inflammatory Conditions and Marma Intervention

Inflammation is a natural process of the body's immune response, often exacerbated into chronic states by lifestyle and environmental factors. Marma Chikitsa provides a nuanced approach to such conditions, promoting healing by balancing the body's energies (doshas), which, if disturbed, contribute to inflammation.

Specific Marma points like Apana Vayu, located in the lower abdomen, and Kshipra, at the hands and feet, are targeted to regulate the inflammatory pathways. Gentle stimulation of these points helps modulate immune responses and enhance toxin removal, which is vital for reducing inflammation levels. This intervention supports not just local but systemic alleviation of inflammatory symptoms, such as swelling and pain, offering a holistic remedy.

Moreover, regular Marma therapy aims to reinforce the body's inherent healing capabilities over time. Patients with chronic inflammatory conditions report significant improvements in their symptoms, attributed to enhanced quality of life. This underscores Marma Chikitsa's potential as a sustainable, non-invasive treatment modality, pivotal for managing complex inflammatory diseases.

Autoimmune Diseases: Balancing Immunity via Marma

Autoimmune diseases present a unique challenge in healthcare, characterized by the body's immune system mistakenly attacking its own tissues. Marma Chikitsa offers transformative insights into restoring balance and modulating the immune response through strategic engagement of Marma points. These points, integral to Ayurvedic healing, serve as junctions of vital life energy that can be activated to harmonize bodily functions.

The practice focuses on specific Marmas that influence the immune system, such as Kshipra, located in the hands and feet, which is associated with enhancing vitality and regulating immune reactions. Gentle stimulation of these points aims to correct Pranic imbalances that contribute to autoimmune pathology. By restoring the flow of prana, Marma Chikitsa helps reestablish the immune system's correct discernment between self and non-self, which is pivotal in autoimmune

conditions.
Patients undergoing this holistic treatment often report a reduction in autoimmune symptoms and a marked improvement in overall well-being. Marma Chikitsa not only alleviates physical symptoms but also addresses emotional and spiritual aspects, which are essential for healing autoimmune disorders.

Diabetes Mellitus and Meda Dhatu Marma Support

Diabetes Mellitus, characterized by the body's inadequate processing of glucose, finds a unique ally in Marma Chikitsa through the stimulation of Meda Dhatu Marma points. These points, integral for regulating fat metabolism and insulin sensitivity, are gently manipulated to enhance the body's glucose management. By focusing on the Meda Dhatu, located primarily in the abdomen, Marma Chikitsa aims to restore balance to the metabolic functions disrupted in diabetes.
Strategic stimulation of these Marmas helps in revitalizing the associated organs like the pancreas and liver, which are crucial for insulin production and glucose storage. This Marma approach not only aids in lowering blood glucose levels but also in reducing dependency on external insulin and other medications.
Patients treated with this protocol report better control over their blood sugar levels and a noticeable improvement in their overall energy and well-being. Embracing this ancient technique could revolutionize the holistic management of Diabetes Mellitus, reducing both the burden of the disease and its associated complications.

Hypertension and Cardiovascular Support Using Marma

Hypertension and cardiovascular disorders, pervasive in their prevalence, often challenge modern medical practices with their persistent, multifactorial nature. Marma Chikitsa introduces a profound dimensional approach into the holistic treatment spectrum, focusing particularly on vital Marma points that regulate cardiovascular function and blood pressure.
One key area is the Hridaya Marma, located in the region of the heart. Stimulating this Marma helps in balancing the circulatory rhythm and stabilizing blood pressure. Techniques involve gentle pressure and rotational movements, synced with regulated breathing to optimize cardiovascular efficacy. Another significant Marma point, the Anahata, influences the smooth cardiac function and emotional well-being, thereby reducing stress-induced hypertension.
This ancient method supports not just symptomatic relief but endeavors to rectify the root causes of the imbalance in the body's energies. Patients undergoing Marma therapy for hypertension commonly report improved vitality and a marked reduction in their dependency on conventional medication, showcasing the potential of Marma Chikitsa as a complementary therapeutic discipline.

Liver Disorders: Detox Marma Points and Timing

The Ayurvedic practice of Marma Chikitsa offers nuanced methodologies for alleviating liver disorders, focusing on the detoxification pathways through specific Marma points. Known as 'gateways' for Pranic energy, these points facilitate the regulation and cleansing of liver functions, which is pivotal in eliminating toxins accumulated from diet and environmental factors. Key Marma points like the Yakrut, located on the torso, are central to liver health. Manipulating the Yakrut Marma harmonizes the liver's energy flow, enhancing bile production and detoxification processes. The timings of these interventions are critical, ideally performed during the early morning or late evening when the body's Pranic flow is in an optimal state for detoxification.

Regular application of Marma therapy on these points reactivates the liver's natural detox mechanisms. Patients with chronic liver ailments report significant improvements in their overall health and energy levels, underscoring the efficacy of this ancient therapeutic system in managing liver disorders through holistic, energy-based interventions.

Kidney Disorders: Guda and Basti Marma Activation

Kidney disorders present a significant health challenge, deeply impacting the Pranic balance within the body. Marma Chikitsa introduces a specialized approach focusing on Guda and Basti Marma points, vital for renal health and functional balance. These points, located at crucial junctures, are stimulated to enhance kidney function and aid in the filtration and elimination processes.

In practice, gentle pressure applied to the Basti Marma, located in the lower back, can improve renal circulation and stimulate the natural detox processes. Similarly, the Guda Marma, situated around the anal region, is targeted to support the lower digestive tract, which shares a critical functional relationship with kidney health.

Regular Marma therapy on these points can diminish symptoms associated with kidney disorders, such as edema and uremia. Moreover, optimizing the Pranic flow through these Marmas helps revitalize the body's intrinsic healing capabilities, offering a holistic approach to kidney health restoration.

Digestive Disorders: Nabhi, Parsruti, and Hridaya

Digestive disorders encompass a range of issues that affect the gastrointestinal tract. Marma Chikitsa, with its precise focus on vital energy points, introduces effective interventions through the Nabhi, Parsruti, and Hridaya Marma points, each associated explicitly with enhancing digestive health.

Nabhi Marma, located around the navel, is considered the center of energy distribution in the body. Stimulating this Marma can regulate the digestive fire (Agni), essential for proper digestion and absorption of nutrients. Techniques involve gentle circular motions that harmonize the intestinal functions and alleviate common digestive complaints such as bloating and constipation.

Parsruti Marma, positioned near the ribs, plays a crucial role in the diaphragmatic movement, which aids in the mechanical aspect of digestion. Activation of this Marma point can help ease respiratory motions that support the digestive process. Simultaneously, Hridaya Marma, situated near the heart, influences the emotional states that are often linked to digestive issues like stress-induced gastritis. Addressing this Marma in conjunction with the others offers a holistic approach to treating digestive disorders by balancing both physiological and emotional well-being.

Respiratory Conditions: Asthma and Bronchitis

Asthma and bronchitis, two prevalent chronic respiratory disorders, garner significant attention in Marma Chikitsa for their management through the stimulation of energy points. The treatment focuses on Marma points that directly influence the respiratory channels and lung tissues, such as the Kshipra and Uru Marma located near the chest and underarms. Gentle manipulation of these sites helps reduce constrictions and enhances the flow of prana, alleviating symptoms such as wheezing and breathlessness.

Specifically, for asthma, the activation of the Prana Vayu, which governs the respiratory system, is crucial. Techniques include subtle pressures along the collarbone and back, areas associated with respiratory functionality. These practices aim to strengthen lung capacity and reduce dependency on inhalers over time.

In cases of bronchitis, Marma therapy focuses on clearing the respiratory tract from mucus accumulation. The stimulation of the Gandhara Marma, situated at the base of the throat, plays a pivotal role in fostering clearer breathing passages, thereby enhancing overall respiratory health. Regular engagement with these Marma points offers a supportive, non-invasive complement to conventional treatments, embodying holistic healing principles.

Thyroid Imbalance: Kanth Marma Sequence

Thyroid imbalance, often manifesting as hypothyroidism or hyperthyroidism, profoundly affects metabolic processes. Marma Chikitsa offers a promising adjunct by focusing on the Kanth Marma, located around the throat, which is pivotal for thyroid regulation.

Gentle stimulation of the Kanth Marma can enhance the thyroid's energetic flow, addressing both underactivity and overactivity. Techniques employed include subtle pressures with soothing circular motions, aimed specifically at rebalancing the thyroid's release of hormones. This is complemented by deep, rhythmic breathing to maximize Pranic distribution throughout the region, facilitating the body's intrinsic healing responses.

These practices not only seek symptomatic relief but strive to harmonize the underlying energy imbalances that contribute to thyroid disorders. Regular sessions help stabilize hormone levels, potentially reducing the need for extensive medical interventions. Patients practicing these techniques report improved metabolic functions and decreased symptoms of fatigue and mood instability, highlighting the effectiveness of Marma Chikitsa in the holistic management of thyroid health.

Chronic Pain Management: Key Marma Points and Tools

Chronic pain, a pervasive ailment, significantly diminishes the quality of life, propelling the need for effective and sustainable relief solutions. Marma Chikitsa, through its profound understanding of energy channels, offers a compelling approach to managing chronic pain. Key Marma points like Ani, located near the joints, and Kshipra, situated at the base of the fingers and toes, are targeted to alleviate localized pain and enhance overall energy flow.

Techniques employed include gentle pressure, sometimes integrated with herbal oils known for their anti-inflammatory properties. This method not only addresses pain but also works on the emotional distress often associated with long-term pain conditions. Regular application facilitates a better range of movement and fosters a deeper healing by reestablishing Pranic

balance within the body.
For chronic conditions like fibromyalgia or neuropathic pain, a specialized sequence connecting Janu (knee) to Gulpha (ankles) Marma points is advised, linking key energy centers to diminish pain transmission. Implementing these Marma practices encourages not just physical ease but also psychological resilience amidst chronic pain scenarios.

Arthritis Protocols: Joint-Based Marma Treatments

Arthritis, a widespread affliction characterized by joint pain and stiffness, finds a promising ally in Marma Chikitsa, utilizing ancient techniques tailored to combat joint inflammation and enhance mobility. The approach harnesses specific Marma points associated with joint health, such as Janu Marma at the knees and Kshipra Marma at the base of the fingers and toes.
By applying gentle pressure on these points, practitioners stimulate the flow of prana, effectively reducing pain and facilitating joint function. This localized treatment not only addresses the physical manifestations of arthritis but also targets the energetic imbalances that exacerbate joint degeneration. Techniques often incorporate herbal oils that possess natural anti-inflammatory properties, enhancing the therapeutic impact.
Regular sessions utilizing these Marma practices promise not just symptomatic relief but also at a deeper, more holistic level of healing, restoring vitality and motion. Such integrative treatment plans are tailored individually, considering the type and severity of arthritis, making Marma Chikitsa a versatile and vital component of arthritis management.

Alzheimer's Disease: Head and Memory Marmas

Alzheimer's disease presents a formidable challenge in the realm of chronic conditions, manifesting as progressive memory loss and cognitive decline. Marma Chikitsa, an ancient Ayurvedic practice, offers a nuanced approach for managing such neurodegenerative disorders through targeted activation of head and memory-related Marma points.
Specifically, the Brahmarandhra and Sthapani Marmas, located at the crown of the head and between the eyebrows, respectively, are pivotal in treatments aimed at cognitive enhancement. Gentle stimulation of these points is believed to facilitate mental clarity and improve neural pathways. Techniques often include soft circular massaging with medicated oils, which are chosen for their properties conducive to nerve health and memory improvement.
Moreover, integrating the Aja Marma, located at the midpoint between the ears, further aids in balancing the subtle energies within the brain, purportedly slowing the progression of the disease. Regular sessions focusing on these critical Marma points can thus play a supportive role in the holistic management of Alzheimer's, potentially alleviating symptoms and enhancing quality of life for afflicted individuals.

Parkinson's Disease: Tremor Reduction Strategy

Parkinson's Disease, known for its debilitating tremors and movement challenges, benefits remarkably from Marma Chikitsa, tapping into the power of energy healing to mitigate symptoms. The focus is notably on Manibandha and Talahridaya Marma points, located at the wrists and center of the palms, respectively, which are crucial for managing limb tremors.

Applying gentle pressure on these points, coupled with calming herbal oils, helps soothe the overactive nerve impulses, aiming to reduce the frequency and intensity of tremors experienced by patients. This Marma practice not only localizes treatment to symptomatic areas but also enhances the overall neurological function, helping in smoother motion and better control. Integrating these sessions bi-weekly with structured breathing exercises further enhances Pranic distribution, promoting a deeper sense of body and mind equilibrium. Patients often report a noticeable improvement in their daily functions and a reduction in tremor-related anxiety, underscoring Marma Chikitsa's potential as a complement to conventional Parkinson's therapies.

Hormonal Imbalance: Marma Role in Endocrine Reset

Hormonal imbalances, whether due to stress, diet, or genetic predispositions, can disrupt bodily functions significantly. Marma Chikitsa addresses these imbalances, focusing on Marma points that influence endocrine activity, thereby promoting hormonal equilibrium.

One pivotal Marma point for this purpose is the Indrabasti, located at the center of the calf. Stimulating Indrabasti helps regulate the adrenal gland's production of cortisol, which in turn supports overall hormonal balance. Techniques involve gentle pressure and circular massages, often enhanced by the application of warm, herbal-infused oils that penetrate deeply to stimulate the internal energies.

In addition, the Nabhi Marma, located around the navel, is central to resetting digestive enzymes and hormones secreted by the pancreas. Regular stimulation assists in optimizing digestion and absorption, key processes that affect hormonal health.

Marma Chikitsa's holistic approach not only aims at symptomatic relief but seeks to restore the body's natural state of balance, enhancing vitality and wellbeing through the ancient wisdom of energy regulation.

Menstrual Irregularities and Reproductive Health

Addressing menstrual irregularities and broader reproductive health concerns, Marma Chikitsa offers specialized treatments focusing on the delicate balance of the reproductive system. Key Marma points such as the Shroni Marma around the pelvic area and the Nabhi Marma near the navel are emphasized to regulate menstrual cycles and enhance fertility.

Practitioners apply gentle pressure to these points, often using calming oils that harmonize hormonal activity and soothe the reproductive organs. This not only aids in normalizing menstrual cycles but also addresses symptoms associated with conditions like PCOS and endometriosis.

Beyond physical treatments, Marma Chikitsa encourages a holistic view, integrating dietary recommendations and lifestyle changes that support women's health. Regular sessions help maintain an energetic balance, crucial for reproductive vitality.

This approach is not just about symptom management but restoring a natural state of health, empowering women in their journey towards holistic well-being and reproductive health.

Uterine Fibroids and Pelvic Marmas

Uterine fibroids, benign tumors forming within or on the uterine walls, are addressed distinctively through Marma Chikitsa, an ancient healing practice focused on energy points. These fibroids, which can cause pain, heavy menstrual bleeding, and fertility challenges, are often treated with Marma points located in the pelvic region, believed to enhance reproductive health and alleviate associated discomfort.

The key Marma points utilized include the Shroni Marma, which is pivotal for pelvic stability, and the Basti Marma, associated with the lower abdomen's vitality. Gentle stimulation of these points aims to rebalance the prana (vital energy) flow, mitigating the energetic disturbances that contribute to fibroid formation and growth. Techniques such as circular massages with medicated oils tailored to reduce inflammation and promote tissue healing are commonly used. These holistic practices not only address the physical symptoms but also aim to restore emotional and hormonal harmony, providing a comprehensive approach to managing uterine fibroids. Regular treatments can improve overall reproductive health, offering a non-invasive alternative to conventional medical interventions.

Prostate Disorders: Basti and Medhra Marma

Addressing prostate disorders, Marma Chikitsa offers distinct avenues for alleviating symptoms and promoting prostate health, particularly through the Basti and Medhra Marma points. Positioned crucially for influencing urogenital functions, these Marma points facilitate energy flow crucial to prostate well-being.

Gentle stimulation of the Basti Marma, located around the sacral region, supports urinary tract efficiency and can help alleviate discomfort related to benign prostatic hyperplasia (BPH). Medhra Marma, positioned at the perineal area, directly influences glandular health, easing symptoms like frequent urination and pelvic discomfort.

Marma practitioners employ herbal oils specifically chosen for their anti-inflammatory and diuretic properties, enhancing the therapeutic impact. Routine stimulation through precise techniques may reduce the need for invasive treatments, offering a holistic alternative focused on restoring bodily harmony and prostate health.

This approach not only helps manage day-to-day symptoms but also integrates the deeper layers of emotional and energetic healing necessary for long-term wellness in prostate management.

Skin Disorders: Immune Balancing Through Marma

Skin disorders, often reflective of internal imbalances, are uniquely addressed through Marma Chikitsa, focusing on restoring immune harmony. Vital Marma points like the Brahmarandhra and Simanta are central to this practice, believed to influence skin health by regulating the body's immune response.

By targeting these specific points located on the head, practitioners apply gentle pressure combined with medicated oils known for their anti-inflammatory properties. This not only soothes irritated skin but also activates the body’s natural healing processes, helping to clear toxins that can exacerbate skin conditions such as eczema, psoriasis, and acne.

Furthermore, the immune system is closely linked to stress levels, and Marma therapy employs

techniques to reduce stress, thereby indirectly benefiting skin health. Regular Marma sessions promote a deeper balance within the endocrine system, which is crucial for maintaining immune homeostasis and overall skin vitality.
Thus, Marma Chikitsa offers a holistic approach to skin health, emphasizing not just external treatment but also internal balance and emotional wellness, fostering an environment for the body to heal itself.

Migraine: Sthapani, Apanga, and Shankha Protocol

Migraines, characterized by severe, debilitating headaches, find a soothing solace in Marma Chikitsa through the strategic application of the Sthapani, Apanga, and Shankha Marma points. These points, located around the forehead and temples, are central in the energetic pathways that influence headache and migraine relief.
The Sthapani Marma, situated between the eyebrows, is considered pivotal for balancing the frontal brain functions and alleviating stress, a common trigger for migraine attacks. Gentle pressure and circular movements at this point help soothe the nervous system, reducing the intensity of headaches.
Similarly, the Apanga Marma, located near the outer corners of the eyes, targets the relief of eye strain and tension around the temples, which are frequently associated with migraines. The Shankha Marma, found near the temples, plays a crucial role in harmonizing the temporal region's Pranic flow, crucial for mitigating pain and promoting relaxation.
Regular treatment involving these points can significantly lessen migraine frequency and pain, offering a holistic alternative to conventional therapies.

Vertigo and Balance Disorders: Marma Application

Vertigo and balance disorders can disrupt daily life, often stemming from deeper energetic imbalances that can be addressed through Marma Chikitsa. This ancient system identifies the vital Marma areas, strategically located around the head and ears, which are known to influence equilibrium directly.
Key points, such as the Indrabasti and Brahmarandhra Marmas, are targeted to stabilize the inner ear's vestibular functions and the central nervous system. Utilizing light pressure paired with specific herbal oils that possess anti-vertiginous properties, practitioners aim to restore the body’s natural sense of balance. These applications not only alleviate dizziness but also enhance the overall sensory pathways that govern spatial orientation.
Since Marma Chikitsa is an essential protocol in Ayurveda, there are also common interactions and recommendations for Yoga Therapy. In treating Vertigo conditions, variations of traditional Yoga postures are indicated. Yoga Vinyasa, based on “Child's Pose” (balasana or shishuasana), can be especially helpful in relieving significant symptoms.
Moreover, emotional stress often exacerbates vertigo symptoms. Marma therapy integrates calming techniques at the mental Marma points to reduce anxiety and stress, facilitating a holistic recovery. With consistent treatment, patients commonly report a rejuvenation in vitality and a significant decrease in episodes of imbalance and disorientation, reclaiming their freedom of movement and quality of life.

Cancer Support: Marma as a Complementary Therapy

In the domain of chronic maladies, cancer particularly benefits from the supplementary application of Marma Chikitsa. This ancient knowledge accentuates specific Marma points purposed to enhance the body's resilience and support the immune system during cancer treatments like chemotherapy and radiation.

Key points such as Kshipra and Talahridaya are gently stimulated to aid in detoxification and the management of treatment side effects. These points are known to help mitigate nausea, fatigue, and other distressing symptoms by fostering a better flow of vital energy (prana) that is often disrupted by conventional cancer therapies. Additionally, the emotional and psychological burden that weighs heavily on cancer patients is addressed through Marma, promoting mental calmness and pain relief.

Regular sessions of Marma Chikitsa can therefore provide a holistic support system, amplifying physical and mental coping mechanisms. It acts not just in symptom management but as an integral part of a broader healing protocol, potentially hastening recovery and improving quality of life.

HIV and Immune Regulation Through Marma Touch

Marma Chikitsa approaches HIV management with a focused intention to enhance immune regulation. Recognizing the vital force (prana) disruptions brought by HIV, this traditional practice targets specific Marma points, like the Kshipra and Adhipati, to fortify the body's immune defenses and improve overall vitality.

The gentle stimulation of these points, located on the limbs and crown of the head respectively, mobilizes the body's natural resilience mechanisms. Herbal oils with antiviral properties, such as neem and turmeric, are often incorporated to augment the efficacy of the treatment, aiming to balance immune function and reduce susceptibility to common infections associated with HIV.

Additionally, Marma therapy provides emotional support, crucial for coping with the psychological aspects of living with HIV. Techniques that release emotional blockages help enhance mental well-being, making this a holistic intervention that addresses the physical and emotional health challenges posed by HIV.

Marma-Based Detox Protocols (Ama Cleansing)

Marma Chikitsa, a profound pillar of Ayurveda, addresses Ama — the concept of toxins that accumulate and disrupt body functions. This subheading explores the specific Marma-based detox protocols designed to cleanse and rejuvenate the body holistically.

In the traditional framework, Ama results from improper digestion and is a root cause for numerous diseases. Leveraging Marma points like the Kukundara and Apana, practitioners affect the body's bioenergetic fields to stimulate detoxification processes. Gentle, precise pressure on these points, coupled with suitable herbal oils, facilitates the elimination of Ama, thus restoring physiological balance.

The Apana Marma point, located near the lower abdomen, is particularly crucial for removing water and earth element accumulations, thereby enhancing digestive fire (Agni). This activation directly supports the detoxification of the gastrointestinal tract and invigorates the body's natural purification systems.

Incorporating Marma detox protocols regularly supports a systemic reset of the body's metabolic mechanisms, improving overall vitality and preventing disease accumulation. This approach embodies a holistic safeguard for maintaining health and longevity.

Summary

Marma Chikitsa, an integral Ayurvedic practice, treats chronic diseases by targeting Marma points—specific sites on the body where vital life forces converge. This ancient method emphasizes restoring balance among the body's energies (doshas) and enhancing the life force (prana). It addresses the root causes of diseases, unlike Western medicine, which often focuses only on symptomatic relief. Marma Chikitsa views patient health holistically, considering each patient's unique constitution and the complex interplay of physical, mental, and emotional factors. Inflammatory conditions, autoimmune diseases, diabetes mellitus, hypertension, cardiovascular, liver, kidney, and digestive disorders, as well as respiratory conditions like asthma and bronchitis, are addressed through specific Marma points, which regulate various physiological pathways and alleviate symptoms. The approach also supports hormonal regulation, manages chronic pain and arthritis, and aids in neurological conditions such as Alzheimer's and Parkinson's Disease, as well as provides cancer support due to its immune-enhancing capabilities. Marma Chikitsa also encompasses mental health, providing relief from stress and enhancing overall well-being. Each treatment is personalized, supporting long-term health benefits and improved quality of life. Regular practice can lead to significant improvements in physiological functions and reduction of dependency on conventional medications. Marma Chikitsa not only alleviates physical symptoms but also addresses the underlying energetic imbalances, offering a comprehensive treatment paradigm for chronic conditions.

References

[1] Lad, Vasant. Textbook of Ayurveda, https://beardedmedia.com/product/textbook-of-ayurveda-vol-1-fundamental-principles-of-ayurveda/

[2] Johari, Harish. Ayurvedic Massage: Traditional Indian Techniques for Balancing Body and Mind, https://www.google.com/books/edition/Ayurvedic_Massage/Q8ryo-SyO3UC?hl=en

[3] Frawley, David. Ayurveda and the mind: the healing of consciousness, https://archive.org/details/ayurvedamindheal00fraw

[4] Subhash Ranade,. Introduction to Kayachikitsa, https://www.google.com/books/edition/A_Textbook_of_Kaya_Chikitsa/FnVEzQEACAAJ?hl=en

Case Study: Comprehensive Management of Chronic Arthritis through Marma Chikitsa

In the holistic realm of Ayurveda, Marma Chikitsa stands out as a profound therapeutic technique targeting the Marma points to balance energy flows and restore health. We explore a detailed case involving a 58-year-old woman, Mrs. Anita Desai, who presented with chronic arthritis, characterized by joint pain, stiffness, and reduced mobility, primarily in her knees and wrists.

Despite conventional treatments, her condition showed minimal improvement, leading her to explore alternative therapies, including Marma Chikitsa.

Upon initial consultation, Mrs. Desai was evaluated using the principles of Ayurveda, which involved assessing her dosha (body constitution) and prakruti (nature). It was determined that her Vata dosha was predominantly imbalanced, contributing to her joint issues. Her treatment protocol was meticulously planned to involve targeted stimulation of specific Marma points like Janu (knees) and Manibandha (wrists), known for their significance in managing joint health and pain relief. Over twelve sessions, each lasting about 45 minutes, gentle pressure was applied using herbal oils tailored for their anti-inflammatory properties.

The therapist focused on not only alleviating the physical symptoms by re-establishing energy flow in affected areas but also on psychological aspects by incorporating stress-reducing techniques. With each session, Mrs. Desai reported a noticeable improvement in pain and flexibility. Additionally, advice on diet and lifestyle changes conducive to managing Vata dosha was provided, emphasizing warm, lubricating foods and regular gentle exercise.

After completing the treatment cycle, Mrs. Desai experienced a significant reduction in symptoms, an enhanced range of motion, and a stronger sense of well-being. These results illustrated Marma Chikitsa's capability to provide comprehensive care by addressing not only the physical dimensions of arthritis but also the underlying energetic imbalances, showcasing its potential as a non-invasive, integrative treatment modality complementing traditional medical approaches.

Case Study: Revitalizing Cardiovascular Health with Marma Chikitsa

The case study explores the journey of Mr. Rohit Verma, a 65-year-old retired bank manager, who began experiencing episodes of hypertension and general fatigue, which are common cardiovascular issues among elderly populations. Despite being on a regimen of antihypertensive drugs, Mr. Verma's blood pressure readings remained inconsistently high, and he reported a decline in his overall vitality and mood. In search of a holistic approach, he turned to Marma Chikitsa under the guidance of a renowned Ayurvedic practitioner.

Marma Chikitsa, revered in Ayurveda for its capacity to balance the body's vital energies, was deemed an appropriate intervention for his cardiovascular concerns. Initial assessment focused on understanding Mr. Verma's doshic constitution which revealed a predominance of Vata and Kapha, known to influence the circulatory and metabolic systems respectively. Specific Marma points such as Hridaya (heart region) and Anahata (chest area) were targeted to optimize his cardiac function and stabilize his blood pressure.

Each session involved gentle stimulations using specialized techniques and herbal oils, known for their efficacy in aiding cardiovascular health. Over several sessions, Mr. Verma reported feeling more energetically aligned, with improved blood pressure readings and reduced dependency on his conventional medications. Emphasis was also placed on integrating dietary adjustments and lifestyle modifications tailored to support his doshic balance, which included incorporating heart-healthy foods and mild aerobic exercises into his daily routine.

This treatment episode not only showcases Marma Chikitsa's potential in managing heart health but also highlights its role in enhancing general well-being. The strategic, holistic approach fostered a profound improvement in Mr. Verma's quality of life, presenting a compelling case for the incorporation of Ayurvedic practices alongside conventional therapies in addressing complex health issues like cardiovascular disease.

Case Study: Holistic Treatment of Type 2 Diabetes Mellitus Through Marma Chikitsa

The case study examines the therapeutic journey of a 52-year-old teacher, Mr. Sunil Kumar, who was diagnosed with Type 2 Diabetes Mellitus. Despite adhering to conventional medication regimens, his glycemic control remained suboptimal, marked by fluctuating blood sugar levels and frequent episodes of fatigue. Intrigued by the holistic promises of Ayurveda, particularly Marma Chikitsa, he consulted an experienced practitioner specializing in chronic care management.

The initial assessment focused on understanding Mr. Kumar's doshic constitution, which revealed an imbalance predominantly in Kapha, correlating with metabolic disruptions typical in diabetes. The practitioner decided to focus on the Meda Dhatu Marma points, which are vital in regulating metabolic pathways and enhancing pancreatic function, thereby crucial for insulin management in diabetic patients. Over several sessions, these points, located primarily in the abdominal area, were stimulated using gentle pressure combined with specific herbal oils known to influence insulin sensitivity and carbohydrate metabolism.

Each session included not only Marma therapy, but also dietary counseling tailored to Mr. Kumar's dosha imbalance, emphasizing low-glycemic, high-fiber foods that are essential in managing diabetes. Furthermore, lifestyle adjustments such as regular exercise, particularly Yoga and mild cardiovascular exercises, were recommended to enhance his overall metabolic rate and assist in better glycemic control.

Progress was monitored through regular follow-ups, during which Mr. Kumar showed considerable improvement in his blood sugar levels and a remarkable reduction in his dependency on insulin injections. His energy levels improved, and he reported feeling a greater sense of well-being. These positive outcomes highlight how Marma Chikitsa, when integrated with conventional diabetes management strategies, can provide a comprehensive and personalized approach to controlling blood glucose levels while also enhancing overall health.

This case study highlights the potential of Marma Chikitsa in managing complex chronic diseases, such as Type 2 Diabetes, through a multifaceted approach. It addresses not only the physical aspects of the disease but also incorporates dietary and lifestyle changes to restore the overall balance of body energies.

Case Study: Targeted Treatment of Chronic Respiratory Conditions with Marma Chikitsa

This case study explores the holistic approach of Marma Chikitsa in managing severe, chronic respiratory conditions, with a focus on asthmatic bronchitis. We will explore the case of Mrs. Geeta Roy, a 47-year-old schoolteacher, who has been enduring asthmatic symptoms compounded by chronic bronchitis. Conventional treatments provided temporary relief, but her symptoms frequently recurred, impacting her quality of life and her ability to perform daily activities.

An initial comprehensive assessment employing Ayurvedic principles revealed an imbalance primarily in her Vata and Kapha doshas, contributing to her respiratory issues. Marma Chikitsa, recognized for its potential to correct energy imbalances through precise point stimulation, was proposed as an integrative treatment strategy. The focus was on significant Marma points, such as Kshipra and Uru, located respectively in the hands and chest area, which are associated with respiratory health.

Each treatment session lasted 45 minutes, during which gentle manipulation of these Marma points was conducted. Herbal oils, specifically chosen for their anti-inflammatory properties and capacity to mitigate mucus production, were applied. Techniques included gentle pressure and circular massage, synchronized with specific breathing exercises aimed at facilitating deeper pranic penetration and respiratory relief.

Throughout several treatments, Mrs. Roy reported a noticeable improvement in her breathing, along with a reduction in wheezing and cough frequency. The integrative approach of Marma Chikitsa not only alleviated her physical symptoms but also addressed associated psychological stress, a complementary factor often exacerbating respiratory conditions.

This case highlights the importance of a holistic treatment approach through Marma Chikitsa, which may lead to sustainable health improvements in chronic respiratory conditions by recalibrating the body's energy flow and enhancing psychological resilience.

Case Study: Integrative Management of Autoimmune Disorders with Marma Chikitsa

The focus of this case study is on the holistic treatment of autoimmune disorders using Marma Chikitsa, explored through the experience of 43-year-old Sarita, suffering from rheumatoid arthritis, an autoimmune condition marked by chronic inflammation and joint pain. Traditional medicine had provided Sarita with symptomatic relief primarily through anti-inflammatory drugs, but she sought a deeper, more sustainable healing approach. She turned to Marma Chikitsa after learning about its holistic benefits in managing autoimmune conditions.

An initial consultation with an experienced Ayurvedic practitioner involved a detailed assessment of Sarita's overall health, lifestyle, and symptoms, as well as an evaluation of her doshas, revealing a significant imbalance in her Vata and Pitta doshas, which are often implicated in inflammatory responses and autoimmune activities. The treatment plan was meticulously crafted to focus on calming these doshas and enhancing the flow of prana, specifically around the affected joints and throughout the immune system.

Specific Marma points, such as Kshipra (located at the base of the thumb and big toe) and Talahridaya (located at the center of the palms and soles), known to influence immune responses and inflammation, were targeted. Sessions involved gentle stimulation of these points through light pressure and application of medicinal oils, specifically chosen for their anti-inflammatory properties. Sarita underwent this therapy twice a week, with each session lasting approximately 60 minutes.

Over the course of the treatment, Sarita reported not only a reduction in joint pain and swelling but also an increased sense of overall well-being and energy. As part of her therapy, dietary recommendations were made to support Sarita's specific doshic balance, incorporating foods with anti-inflammatory properties and avoiding those aggravating autoimmune responses.

This integrative approach, facilitated by Marma Chikitsa, which focuses on both physical alignment and doshic harmony, provided significant insights into the holistic management of autoimmune disorders. It demonstrated effective synergy with conventional treatments, suggesting a promising approach for patients seeking comprehensive care in managing complex health conditions, such as autoimmune disorders.

Case Study: Reviving Renal Function and Managing Chronic Kidney Disorder through Marma Chikitsa

In the domain of alternative medicine, Marma Chikitsa adopts a singular stance, particularly when dealing with chronic ailments like kidney disorders. This case study unfolds the therapeutic journey of Mr. Ashok Patel, a 62-year-old retired schoolteacher diagnosed with chronic kidney disease (CKD), whose health gradually deteriorated despite undergoing conventional treatment regimens, including medication for controlling hypertension and maintaining fluid balance.

Following a detailed initial assessment according to Ayurvedic principles, which involved a thorough evaluation of Mr. Patel's doshic patterns and prakruti (his inherent constitution), it was discerned that an imbalance in the Vata and Pitta doshas might be affecting his renal health. Consequently, the plan was to harness specific Marma points, notably the Basti (located in the lower back region) and Guda (associated with the anal and lower pelvic region), which are vital for renal health, to improve his condition.

Over the course of twelve 40-minute sessions of Marma Chikitsa, gentle stimulation was applied to these points. Herbal oils infused with rejuvenating properties were used methodically to enhance the treatment's efficacy. These sessions were interspersed with insights on lifestyle adjustments geared towards maintaining a balance between the Vata and Pitta doshas, including dietary changes that incorporate renal-protective foods and moderate hydraulic exercises.

Progressively, Mr. Patel reported improvements, indicated by better creatinine levels and reduced urea in his blood tests. The soothing impact of Marma Chikitsa on his nervous system also offered him relief from anxiety, which is often influential in exacerbating CKD symptoms. He found a notable uplift in energy levels and began enjoying walks and light activities, which previously were marred by fatigue.

Thus, this case illustrates the effectiveness of Marma Chikitsa in dealing with chronic conditions by not only addressing the somatic symptoms but also by realigning the patient's energy fields and emotional state. The holistic approach provided by Marma Chikitsa, which integrates physical healing with emotional and energetic balancing, highlights its potential as a complementary therapy in managing and potentially reversing the debilitating impacts of chronic kidney disorders.

Case Study: Rejuvenating Mental Health and Emotional Well-being Through Marma Chikitsa

Exploring the profound implications of Marma Chikitsa on mental health, this case study delves into the therapeutic journey of a 34-year-old software engineer, Mr. Aarav Gupta, who was grappling with chronic stress, anxiety, and symptoms of depression. Despite undergoing various conventional therapies, including medication and counseling, Mr. Gupta found temporary relief, but his symptoms recurrently intensified due to high job demands and personal life pressures. This led him to seek a holistic alternative, introducing him to the ancient practice of Marma Chikitsa.

An initial assessment by a seasoned Ayurvedic practitioner determined an imbalance predominantly in Mr. Gupta's Vata and Pitta doshas, known to govern the nervous system and emotional responses. The customized treatment plan focused on Marma points like Anahata (heart region) and Ajna (forehead region), which are instrumental in addressing psycho-emotional imbalances. Each session involved gentle stimulation of these points, complemented by the application of soothing herbal oils, aimed to calm the sensory system and revitalize the mind.

Over the course of twenty sessions, each lasting approximately 30 minutes, significant emphasis was placed on synchronizing Marma therapy with mindful breathing techniques. These practices were designed to deepen the therapeutic effects by enhancing pranic distribution and fostering mental clarity. Mr. Gupta was also guided in adopting lifestyle changes including a Vata-Pitta pacifying diet, regular sleep patterns, and daily meditation, which integrated seamlessly with the Marma therapy to enrich his overall well-being.

Post-treatment evaluations highlighted a notable enhancement in Mr. Gupta's emotional resilience, a marked decrease in anxiety levels, and substantial improvements in sleep quality and concentration. This case vividly underscores the potential of Marma Chikitsa not just in relieving psychological symptoms, but in fundamentally restoring emotional and mental harmony, offering a robust framework for managing modern mental health challenges.

Case Study: Enhancing Digestive Health via Marma Chikitsa

The case in focus examines the holistic application of Marma Chikitsa to treat chronic digestive disorders, particularly in the context of a 45-year-old male patient, Mr. Rajesh Sharma, who had been suffering from irritable bowel syndrome (IBS) and chronic indigestion. Despite several medical interventions and lifestyle adjustments, his symptoms of bloating, irregular bowel movements, and abdominal pain persisted, compelling him to explore alternative treatments like Marma Chikitsa.

A thorough initial evaluation, based on Ayurvedic principles, identified an imbalance primarily in Mr. Sharma's Vata dosha, which is characteristically linked to digestive irregularities. The tailored treatment plan targeted specific Marma points, primarily Nabhi (around the navel) and Parsruti (near the ribs), which are integral to digestive health. Each session, lasting around 40 minutes, involved gentle stimulation of these points using medicinal oils recognized for their digestive properties.

Over a course of several weeks, Mr. Sharma experienced significant improvement in his digestive functions. The practitioner also focused on the Hridaya Marma (heart region) to address related anxiety and emotional stress that Mr. Sharma reported exacerbated his digestive issues. Complementary dietary advice was provided, emphasizing warm, cooked foods that are easier to digest, and lifestyle recommendations were established to support regularizing sleep and exercise routines, thereby enhancing overall digestive health.

Progress was evident as Mr. Sharma's symptoms gradually diminished. He reported less bloating, more regular bowel movements, and a significant reduction in abdominal pain. The strategic use of Marma Chikitsa not only provided symptomatic relief but also worked on a deeper level to restore and rebalance his body's vital energies. This case highlights the effectiveness of Marma Chikitsa in managing and potentially resolving chronic digestive disorders through a meticulous, personalized approach that focuses on restoring energy balance and promoting holistic wellness.

Case Study: Advanced Management of Alzheimer's Disease through Marma Chikitsa

The integration of Marma Chikitsa in treating Alzheimer's disease provides a unique lens through which we explore the therapeutic journey of Mrs. Lalitha Reddy, a 72-year-old retired school principal diagnosed with early-stage Alzheimer’s. Despite conventional treatments involving medications known to slow disease progression, Mrs. Reddy's cognitive decline continued, accompanied by mood swings and increased forgetfulness, profoundly affecting her daily life and emotional well-being.

Upon consultation, an experienced Ayurvedic practitioner assessed Mrs. Reddy's individual constitution and doshic imbalances, identifying significant Vata and Pitta disturbances affecting her mental functions. The treatment strategy formulated involved specific Marma points known to influence cognitive faculties and emotional health, including Brahmarandhra (the crown of the head) and Sthapani (the forehead).

Each session commenced with gentle stimulation of these Marma points, using therapeutic herbal oils chosen for their properties that support neural activity and calm the mind. Additionally, Sankha (near the temples) and Aja (at the mid-point on the ears) Marma points were activated to further support memory retention and alleviate anxiety.

Structured into twice-weekly sessions spanning 40 minutes, the treatment plan was complemented by dietary recommendations rich in nuts, green leafy vegetables, and berries, which are known for their neuroprotective properties. Also, lifestyle adaptations such as meditative walks in nature and controlled breathing exercises were integrated to enhance overall pranic distribution.

Over several weeks, Mrs. Reddy showed noticeable improvements in memory retrieval and a reduction in confusion. The sessions also fostered a calming effect, stabilizing her mood swings and improving sleep patterns. Her family reported a happier demeanor and increased social interaction, highlighting the profound impact of Marma Chikitsa on not only her cognitive abilities but also her emotional and psychosocial health.

This comprehensive treatment approach of Alzheimer’s through Marma Chikitsa, alongside conventional therapies, underlines the potential for Ayurvedic practices to significantly enhance quality of life, even in neurodegenerative diseases where mainstream medicine often finds limitations.

Case Study: Holistic Management of Menstrual Irregularities through Marma Chikitsa

This case study delves into the detailed account of Ms. Neeta Singh, a 33-year-old software developer, who experienced severe menstrual irregularities and associated symptoms such as pain, fatigue, and emotional distress. Traditional treatments, including hormonal therapies, provided temporary relief but did not address the underlying issues effectively, prompting Ms. Singh to explore alternative forms of healing such as Marma Chikitsa.

An initial Ayurvedic assessment highlighted an imbalance in Neeta's Pitta and Vata doshas, which are crucially linked to reproductive health and overall vitality. The practitioner decided to target specific Marma points known to influence the reproductive system, such as the Shroni and Nabhi Marma, situated around the pelvic area and navel, respectively, to restore harmony and alleviate discomfort.

Each session, which lasted approximately 60 minutes, employed gentle manipulation of these key Marma points using therapeutic herbal oils known for their benefits in regulating hormonal activity and soothing pain. The treatment plan also incorporated lifestyle and dietary recommendations tailored to pacify the aggravated doshas, including the integration of cooling and nourishing foods, as well as stress-reduction techniques such as yoga and meditation.

Over a series of twelve treatments, Ms. Singh noted significant improvement in her menstrual cycle regularity and a substantial decrease in pain. Additionally, positive shifts in her emotional well-being were observed, attributed to the holistic approach of Marma Chikitsa, which not only focused on physical health but also encompassed the mental and spiritual dimensions.

This case exemplifies how Marma Chikitsa can be effectively utilized to manage complex gynecological conditions, such as menstrual irregularities, by addressing both the symptomatic expressions and the root energetic imbalances. It demonstrates the scope of Marma Chikitsa as a viable, non-invasive therapy that enriches the quality of reproductive health and supports overall well-being.

Review Questions

1. A 47-year-old female patient presents with chronic hypertension and seeks alternative treatments to complement her conventional medication regimen. She is introduced to Marma Chikitsa, which targets the Hridaya Marma point located near the heart. What is the primary therapeutic benefit expected from stimulating this Marma point?

A) A) Enhanced digestion
B) B) Increased insulin sensitivity
C) C) Stabilization of blood pressure
D) D) Improvement of respiratory function

Answer: C

Explanation: Stimulating the Hridaya Marma point, located near the heart, primarily helps balance the circulatory rhythm and stabilize blood pressure. This technique is particularly beneficial for patients with hypertension, as it involves gentle pressure and rotational movements, integrated with regulated breathing to optimize cardiovascular efficacy, thereby aiding in blood pressure management.

2. A 65-year-old male with Type 2 Diabetes Mellitus has been recommended Marma Chikitsa to help manage his condition. The practitioner decides to focus on the Meda

Dhatu Marma points. What is the primary effect expected from manipulating these points?
A) A) Decrease in blood sugar levels
B) B) Reduction in prostate enlargement
C) C) Increase in immune function
D) D) Improvement in liver detoxification
Answer: A
Explanation: Manipulation of the Meda Dhatu Marma points, located primarily in the abdomen, focuses on restoring balance to the body's metabolic functions, which are crucial in managing Diabetes Mellitus. These points help in enhancing glucose management by revitalizing the pancreas and liver functions, reducing blood sugar levels, and dependency on external insulin. This intervention targets the core metabolic imbalance contributing to diabetes.

3. During a Marma Chikitsa session aimed at managing autoimmune diseases, a practitioner stimulates specific Marma points on a patient complaining of Systemic Lupus Erythematosus (SLE). Which points are likely targeted to modulate the immune system and reduce symptoms?
A) A) Kshipra Marma on hands and feet
B) B) Hridaya Marma on the chest
C) C) Yakrut Marma on the torso
D) D) Guda Marma around the anal region
Answer: A
Explanation: Kshipra Marma points, located on the hands and feet, are often stimulated in cases of autoimmune diseases to modulate the immune responses. The strategic engagement of these points aims to regulate the immune system's functions, harmonizing vital energy and reducing autoimmune reactions. Thus, enhancing vitality, it helps the body in correctly distinguishing between self and non-self, which is crucial in managing autoimmune conditions like SLE.

4. A patient suffering from chronic kidney disorders seeks Marma Chikitsa as a complementary treatment. The practitioner plans to stimulate specific Marma points focused on renal health. Which Marma points are most appropriate for this purpose?
A) A) Guda and Basti Marma
B) B) Meda Dhatu and Yakrut Marma
C) C) Sthapani and Brahmarandhra Marma
D) D) Nabhi and Hridaya Marma
Answer: A
Explanation: In the treatment of kidney disorders, the Guda and Basti Marma points are specifically targeted. The Basti Marma, located in the lower back, helps to enhance renal circulation and stimulate natural detox processes, crucial for kidney health. The Guda Marma, positioned around the anal region, supports the lower digestive tract, enhancing renal function. Regular therapy on these points can improve symptoms related to kidney issues such as edema and uremia.

5. A client with persistent liver disorders is recommended Marma Chikitsa to facilitate liver detoxification. Which Marma point is primarily focused upon to enhance liver function and bile production?
A) A) Hridaya Marma
B) B) Yakrut Marma
C) C) Indrabasti Marma
D) D) Kshipra Marma

Answer: B
Explanation: The Yakrut Marma, placed on the torso, is particularly significant for liver health. Stimulating the Yakrut Marma harmonizes the liver's energy flow and enhances its functions such as bile production and detoxification processes. The ideal timing for these interventions, such as early morning or late evening, maximizes the body's natural detox capabilities, aiding those with chronic liver ailments to see improvements in their health and energy levels.

CHAPTER EIGHT: Marma Chikitsa for Mental and Emotional Healing

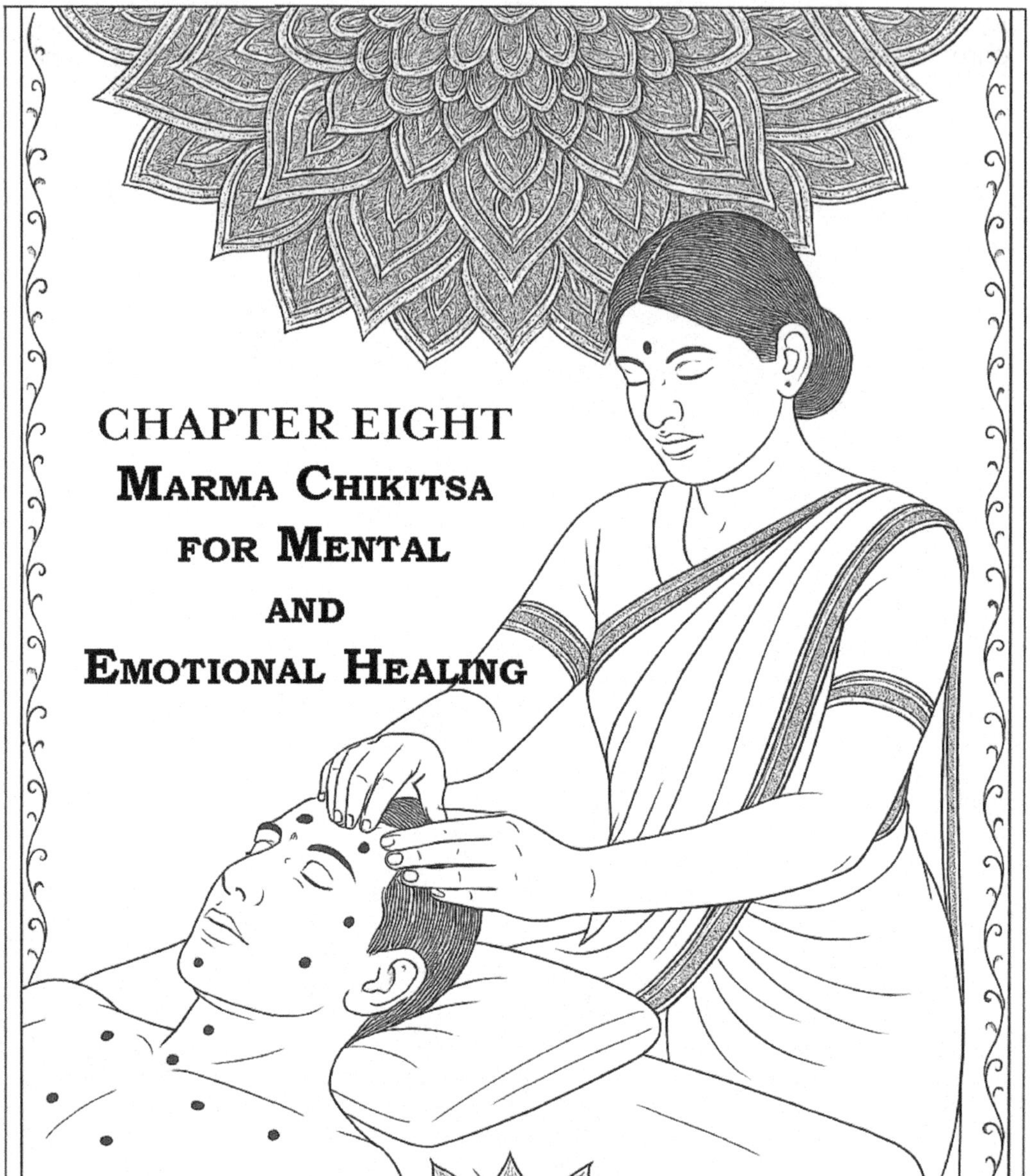

Ayurveda's Concept of the Mind and Manas

In Ayurveda, the mind is conceived as an entity independent yet intimately linked to the physical body, functioning through three fundamental qualities: Sattva, Rajas, and Tamas. These qualities correspond to harmony, activity, and inertia, shaping mental and behavioral tendencies. 'Manas,' often translated as the mind, holds the prerogative of processing sensory and emotional stimuli, determining how we perceive and react to our environments.
Central to Ayurvedic psychology is the understanding that Manas operates through the subtle channels of Prana, the life force, asserting significant influence over both health and disease. It is believed that imbalances in Manas can lead to psychological disturbances, requiring rebalancing through tailored approaches such as Marma Chikitsa. This ancient practice focuses on specific body points that, when stimulated, can directly recalibrate the mind's pranic flow. Marma Chikitsa for mental and emotional healing targets these sensitive points, aiming to restore the equilibrium of Manas. It integrates physical touch with energetic and spiritual healing, designed to treat the mind holistically. This intricate interplay between mind and body underscores the sophisticated nature of Ayurvedic medicine, emphasizing the profound connection and understanding between the two.

Sattva, Rajas, and Tamas – The Three Gunas: Mental Doshas

Classic Ayurveda states that the ego, which manifests at birth, has three principal characteristics, and it has three principal defilements called Gunas. My professors in India referred to them as the three evils. The three egos, three pernicious influences, three defilements. The three distortions of that which was perfect, that which is not perfect anymore. They also referred to them as the three fractures or the three broken aspects.
Deeply embedded within Ayurvedic teachings are the concepts of Sattva, Rajas, and Tamas. Known as the mental doshas, these qualities are not merely traits but dynamic forces that influence cognitive and emotional equilibrium.
Satvas/ Satvic Principle:

Satvas express lightness, essence, understanding, purity, clarity, compassion, and love. It activates the senses and is responsible for the perception of knowledge. If you want to know more about the characteristics or qualities of, for example, the Satvic principle, read and study Brahma. Look at icons, symbols, pictures, and images of Brahma. Explore who Brahma was. What did Brahma do? We also call the Satvic principle the sun, or the solar principle. The sun principle is also vital. Satvas and Tamas are related as two halves of one coin. The principles of composting, degeneration, deterioration, and deconstruction of the Tamasic are not possible without the sun's energy.
Satvas relates to the five motor organs, which we refer to as the organs of action. They are mouth, hands, feet, reproductive organs, and excretory organs. The organs of action are how we implement our consciousness in the real world. It is how we extend and affect the world without being conscious of it. They enable us to eat, reach, run, reproduce, and evacuate. They facilitate what we can take in, let go of, grab, or hold, and throw. These are the tools that consciousness uses to interact with the environment in which we exist.
Interestingly, the mind is also Satvic. The mind is both an organ of action and cognition. The first thing I want you to notice about the mind is that, according to Ayurvedic theory, the mind is not considered special. It is no different than the excretory organs. Sometimes the mind acts as an excretory organ. The mind is not very different than any of the other organs of action and

cognition.
It is not special, it is not superior, and there is no place in Ayurveda where it states that the mind of the brain is in charge. Its function is like that of all the other organs of cognition or action. It serves either as an interface to take in information or to direct external action. However, it is not necessarily where consciousness resides. Consciousness is not contained or in or constrained to your brain. We now have science that supports this understanding.
Sattva typifies purity, knowledge, and harmony, fostering peace and spiritual growth. It influences individuals towards ethical and compassionate behavior and is intensified by practices that cultivate calm and clarity.
Conversely, Rajas represents activity and movement. It is fueled by desires and can lead to restlessness and impulsiveness if uncontrolled. This quality is necessary for action and change, yet its excess can disrupt mental calmness. Managing Rajas involves balancing routine and stimulation to maintain a compelling dynamism without overwhelm.
Tamas is inertia, often manifesting as resistance or heaviness in the psyche. This quality, while essential for rest, can become predominant and induce lethargy and apathy. Overcoming excessive Tamas requires engaging in stimulating activities that awaken and invigorate the mind, ensuring it does not stagnate but remains rejuvenated for constructive engagement.

The Rajasic quality is a kinetic protective force. It is the active and vital life force (Prana) which drives or directs both the organic and inorganic realms to satvas and tamas. It represents movement, action, stimulation, and the vital life force. It can also simply aggressiveness and extroversion. Rajas is the most active of the gunas. All desires, wishes, ambitions, and imaginations are influenced here.
The five sense faculties, which we call organs of cognition, are the ears, skin, eyes, tongue, and nose. Cognition is "the mental action or process of acquiring knowledge and understanding through thought, experience, and the senses." Cognition is the process we are engaged in; we take in information from our environment, make note of it, and then compare that information with our experiences and memories. Our sense faculties serve as the interface between external reality and internal reality. Without these, we are just a ball of goo as far as our understanding of the world. The body parts, the ears, skin, eyes, tongue, and nose represent Satvic qualities, and in balances that relate to these body parts, they are particularly Satvic. How do I know that? Because that is what is on the chart. That is the traditional listed correlation.
Tamas is characterized by ignorance, inertia, heaviness, and resistance. It produces disturbances in the perception process and mental activities. Delusion, false knowledge, laziness, apathy, sleepiness, and drowsiness are all symptoms of it.
Tamas has the equivalent of Tanmatras. They are called Bhutas: sound, touch, sight, taste, and smell. Sound is the Guna of the Ether element (Akash). Touch is the Guna of the Air Element (Vyo). Sight is the Guna of Fire element (Teho). Taste is the Guna of Water element (Apo). Smell is the Guna of the Earth element (Patavi/ Prythvi), depending on how you say it. Ether, Air, Fire, Water, and Earth, of course, are the principal elements of Ayurveda.
Notice that before the five elements, we have the senses of sound, touch, sight, taste, and smell. The way that we interact with the five elements of the Classical Indian Ayurveda elements, or the "*Thaat Thang Sii*" which are the four Thai Ayurveda elements, is through our senses.

Stress and Anxiety Management Using Marma

Marma Chikitsa offers a transformative approach to managing stress and anxiety, deeply rooted in Ayurvedic wisdom. This technique focuses on the body's vital energy points, or Marma points, which, when stimulated, can significantly alleviate mental strain and emotional unrest.
One potent point for addressing stress is the 'Manipuraka', located in the solar plexus region. Manipulation of this Marma helps in regulating the flow of energy associated with the fire element, which governs digestion and personal power. The calming of this center can lead to a subdued response to stressors, promoting a state of balance and inner peace. Alongside the 'Anahata', or heart Marma, is targeted to release pent-up emotions, enhancing emotional resilience, and providing relief from anxiety.
Additional techniques include the use of aromatic oils, which enhance the efficacy of Marma manipulation. These, combined with breathing exercises, create an integrated healing experience that not only reduces symptoms but also addresses the root causes of stress and anxiety, fostering long-lasting well-being.

PTSD and Trauma Healing Through Energetic Touch

Marma Chikitsa harnesses the power of energetic touch to facilitate profound healing in individuals suffering from PTSD and trauma. By meticulously stimulating specific Marma points, this therapy aims to release psychological blockages rooted in traumatic experiences. These points, when gently pressed, activate the body's innate healing mechanisms, encouraging a flow of prana that can cleanse and revitalize the mental and emotional bodies.
This focused manipulation is particularly centered on the Hridaya, or the heart Marma, known for its capacity to unburden the heart of emotional weight. The subsequent release helps reduce fear and establish a sense of security and trust, which are fundamental to trauma recovery. Additionally, the Adhipati Marma, located at the crown of the head, is targeted to calm the mind and restore mental clarity, an essential aspect of healing the remnants of psychic disturbances. Throughout the session, the practitioner may incorporate soothing essential oils, such as lavender or sandalwood, which significantly amplify the calming effect, thereby fostering a nurturing environment for emotional recovery. This integrative approach not only heals physical manifestations of trauma but also reestablishes mental peace and emotional resilience.

Depression: Pranic Rebalancing and Activation Points

In the realm of Marma Chikitsa, treating depression transcends conventional methods, focusing instead on pranic rebalancing through specific activation points. These points, pivotal in Ayurvedic therapy, are believed to directly influence the flow of prana, the vital life force, equilibrating the energies that govern emotional states.
The Prana Vayu, located in the chest region, is crucial for psychological balance. Stimulating this Marma point helps alleviate the heaviness of depression by enhancing upward and outward movement of energy, promoting feelings of lightness and clarity. Similarly, the Manas Marma, located at the crown of the head, plays a crucial role in clearing mental fog and emotional turmoil. Activation of this point is often paired with mindfulness techniques to intensify its therapeutic effects.
Additionally, the Anandabhairava Marma, found around the heart area, is targeted to release

emotional blockages, fostering an inner sense of joy and vitality. Through gentle pressure and circular motions, this point catalyzes the release of serenity-inducing prana, gradually restoring emotional equilibrium and mitigating depressive symptoms.

Emotional Detox with Sthapani, Apanga, and Hridaya

Marma Chikitsa, in its approach to emotional detoxification, focuses on rejuvenating the mind and spirit by harnessing the therapeutic powers of the Sthapani, Apanga, and Hridaya Marma points. These points are central to releasing emotional toxins that may have stagnated in the mental and emotional layers of the body. The Sthapani, located in the center of the forehead, directly influences the pineal gland, which is crucial for emotional regulation. Stimulating this Marma can help clear mental clutter and foster emotional clarity.

Moreover, the Apanga point, located at the outer corners of the eyes, plays a significant role in processing emotional experiences. Gentle stimulation of Apanga can alleviate emotional strain, soothing the eyes, which often bear the weight of emotional stress. This practice encourages a softening of the gaze, which can lead to a broader perspective on life's challenges.

Then there is the Hridaya, the heart Marma, essential for emotional release and detox. Engaging with this point invites profound shifts in heart energy, potentially releasing deep-seated emotions such as guilt, sadness, and fear. Through this detox, one experiences a heart unburdened by old emotional pains but invigorated with renewed passion and joy.

Cognitive Decline: Preventive Marma Practices

As aging progresses, concerns regarding cognitive decline often arise – a concern aptly addressed through Marma Chikitsa's preventive strategies. This ancient practice enriches neural health by stimulating specific Marma points, believed to enhance memory and cognitive functions. Ayurveda identifies points such as Brahmarandhra and Ajna, located on the head, as pivotal in maintaining neural agility. Gentle stimulation of these sites can boost cerebral circulation and facilitate mental clarity.

Additionally, the practice incorporates dietary recommendations and herbal remedies that support cognitive health. Ingredients like Brahmi, known for their neuroprotective properties, are often prescribed. These natural supplements, when combined with targeted Marma therapy, form a holistic regimen to combat cognitive decline.

Moreover, lifestyle adjustments play a crucial role. Regular practice of Marma, combined with adequate sleep, meditation, and mentally stimulating activities, forms a comprehensive approach. Thus, Marma Chikitsa not only preserves cognitive functions but also enhances overall mental resilience and vitality, laying a foundation for a mentally enriched aging process.

Enhancing Memory and Focus Through Avarta and Adhipati

The ancient wisdom of Marma Chikitsa encompasses techniques not only for physical healing but also for cognitive enhancement and mental well-being. Central to this is the stimulation of the Avarta and Adhipati marma points, which are vital energy centers directly linked to memory and concentration. The Avarta, located just above the eyebrows, serves as a gateway to clearer thinking and focus. Manipulation of this point can dissolve mental clutter, empowering sharper

cognition and alertness.
The Adhipati, located at the crown of the head, is considered the supreme center influencing cerebral functions. Stimulating this Marma harmonizes the mental faculties, recharging the brain's capability to process information and retain knowledge. This stimulation is believed to facilitate a deeper connection between the mind, body, and spirit, thereby enhancing neural pathways that are essential for memory retention and focus.
Together, these Marma points form a dynamic duo in Ayurvedic therapy. Regular stimulation can lead to improved cognitive functions, aiding in the battle against memory lapses and concentration issues, and fostering a vibrant, alert state of mind.

Panic Attacks: First-Response Marma Points

Panic attacks, those sudden surges of overwhelming anxiety and fear, can be intensely destabilizing. Marma Chikitsa offers a beacon of relief through the strategic activation of first-response Marma points. These select points, known for their ability to quickly reduce panic symptoms, can be gently stimulated to pacify the racing mind and restore a sense of control. Prominently, the Adhipati Marma, located at the crown of the head, plays a crucial role. Its stimulation helps in calming the storm of thoughts, ushering in clarity and peace. Another vital point is Hridaya, situated at the heart. This Marma point is central in soothing rapid heartbeats, a common manifestation during panic attacks, fostering tranquility in its stead.
Additionally, the Gandhara Marma, located in the throat area, encourages smoother breathing and helps alleviate the choking sensation often associated with panic attacks. By integrating these practices promptly in response to panic symptoms, individuals can experience an immediate easing of their distress, effectively grounding themselves back in a calmer state.

Anger and Irritability Release via Urvi and Kurpara

Marma Chikitsa, revered for its profound healing capabilities, extends its therapeutic reach to alleviating anger and irritability through the targeted activation of the Urvi and Kurpara Marma points. These unique points, strategically situated on the arms and elbows respectively, serve as vital conduits for regulating the fiery energy associated with anger. Gentle stimulation of the Urvi Marma helps balance the intricate energy flow, soothes intense emotions of anger, and brings about a state of calm and centeredness.
Additionally, the Kurpara, located at the elbow, when activated, influences the body's ability to release tension and frustration, which are common precursors to irritability. The application of precise pressure and rotational movements on this point can significantly diminish irritability, fostering a more composed and balanced emotional state.
By integrating these practices into regular wellness routines, individuals can achieve a more harmonious balance of emotions. This leads not only to personal well-being but also to improved interpersonal relationships, enhancing overall quality of life and interaction.

Grief and Loss: Supportive Heart-Centered Marma

Marma Chikitsa offers compassionate relief to those grappling with grief and loss by nurturing the heart-centered Hridaya Marma point. Situated at the core of the chest, this vital energy center serves as a conduit for emotional healing, particularly the deep-seated shadows cast by loss. Gentle stimulation of Hridaya promotes an emotional release, allowing for a ripple of relief to spread across the heart's energetic field, facilitating the transition from sorrow to acceptance with greater ease.

This practice not only alleviates symptoms but also seeks to restore the emotional equilibrium disrupted by grief. The activation of Hridaya invites a reconnection to emotional resilience, helping individuals rediscover their inner strength amidst vulnerability. It is a profound journey back to wholesomeness through the tender touch of Ayurvedic wisdom.

Furthermore, associated rituals and meditative practices enhance this healing, advocating a holistic approach. Regular engagement with these Marma points nurtures a sustained healing, embedding a sense of peace and emotional clarity that shields against future emotional turmoil.

Guilt and Shame: Energy Clearing Via Urah and Basti

Marma Chikitsa unveils profound strategies for addressing deep-seated emotions, such as guilt and shame, by focusing on the Urah and Basti Marma points. These points, located around the chest and lower back respectively, are crucial in the energetic processing of emotional wounds. Gentle manipulation of Urah helps unblock the heart's energy, releasing pent-up feelings of guilt and fostering self-forgiveness. This action rekindles the vital pranic flow, crucial for emotional detoxification.

Furthermore, Basti's stimulation helps dispel the debilitating energy of shame, reinforcing the individual's sense of grounding and personal strength. This specific point works by releasing stored negative energies in the lower spine, which often correlate with feelings of unworthiness and humiliation.

Integrating these Marma practices provides a dual approach to healing, ensuring a comprehensive emotional cleanse. Implemented regularly, these techniques not only alleviate guilt and shame but also enhance emotional resilience, thereby contributing to overall mental and emotional well-being.

Inner Child Healing Through Specific Marma Sequences

Marma Chikitsa opens a unique pathway to healing the inner child, a concept that addresses unresolved childhood emotions that often persist into adulthood. Through specific Marma sequences, practitioners seek to release these dormant emotional blockages, facilitating a journey toward emotional maturity and healing.

Key Marma points, such as Anahata and Manipura, are targeted to awaken and soothe the inner child. Anahata, located at the heart, is gently stimulated to open the emotional heart space, allowing the release of suppressed feelings such as sadness or fear. Manipura, located at the solar plexus, is activated to instill feelings of personal power and resilience, which are essential for self-acceptance and growth.

This therapeutic approach combines gentle touches and mindful awareness, guiding individuals through a reconnection with their younger selves. By nurturing the inner child, Marma Chikitsa facilitates profound healing from past traumas, thereby enhancing emotional freedom and overall well-being.

Regular practice reinforces emotional resilience, equipping individuals to handle future stresses more effectively and contributing to a balanced and harmonious life.

Self-Worth and Confidence Marma Protocols

In the realm of Marma Chikitsa, enhancing self-worth and confidence can significantly shift an individual's interface with the world. The selected Marma points, such as Brahmarandhra and Manipura, are pivotal in energizing and grounding one's self-esteem. Gently stimulating the Brahmarandhra, located at the crown, invigorates the body's spiritual gateway, fostering a connection with one's higher self and clarifying personal purpose and values.

Manipura, the solar plexus Marma, is another critical point for enhancing self-assurance. Positioned at the core of the torso, its activation strengthens inner resolve and power, radiating outward confidence. Techniques involve precise, rhythmic pressure that stimulates emotional and energetic rebirth, cleansing doubts and insecurities.

Additionally, engaging the Anahata, or heart Marma, aligns emotional energies, promoting feelings of love and self-acceptance. Regular practice of these protocols fortifies a positive self-image and robust confidence, essentials for a fulfilling life.

Addiction Recovery Support: Marma and Detox Points

Marma Chikitsa offers transformative support for addiction recovery by harnessing specific Marma and detox points to restore the body's natural equilibrium. These points act as gateways to more profound healing, directly influencing the subtle energy pathways that govern emotional and physical dependencies. Activation of vital points such as the Mooladhara chakra at the base of the spine helps stabilize foundational energies, providing a sense of grounding necessary in early recovery stages.

Further, the stimulation of Manas Marma, located on the head, addresses the mental cravings and psychological aftermath of addiction. This crucial point promotes clarity and neurological balance, easing the transition from dependency to sobriety. Regular manipulation of these Marma points detoxifies the body, clears the mind, and lifts the spirits, aligning the addict along a path of holistic health and emotional resilience.

Alongside these treatments, supportive lifestyle adjustments and Ayurvedic dietary recommendations reinforce the body's ability to heal and detoxify. This comprehensive approach empowers individuals, fostering not only recovery but also a sustained state of wellness and vitality.

Bipolar Symptoms and Energy Rebalancing

Marma Chikitsa addresses the complex emotional oscillations associated with bipolar disorder through targeted energy rebalancing. By focusing on critical Marma points like Manas and Ajna, practitioners aim to stabilize mood swings and promote mental clarity. The Manipura point, pivotal in enhancing personal power and emotional steadiness, is also crucial in managing bipolar symptoms.

The activation of Manas, located at the crown of the head, directly influences neurological harmony, reducing episodes of extreme highs and lows. This is complemented by Ajna, the third-eye point, which is instrumental in fostering emotional insight and self-awareness, essential for recognizing and managing personal triggers.
Furthermore, regular stimulation of the Surya and Chandra Marma, which represent solar and lunar energies, helps achieve emotional equilibrium, a vital aspect in managing bipolar disorder. These practices, combined with structured lifestyle routines, significantly aid in reducing the intensity and frequency of bipolar episodes, setting a foundation for sustained mental health and well-being.

Autism and Sensory Regulation via Marma

In Marma Chikitsa, addressing sensory regulation in individuals with autism involves a nuanced application of specific Marma points to harmonize sensory inputs and soothe the nervous system. This practice focuses on enhancing the sensory processing capacities that are often disrupted in autism, creating a more balanced internal environment.
Key Marma points such as Talahridaya and Gandhara are considered pivotal for their roles in calming overstimulated senses and fostering a sense of emotional security. Stimulation of Talahridaya, located on the palms, directly impacts hand sensitivity—a common issue in autism—thereby moderating the response to tactile stimuli. Gandhara, located near the throat, is gently activated to aid in verbal expression and communication, areas that are frequently challenging for individuals on the autism spectrum.
These techniques not only soothe and realign disrupted energies but also promote overall well-being, making daily interactions more manageable. Regular practice is recommended to achieve optimal sensory integration and emotional tranquility, which are crucial for enhancing the quality of life in individuals with autism.

Schizophrenia: Subtle Energy Point Modulation

Marma Chikitsa provides a profound approach for managing schizophrenia through subtle energy point modulation, a practice that helps restore mental balance and clarity. Important Marma points, such as Brahmarandhra and Ajna, are emphasized for their capacity to influence cognitive functions and emotional regulation. Activation of Brahmarandhra, located at the crown of the head, aims to clear mental fog and confusion often encountered in schizophrenia. Additionally, the Ajna point, or the third eye, facilitates insight and awareness, critical for those experiencing schizophrenic symptoms. This point's stimulation supports a deeper connection to one's inner thoughts and a better understanding of external realities, which are often obscured by the condition.
Holistic integration of these treatments with traditional therapies can enhance outcomes, providing a comforting, non-invasive supplement to conventional care. Regular Marma therapy sessions are recommended to maintain mental stability and nurture a calmer, more balanced emotional state.

Social Withdrawal and Isolation Relief

Marma Chikitsa's approach to alleviating social withdrawal and isolation involves a compassionate application of Marma points to re-establish connection and emotional openness. Vital points, such as Anahata (the heart center) and Ajna (the third eye), play a pivotal role in this healing. Activation of Anahata promotes an outpouring of empathy and self-compassion, vital for overcoming feelings of loneliness and detachment. Simultaneously, stimulation of Ajna enhances self-awareness and understanding, key components in navigating social interactions more effectively.

Furthermore, the manipulation of connected Marma points like Indrabasti and Shankha, located around the neck and shoulders, specifically addresses the physical manifestations of social reluctance, such as a closed posture or a downtrodden gaze. By relieving these tensions, Marma Chikitsa opens the physical gateway to improved interaction, inviting a sense of belonging and community engagement.

These Marma practices are supplemented by guided meditations focusing on social connectivity, fostering a sense of unity with the surrounding world. Regular sessions encourage sustained emotional recovery and reintegration into social settings, paving the way for enriched interactions and a more vibrant community life.

Sleep Disorders and Nervous System Calming

Marma Chikitsa provides a serene approach to managing sleep disorders, addressing both the symptoms and the underlying energy imbalances that exacerbate them. Central to this practice are Marma points, which are known to influence sleep patterns and calm the nervous system, such as Anja (located between the eyebrows) and Sthapani (at the center of the forehead). The gentle stimulation of these points helps regulate the pineal gland, which produces melatonin, a crucial hormone for maintaining healthy sleep cycles.

Additionally, calming the Vata dosha, often responsible for disturbances in sleep, involves focusing on calming points along the spine and the base of the skull. These areas, rich in nerve endings, directly affect the central nervous system's ability to relax and enter a state conducive to deep, restorative sleep.

By incorporating these specialized Marma treatments with herbal remedies and Ayurvedic nutrition, practitioners work to create a holistic environment that nurtures the body's natural tendency toward balance and rest, promoting a peaceful night's sleep and a rejuvenated waking state.

Breath-Based Emotional Reset

Marma Chikitsa's breath-based emotional reset harnesses the power of controlled breathing to realign the body's pranic energy, offering profound relief for emotional distress. This practice focuses on specific breathing techniques, coupled with gentle activation of Marma points, such as Anahata (the heart center) and Vishuddha (the throat chakra), which are pivotal in managing emotional flows and facilitating emotional release.

By guiding the breath consciously through these points, a practitioner can help stabilize fluctuating emotions, clear the mental clutter, and soothe the spirit. This process not only detoxifies the mind but also enhances mental clarity and emotional resilience. The rhythmic nature of breathwork, integrated with Marma therapy, instills a deep sense of peace and groundedness, which is crucial for emotional recovery.

Regularly incorporating these techniques can transform acute emotional episodes into opportunities for growth and self-awareness. This therapeutic approach promotes a recalibrated emotional state, enabling individuals to resume their daily activities with renewed vigor and a more optimistic outlook.

Sound and Music for Mood Regulation

The therapeutic use of sound and music in Marma Chikitsa offers a unique conduit for mood regulation and emotional balance. Harnessing the vibrational properties of sound, practitioners implement specific tones and rhythms to resonate with Marma points, facilitating the harmonization of mind and body energies. This approach is rooted in the ancient understanding that sound frequencies can directly influence the body's energetic fields, promoting emotional release and stability.

Particularly, classical ragas and instrumental sounds are chosen for their frequencies, which align with the energetic vibrations of emotional centers in the body. For example, calming music might be used to gently stimulate the Hridaya Marma point at the heart, soothing feelings of anxiety and fostering a sense of peace. Conversely, stimulating beats might target the Adhipati Marma on the crown to uplift and energize mood during moments of depression.

Incorporating sound therapy into Marma Chikitsa not only augments the physical manipulation of energy points but also enhances the overall therapeutic experience, allowing for a deeper emotional healing process. Such integration invites a restoration of balance, ultimately contributing to a more vibrant and regulated emotional state.

Visualization Techniques in Marma Mental Health

Visualization techniques in Marma Chikitsa provide a transformative approach to mental health, integrating vivid imagery with the body's energetic pathways. Such practices involve patients visualizing healing energies flowing through Marma points, promoting mental clarity and emotional stability.

In practice, visualizing light or energy moving from the Hridaya point in the chest to the Ajna, or third eye, can help alleviate feelings of anxiety and depression. This visualization supports the flow of pranic energy to areas burdened by mental stress, facilitating a natural healing process of the mind as the mind engages with these positive images, a synchronization of thought and energy occurs, thereby enhancing emotional resilience.

Moreover, visualization can be tailored to individual needs, addressing specific mental health issues such as fear, insomnia, or persistent negative thoughts. Guided sessions foster the development of beneficial mental habits and enhance self-perception, which are essential for overcoming psychological barriers. The continued application of these techniques aims to promote a lasting, balanced state of mental well-being.

Affirmation with Touch: Integration Strategy

In the holistic landscape of Marma Chikitsa, the technique of 'Affirmation with Touch' merges physical touch with mental reinforcement, targeting both psychological and energetic layers of healing. This nuanced method harnesses the power of affirmations — positive, structured statements — while simultaneously applying gentle pressure to specific Marma points. This dual action facilitates a deeper integration of healing and grounding affirmations into the consciousness.
Touch, an elemental human experience, is amplified by the strategic localization and stimulation of Marma points. For example, when affirming emotional resilience, simultaneous manipulation of the Hridaya (heart) Marma may enhance feelings of courage and inner strength. The tactile aspect not only supports the embedding of positive mental narratives but also catalyzes a more potent and immediate physiological response, reinforcing the therapeutic effects.
Each session is tailored to reflect the individual's unique emotional and mental health needs through personalized affirmations. This person-centric approach ensures that the affirmations resonate personally, maximizing the therapeutic potential of each interaction and promoting long-term mental health and emotional balance.

Summary

Chapter 7 of the book explores Marma Chikitsa, an Ayurvedic therapeutic technique intended for mental and emotional healing. Starting with the understanding of the mind in Ayurveda, governed by the qualities Sattva, Rajas, and Tamas, the chapter details how these qualities influence psychological processes and behaviors. Manas (mind) in Ayurveda is crucial as it processes sensory and emotional stimuli, which in turn affect both health and disease. Marma Chikitsa focuses on specific body points that help recalibrate the mind's pranic flow when stimulated, offering solutions for dealing with stress, anxiety, PTSD, depression, and more. Techniques such as stimulating points like the Manipuraka and Anahata Marma are highlighted for managing stress and alleviating emotional distress. Marma Chikitsa is portrayed not just as a physical interaction with the body's Marma points but also incorporates spiritual and energetic healing dimensions, aiming at a holistic treatment approach. This is further exemplified in how it addresses PTSD by easing symptoms and the underlying psychological causes through energetic touch. Marma Chikitsa also extends its benefits to cognitive functions, particularly aiding in memory enhancement and focus by stimulating points such as Avarta and Adhipati Marma. It also shows remarkable efficacy in assisting patients with psychological conditions such as bipolar disorder and schizophrenia by helping stabilize mood and clear mental fog. Moreover, the chapter outlines the effectiveness of Marma Chikitsa in addiction recovery and managing sensory irregularities in autism. Incorporated treatments are not confined to touch but integrate aromatherapy, sound therapy, and visualization techniques to amplify the healing process. In summary, this chapter provides a comprehensive insight into how Marma Chikitsa serves as an integral component of Ayurveda in promoting mental health, emotional balance, and cognitive vitality.

References

[1] Kulkarni, P.H., & Kaushik, J.S. (2012). Marma Therapy for Stress Management. Journal of Ayurveda and Integrative Medicine. https://www.jaim.in/article.asp?issn=0975-9476;year=2012;volume=3;issue=4;spage=192;epage=198;aulast=Kulkarni

[2] Rath, C.C. (2014). Understanding Ayurvedic Prana Management for Mental Health. AyuJournal. https://www.ayujournal.org/text.asp?2014/35/2/123/146974

[3] Tripathi, B. (2010). Marma Science and Principles of Marma Therapy. Journal of Ayurveda and Holistic Medicine. http://www.jahm.in/index.php/JAHM/article/view/102

Case Study: Holistic Approach to Managing Chronic Stress with Marma Chikitsa

Emma, a 38-year-old marketing director, experienced chronic stress due to the high demands of her job and balancing her family life. She often reported a significant decline in her physical health, emotional stability, and cognitive sharpness, feeling overwhelmed with anxiety and frequent tension headaches. These symptoms not only affected her work performance but also her interpersonal relationships and self-esteem. Emma sought an alternative approach after conventional stress management strategies provided only transient relief.

Upon consulting with an Ayurvedic practitioner, Emma was introduced to Marma Chikitsa, a traditional Indian therapy that focuses on the body's vital energy points to heal and balance life energies. The practitioner explained that this technique could address her stress holistically, harmonizing her bodily energies troubled by the excessive Rajas (activity) and fostering the Sattva (harmony) for mental clarity and peace.

Her treatment sessions included the precise stimulation of several key Marma points: Anahata (heart), Manipura (solar plexus), and Sthapani (forehead), which are primary centers affected by stress. Each session began with gentle stimulation of these points combined with specific aromatic oils to calm her nervous system. The practitioner also advised Emma on dietary changes and incorporated breathing exercises to complement the Marma therapy, enhancing overall effectiveness.

Over several weeks, Emma noticed a significant improvement in her symptoms. The subtle yet profound activation of Marma points helped reduce her anxiety levels and improve her emotional responses to stress. Sessions focusing on the Manipura Marma helped boost her confidence and personal empowerment, which are crucial in navigating her demanding job.

This case exemplifies how Marma Chikitsa offers a comprehensive approach to stress management, addressing not only symptoms but also identifying and rectifying underlying imbalances in the body's energy channels. Those seeking alternatives to conventional methods may find in Marma Chikitsa a pathway to sustained mental, emotional, and physical health.

Case Study: Revitalizing Emotional Balance in PTSD Recovery with Ayurvedic Marma Therapy

John, a 45-year-old veteran, struggled significantly with post-traumatic stress disorder (PTSD) since returning from military service. His symptoms included severe anxiety, flashbacks, social withdrawal, and insomnia, which profoundly impacted his daily functioning and quality of life. Traditional treatments such as medication and cognitive-behavioral therapy provided some relief, but John still felt disconnected and continually battled with emotional numbness and frequent mood swings.

Seeking a more integrative approach to his condition, John turned to Marma Chikitsa, drawn by its emphasis on restoring mental and emotional health through balancing the body's energy. During his initial consultation, the practitioner highlighted how PTSD disrupts the flow of Prana (life energy) through the body's subtle channels and that Marma therapy could help in recalibrating his emotional and energy pathways, thus aiding in healing trauma.

His treatment involved stimulation of specific Marma points known to affect emotional and psychological health, such as the Hridaya (heart), Anahata (associated with emotional balance), and Manas (mind) points. Careful and mindful stimulation of these points aimed to release blocked energy and facilitate a smoother flow of Prana, which is often stagnated in individuals suffering from trauma. The practitioner also incorporated aromatic oils known for their calming properties, such as lavender and chamomile, which are believed to enhance the therapeutic effects.

Over several months of consistent therapy, John reported meaningful improvements. He noticed a decrease in his anxiety and flashbacks, a better quality of sleep, and a gradual return to social activities. The sessions dedicated to the Hridaya and Anahata Marma points were particularly transformative, alleviating his emotional numbness and helping him reconnect with his feelings and loved ones.

John's case is a prime example of how Marma Chikitsa, as a complementary therapy, can be pivotal in managing and recovering from PTSD. It illustrates the potential of Ayurvedic practices in addressing not just the symptoms, but the energetic disruptions caused by traumatic experiences, facilitating holistic healing and emotional resilience.

Case Study: Comprehensive Marma Therapy for Anxiety and Depression in a High-Performance Professional

Sara, a 32-year-old software engineer, found herself grappling with escalating symptoms of anxiety and depression, which began to compromise her work performance and personal relationships. Despite her successful career, Sara experienced frequent episodes of overwhelming fear and a persistent sense of hopelessness that made day-to-day functions daunting. Traditional psychotherapy and medication offered some relief, but they did not fully address the root causes of her emotional disturbances, leading Sara to explore alternative treatments.

At the recommendation of a colleague, Sara consulted an Ayurvedic practitioner specializing in Marma Chikitsa. During her initial assessment, the practitioner identified imbalances in Sara's Prana Vayu (vital energy), which were thought to contribute to her mental health issues. The practitioner explained that these imbalances could be addressed through targeted stimulation of specific Marma points associated with emotional regulation—namely, Manas (for mental clarity), Hridaya (for emotional balance), and Sthapani (for spiritual insight).

Her treatment regimen was designed not only to handle the symptoms but also restore her overall mental well-being. Each session involved precise stimulation of these points, combined with the application of herbal oils tailored to induce relaxation and improve mood. Additionally, the practitioner integrated a holistic lifestyle approach that included dietary modifications, yoga, and meditation to enhance the efficacy of the treatments.

Over the course of several months, Sara reported noticeable improvements. Her anxiety episodes became less frequent and intense, and her depressive moods started to lift, allowing her clearer thinking and better emotional resilience. The sessions focusing on the Hridaya Marma were particularly effective in fostering a renewed sense of emotional connection and well-being. Through regular Marma therapy and lifestyle adjustments, Sara regained a balanced state of mind, illustrating the potential of Marma Chikitsa to provide deep, transformative healing for those dealing with complex mental health challenges.

Case Study: Integrative Marma Therapy for Enhancing Corporate Leadership Skills and Mental Resilience

Michael, a 50-year-old corporate executive at a leading tech firm, was facing challenges in maintaining his leadership effectiveness amidst rapidly evolving market conditions and high team turnover. His role required constant innovation and emotional intelligence to keep his team aligned and motivated. However, Michael had been having trouble in decision-making, reduced creativity, and symptoms of emotional burnout. Seeking an alternative approach to conventional leadership coaching, he turned to Marma Chikitsa to explore holistic enhancements to his professional skills and personal well-being.

Michael initially consulted with an experienced Ayurvedic practitioner who specialized in Marma therapy for professional and cognitive enhancement. The practitioner explained how Marma points could be stimulated to optimize his mental sharpness and emotional resilience, crucial traits for effective leadership. The therapy sessions targeted specific Marma points, such as the Brahmarandhra and Ajna to enhance cognitive function, and the Manipura to boost confidence and personal power.

Each session involved the gentle stimulation of these points, combined with the application of invigorating aromatic oils such as peppermint and rosemary, which are known for their uplifting and mental clarity properties. The practitioner also advised Michael on nutritional strategies to sustain high energy levels and focus during long work hours. The integration of these treatments was designed to holistically improve Michael's leadership by enhancing his intuitive decision-making and stabilizing his emotional responses.

Over several weeks, Michael noted significant improvements in his mental clarity, ability to manage stress, and communication more effectively. His creative solutions to problems reflected a renewed vigor. Subsequent reflections with his team indicated higher motivation and better collaborative energy, critical indicators of improved leadership. These results highlighted how Marma Chikitsa can be strategically used to enhance professional capabilities, thereby supporting career advancement and personal growth in highly demanding roles.

Case Study: Resolving Chronic Insomnia and Enhancing Sleep Quality through Marma Chikitsa

Linda, a 43-year-old schoolteacher, had been battling chronic insomnia for over five years. Despite trying various medications and behavioral therapies, the issue persisted, significantly affecting her daily functioning and overall quality of life. Her inability to sleep was accompanied by anxiety, stress, and fatigue, making her unable to concentrate during work hours and irritable at home. Recognizing the limitations of her current treatment methods, Linda sought a more integrative and holistic approach to address her sleep disturbances.

Linda's therapy began with an in-depth consultation with an Ayurvedic practitioner who specialized in Marma Chikitsa. The practitioner assessed Linda's overall health, lifestyle, and the nature of her sleep problems. Based on the initial assessment, it became evident that Linda's Vata dosha was deranged, leading to an imbalance that primarily manifests as restlessness and sleep disruption. The practitioner explained that Marma Chikitsa could offer a profound recalibration of her body's energy system, specifically targeting points that influence the nervous system and sleep-wake cycle.

During the therapy sessions, specific Marma points related to calming the mind and inducing sleep were activated, namely Anja (located between the eyebrows) and Sthapani (on the forehead). Gentle pressure was applied to these points using soothing oils, such as jasmine and lavender, which are known for their sedative properties. Linda was also guided through a series of breathing exercises designed to reduce mental chatter and prepare the body for sleep.

Simultaneously, lifestyle modifications were introduced, including dietary adjustments and a pre-sleep routine that included herbal teas and warm baths to decrease Vata's cold and erratic nature. Over the weeks, Linda reported a noticeable improvement in her ability to fall asleep and the quality of her sleep. She experienced fewer awakenings and felt more refreshed and energized during the day. This case highlights the efficacy of Marma Chikitsa in treating sleep disorders, such as insomnia, by addressing both the symptoms and the underlying energy imbalances, demonstrating its value as a valuable alternative to conventional sleep therapies.

Case Study: Navigating Menopause Transition with Marma Chikitsa

Claire, a 52-year-old executive at a tech startup, began experiencing severe menopausal symptoms, including hot flashes, night sweats, mood swings, and a noticeable decline in her memory and concentration abilities. These symptoms began to affect her performance at work and her overall quality of life. Traditional hormone replacement therapy offered some relief, but Claire was concerned about the long-term effects and sought a holistic approach to manage her symptoms.

Upon consulting with an Ayurvedic practitioner, Claire was introduced to Marma Chikitsa, a therapeutic approach that focuses on vital energy points in the body to restore balance and health. The practitioner explained how hormonal fluctuations during menopause could disrupt Claire's natural energy balance, particularly affecting her Prana Vayu (responsible for vital life energy), Sadhaka Pitta (governing intellect and emotions), and Avalambaka Kapha (supporting stability and lubrication). Marma Chikitsa could target specific energy points to stabilize these fluctuations and ease her symptoms.

Her treatment sessions were structured around stimulating Marma points, such as Brahmarandhra and Manas (both located on the head for mental clarity and emotional stability), Gandhara (on the throat for hormonal balance), and Hridaya (the heart Marma for emotional health). Each session included gentle pressure over these points using herbal oils such as Brahmi for cognitive function and cooling oils like Sandalwood to counter hot flashes. Noticeable relief from mood fluctuations and mental issues was a crucial target in Claire's ongoing sessions.

Over time, Claire found significant relief from her symptoms. The customized holistic approach of Marma Chikitsa not only alleviated the physiological symptoms but also improved her emotional resilience. This integrative treatment helped her maintain her executive responsibilities with greater ease and higher functioning, revealing the potent potential of Marma therapy in managing menopause holistically.

Case Study: Transformative Emotional Healing Through Marma Chikitsa in a Bereaved Individual

Isabella, a 34-year-old graphic designer, faced profound grief following the sudden loss of her spouse. The emotional toll was significant, manifesting physically as frequent migraines and emotionally as prolonged sadness and detachment from her social circles. Despite attempts at traditional counseling and support groups, Isabella struggled with processing her grief, which began to impact her professional performance and personal life, making her feel isolated and stuck in a cycle of despair.

Recognizing the need for a holistic approach to address her emotional and physical symptoms, Isabella turned to an Ayurvedic practitioner specializing in Marma Chikitsa. The practitioner explained that grief could disrupt the flow and balance of Prana (life energy) throughout the body, specifically affecting the Anahata (heart) and Hridaya (the deeper heart) Marma points, which are key centers for emotional processing and release.

Isabella's sessions were designed to focus on these central points, facilitating emotional release and energy rebalancing. Each session involved gentle stimulation of the Anahata and Hridaya Marmas with soothing essential oils, such as rose and jasmine, which are known for their heart-soothing properties. The practitioner also incorporated chanting and sound therapy to enhance the vibrational healing impact, aiming to soothe her emotional heart and reconnect her with feelings of love and acceptance.

Over several months, Isabella experienced a noticeable shift. The therapy sessions not only helped in reducing her physical symptoms but also provided her with emotional relief. She reported feeling lighter and began to engage more with her surroundings, rekindling interests in activities she had previously enjoyed. The focused, gentle pressure applied to the heart-centric Marma points during each session allowed her to release pent-up grief gradually, facilitating healing that was not achieved through conventional methods alone.

This case demonstrates the effectiveness of Marma Chikitsa in managing deep-rooted emotional pain, offering a pathway for transformative healing through the strategic manipulation of energy points, providing a profound emotional detox, and instilling renewed vitality and joy in life.

Case Study: Enhancing Cognitive Performance in Ageing Academics Through Marma Chikitsa

Dr. Alan, a 65-year-old university professor, had been noticing a gradual decline in his cognitive abilities, characterized by memory lapses, difficulty in concentrating during lectures, and a slower pace in academic writing. These changes began to impact his confidence and productivity, raising concerns about his ongoing capabilities in his demanding academic role. Traditional approaches, such as cognitive exercises and pharmaceutical interventions, had offered only limited improvements. Dr. Alan was introduced to Marma Chikitsa by a colleague who had experienced beneficial effects in managing stress and cognitive decline.

During his first consultation with an Ayurvedic practitioner, Dr. Alan learned about the connection between specific Marma points and cognitive functions. The practitioner explained that Marma Chikitsa could enhance neural efficiency by stimulating points that govern mental clarity and memory retention, specifically the Brahmarandhra and Ajna. These points are believed to directly impact the higher cognitive faculties and assist in balancing the subtle energy flows within the brain, which are necessary for mental processes.

The treatment involved gentle stimulation of these Marma points using sesame oil, known for its high magnesium content and beneficial effects on nerve function. Additionally, Dr. Alan was instructed in lifestyle adjustments to support the treatment, including dietary changes rich in omega-3 fatty acids and antioxidants, regular sleep patterns, and mindfulness meditation to enhance mental clarity.

After several months of consistent Marma therapy combined with lifestyle adjustments, Dr. Alan reported noticeable improvements in his cognitive functions. He experienced fewer memory lapses, an increased ability to concentrate for extended periods, and a quicker thought process when engaged in academic discussions or writing. The sessions focusing on the Brahmarandhra and Ajna points were particularly effective, contributing to a significant boost in his mental resilience and academic performance. This case illustrates how Marma Chikitsa, by targeting specific energy points, can be an effective complementary therapy in managing age-related cognitive decline, enhancing not only mental faculties but also overall quality of life for aging professionals.

Case Study: Advanced Marma Therapy for Management of Chronic Fatigue Syndrome

Mia, a 29-year-old software developer, had been battling Chronic Fatigue Syndrome (CFS) for over two years. Her condition, manifesting as persistent tiredness, muscle pain, and difficulty in focusing, was severely impeding her daily activities and work. Traditional medical treatments had so far only provided minimal relief, and Mia started looking for alternative therapies to improve her condition.

Upon a friend's suggestion, Mia turned to Marma Chikitsa, attracted by its promise of balancing the body's energies and enhancing overall well-being without the side effects of conventional medication. She consulted with an experienced Ayurvedic practitioner who specialized in managing chronic ailments through Marma therapy. The practitioner explained how CFS could be associated with vital energy (Prana) blockages and significant Vata dosha imbalances, which could be addressed effectively with Marma Chikitsa.

Mia's treatment began with a thorough assessment of her Prakruti (constitutional type) and Vikruti (current state of imbalance). The sessions focused on stimulating the specific Marma points associated with energy renewal and pain relief, such as Surya, Prana Vayu, and Manas. Techniques involved gentle pressure, suitable aromatic oils like rosemary for mental clarity, and lavender for relaxation, creating a tailored therapeutic experience aimed at managing her symptoms.

Each session also integrated dietary recommendations, yoga poses, and breathing exercises specifically chosen to enhance the effects of the Marma treatment and support energy levels. This holistic approach aimed to revitalize Mia's life energy and address the root causes of her fatigue rather than just alleviating symptoms.

After regular therapy for several months, Mia reported a noticeable improvement in her energy levels and a significant reduction in muscle pain. She experienced increased mental clarity and found herself more engaged in her daily activities. The comprehensive nature of Marma Chikitsa, along with continuous lifestyle adjustments, led not only to improvements in her specific symptoms but also to a greater sense of balance and well-being, showcasing the therapy's potential in managing and possibly overcoming challenges associated with Chronic Fatigue Syndrome.

Case Study: Revitalization Through Marma Chikitsa Following Long-Term Emotional Burnout

Alicia, a 47-year-old social worker, had been experiencing profound emotional burnout after decades of dealing with high-stress situations and helping clients navigate traumatic experiences. Her dedication, while admirable, led to a noticeable decline in her physical health, manifesting as chronic fatigue, insomnia, and recurrent headaches. Emotionally, Alicia felt drained, with a pervasive sense of numbness and disconnection from her personal joys and hobbies.

Recognizing the need for a holistic intervention, Alicia sought out Marma Chikitsa, intrigued by its principles of rebalancing life energy and its potential for deep emotional healing. During her initial consultation, the Ayurvedic practitioner recognized signs of severe Prana Vayu disruption and recommended a tailored Marma therapy regimen targeting key points believed to foster emotional and energetic rejuvenation.

Alicia's treatment focused on the Manas and Hridaya Marma points, vital centers for mental health and emotional processing. The sessions involved delicate stimulation of these points, supplemented with aromatic oils such as rose and geranium, which are known for their uplifting and heart-soothing properties. The practitioner also incorporated Shirodhara—a form of Ayurvedic therapy that involves gently pouring liquids over the forehead, which is particularly effective in calming the mind and reducing stress.

Over the course of treatment, Alicia began noticing a gradual return of her energy levels. Her sleep improved significantly, indicating a restoration of the natural balance of her Vata dosha, often disrupted in cases of insomnia. Emotionally, the continuous focus on the Hridaya Marma helped her reconnect with her feelings, alleviating the numbness. She reported feeling more grounded and began to engage in personal hobbies, finding joy in painting and gardening, activities she had neglected for years.

This case highlights how Marma Chikitsa, by targeting specific energy pathways and points, can facilitate profound healing. It highlights not only the therapeutic benefits of tailored Marma point stimulation but also the importance of integrating sensory therapies, such as aromatic oils and Shirodhara, to enhance the overall emotional and physical healing process, making it a comprehensive approach to tackling conditions like emotional burnout.

Review Questions

1. A 58-year-old woman presenting with chronic depression and feelings of mental heaviness visits a practitioner experienced in Ayurvedic Marma Chikitsa. After assessing her symptoms, the practitioner decides to focus on stimulating specific Marma points known to alleviate such conditions. Which Marma point, known for its role in alleviating the heaviness of depression and promoting feelings of lightness and clarity, is most likely targeted by the practitioner?

A) A. Brahmarandhra Marma
B) B. Prana Vayu Marma
C) C. Anandabhairava Marma
D) D. Manas Marma

Answer: B

Explanation: The Prana Vayu Marma, located in the chest region, is crucial for psychological balance. Stimulating this Marma point helps alleviate the heaviness of depression by enhancing upward and outward movement of energy, promoting feelings of lightness and clarity. Its activation is often paired with mindfulness techniques to intensify therapeutic effects, making it a suitable choice for the symptomology described.

2. A therapist working with an individual suffering from PTSD opts to use Marma Chikitsa to aid in their client's recovery. The therapist concentrates on a specific Marma known to unburden the emotional weight of the heart. Which Marma point is specifically used to diminish fear and establish a sense of security during the session?

A) A. Adhipati Marma
B) B. Hridaya Marma
C) C. Manipura Marma
D) D. Sthapani Marma

Answer: B

Explanation: The Hridaya, or heart Marma, is focused on during sessions targeting emotional disturbances like PTSD because it is known for its capacity to unburden the heart of emotional weights. Stimulating this point helps alleviate fear and foster a sense of security and trust, which are essential for trauma recovery.

3. During a session focusing on managing high levels of stress, which Marma point is primarily targeted to regulate energy associated with the fire element, which governs digestion and personal power, and consequently calms the solar plexus area, leading to a subdued response to stress?

A) A. Manipuraka Marma
B) B. Anahata Marma
C) C. Surya Marma
D) D. Ajna Marma

Answer: A

Explanation: The Manipuraka Marma, located in the solar plexus region, is particularly important in stress management. This Marma is involved in regulating the flow of energy associated with the fire element, which governs digestion and personal power. The calming of this center leads to a subdued response to stressors, providing balance and inner peace, which are essential for managing stress efficiently.

4. To enhance memory and focus, a student of Ayurveda is advised to seek Marma Chikitsa treatment, focusing on the Marma point located just above the eyebrows, known for its relation to clearer thinking and focus.

A) A. Hridaya Marma
B) B. Manipura Marma
C) C. Adhipati Marma
D) D. Avarta Marma
Answer: D
Explanation: The Avarta Marma, situated just above the eyebrows, plays a central role in cognitive enhancement. The manipulation of this Marma serves as a gateway to clearer thinking and focus. By dissolving mental clutter, it empowers sharper cognition and alertness, making it imperative for students seeking improvement in memory and focus through Marma Chikitsa.

5. Identify the Marma point that is primarily employed in an emergency for counteracting the immediate effects of a panic attack, known to calm the storm of thoughts and restore tranquility quickly.
A) A. Brahmarandhra Marma
B) B. Adhipati Marma
C) C. Anahata Marma
D) D. Gandhara Marma
Answer: B
Explanation: The Adhipati Marma, located at the crown of the head, plays a crucial role in calming down the mental and emotional upheaval during a panic attack. Its stimulation helps calm the storm of thoughts and usher in a state of peace and clarity rapidly, making it an essential first-response Marma in such emergencies.

CHAPTER NINE: Advanced Marma Protocols and Therapeutic Sequences

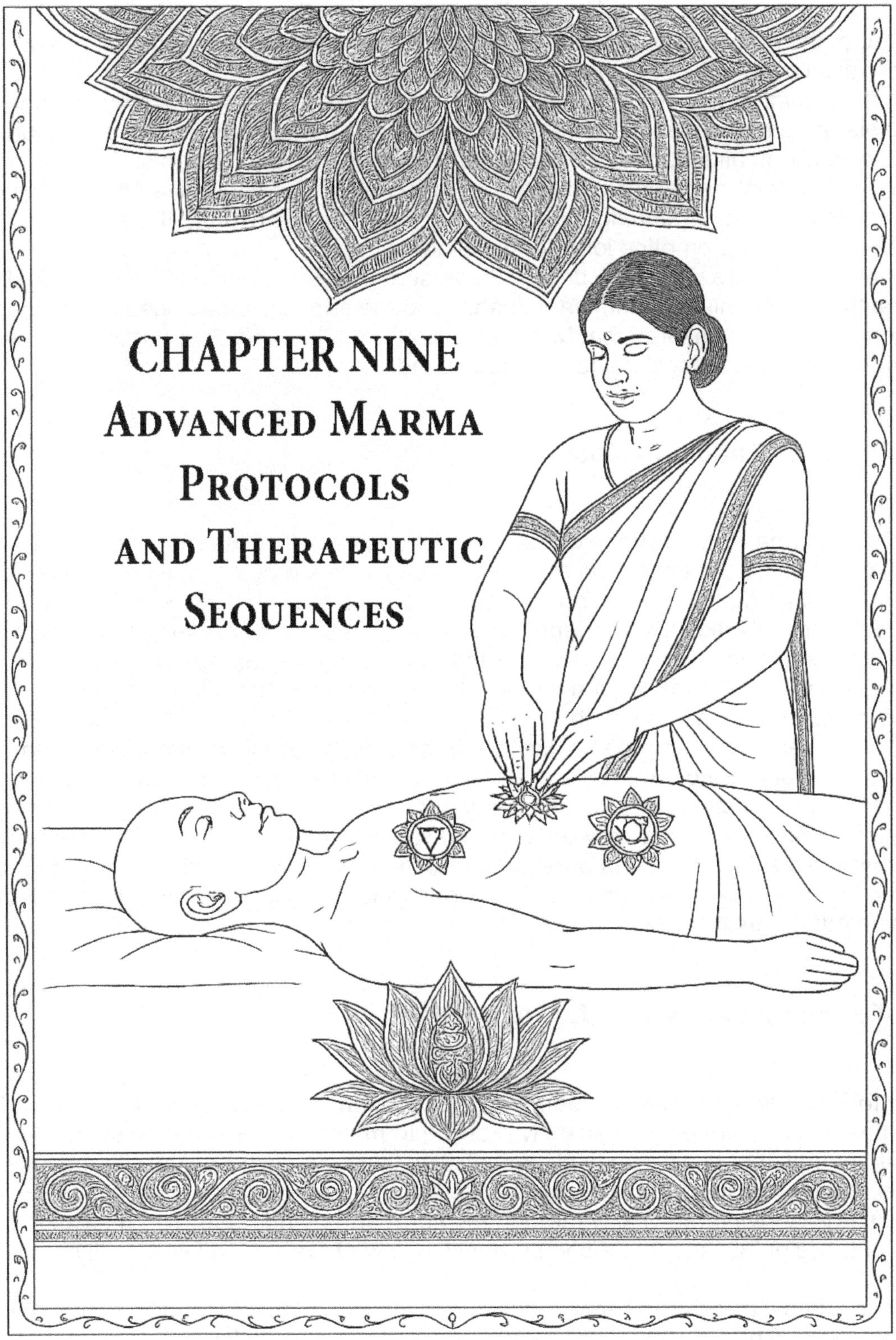

Understanding Therapeutic Sequencing in Marma

Therapeutic sequencing in Marma is a nuanced approach tailored to amplify the healing effects by strategically ordering Marma point stimulation. It ensures that the energy flow, or prana, moves through the body in a manner that maximizes the therapeutic outcomes for both physical and emotional ailments.

The sequences commence with preparatory techniques that warm up the body, making the Marma points more receptive. The core of the sequence involves detailed manipulation of specific Marma points aligned with the patient's unique health requirements. This could range from detoxification to strengthening specific organ systems. The sequence typically culminates with techniques aimed at grounding and stabilizing the energy, ensuring the stability of therapeutic effects and promoting long-term wellbeing.

Professional practitioners rigorously design these sequences, factoring in the individual's current health, medical history, dominant dosha, and the specific imbalances being addressed. This personalized touch ensures that Marma therapy is not just effective but also deeply aligned with the individual's physiological and energetic needs.

Full-Body Marma Reboot Protocol

The Full-Body Marma Reboot Protocol is a comprehensive and revitalizing sequence designed to align and rejuvenate the entire body's energy system. This protocol initiates by gently stimulating the major Marma points from toe to head, systematically awakening the body's inherent healing capabilities. By sequentially activating these critical energy junctions, the protocol supports the unobstructed flow of prana, enhancing overall vitality and organ function. Central to this sequence is the integration of subtle bodywork with rhythmic breath synchronization, creating a synergy that deeply infuses each Marma point with revitalized energy. Practitioners focus on areas typically burdened by stress and stagnation, promoting detoxification and balancing the body's doshas. This meticulous approach not only revitalizes physical health but also sharpens mental clarity and emotional equilibrium.

Following this protocol promises a sweeping renewal, manifesting in smoother energy flow, reduced physical discomfort, and improved mental focus. Regular practice can lead to sustained health benefits, making it an essential routine for anyone seeking comprehensive well-being in a holistic Ayurvedic context.

Head-to-Toe Marma Activation for Daily Health

The Head-to-Toe Marma Activation sequence, also known as "*Shavayatra*" or the "Wind Gates Traveling Exercise," offers a dynamic daily practice to maintain and enhance overall health. Designed to energize the entire body systematically, this sequence begins with the lower extremities, gently stimulating Marma points that govern grounding and stability, progressively moving upwards to invigorate vitality through the core, arms, and head. The meticulous activation of these points ensures a comprehensive flow of prana, fortifying bodily functions and enhancing mental clarity.

Each point is addressed with precision, considering individual health conditions and daily exposure to stress. This not only recharges the physical body but also clears mental fog, setting a tone of calm alertness for the day. Regular practice can significantly enhance daily

performance, resilience to stress, and overall well-being.
By integrating breathwork and meditative focus, the sequence transforms into a potent tool for preventive healthcare and rapid rejuvenation. It culminates in a harmonizing effect, synchronizing bodily rhythms with natural energy flows, essential for lasting health and vitality. Shavayatra is also an excellent way to become familiar with, or learn and develop comfort in, the totality of the Marma Points, which can be intimidating.
A series of self-exercises which will lead to a personal awareness of these gates and the wind that courses through them. This information should be helpful to both you, the practitioner, and your client. I have always maintained that the Thai Ayurveda arts are practical. Even in the most esoteric theories, we find practical examples. The Shavayatra exercise itself is a variation of the Shamatha or 'Calm Abiding' meditation. The specific object of observation or mindful focus is the Marma (wind gates) themselves.
There are many benefits to exercise. As the practice is perfected, the overt effects of aging, degeneration, and deterioration are reduced or avoided. The free flow of all circulation, Prana and Chi, is enhanced with corresponding benefits to all the lines, meridians, and chakras, as well as the organs and soft tissue. It is said that this practice can lead to a greater harmony between the opposing energies of the Sun and the Moon, freeing the essential nectar of the Kundalini Shakti to rise along the Sen Sumana (Sushumna Nadi). This exercise may produce a lot of heat and vibration, indicating a release of energy. You may expect to experience a heightened awareness and connection to emotional states. As the exercise is mastered, you can expect to develop an understanding of the expansiveness of the self. The practice is calming and enlivening at the same time. The heart rate will diminish, and the respiration will become deeper. Fluids will move, and you may experience a toning effect on the digestive and sex organs.
Remember, your greatest ally in any relaxation exercise is the proper use of the breath. Slow, not forced, natural rhythmic breathing will take you wherever your mind can see for you to go. I recommend Shavayatra, also known as the Mother's Breath. This is a pranayama method based on a seven/ one/ seven (7 / 1 / 7) count. If this is unfamiliar to you, do not despair. Simply breathe in fully without straining for a count of seven. Hold the breath stationary without straining or locking the throat for one complete count. Then, breathe out slowly for a full seven count. Once you complete your exhalation, leave it out again, without straining or locking the throat for one complete count. Repeat the breath pattern until it is a natural breathing rhythm without undue effort for the duration of the exercise.
Savasana is essentially a methodical movement through the body, first tensing, then rolling and releasing each part while breathing. First, address the parts of the body most distant from the trunk or spine, and then move closer to the core of the body. For example, begin by stretching and tensing the toes of the left foot, and then wiggle them a little to release them. Then, tense and flex the whole foot. Follow this by rolling it to release any tension. Move to the other foot and repeat. Now move one leg up, then the other. Stretch and hold the entire leg up and out as far as you can for a count of five. Then, drop it hard and gently roll it back and forth a few times, being careful not to do it too vigorously. Repeat with the other leg. Move on to the fingers, hands, and arms, and treat them individually, just as you did the feet. Now lift and separate all the arms and the legs and tense them as hard as you can for a five count before dropping as before. Roll and release. Move up the torso. First, squeeze the buttocks and then release. Follow this same process with the abdomen, only after you tense it, push it out, and make it as large as possible, then release. Do the chest, shoulders, neck, and face, including the mouth and eyes, before moving to the next section.
The object is to see the points more than to be concerned with affecting them in any way; to be with the points which represent so many of the correlations between the mind, body, and psyche continuum. Begin with number one at the midmost point of the perineum. Focus on this point for a few moments without straining, allowing your mind to consider the space. Move

upward and continue with each point, in turn, as you make your way around the course. Each time, allow your attention to remain for approximately two breaths. The first few times, it may be challenging to maintain a meditative state as you consider all the points. Each time you notice that you have drifted off track, simply bring your attention back to the next gate and continue. As with all Thai Ayurveda forms, begin with an emphasis on the flow rather than the precision of the technique. For example, it is okay to visualize the general location of the gate at first. Avoid trying to be too specific, as your practice will deteriorate into just looking for points. After a few days of practice, you will notice fewer distractions and more discursive thinking, along with a greater sense of ease and flow. Remember to continue the Pranayama breathing, rhythmic and full, throughout the exercise. For a more detailed description of the Shavayatra Wind Gates (*Thai Lom*)Traveling Exercise and the Thai Ayurveda traditional variation of the "Head to Toe Marma Activation" exercise, see the book **"Ayurveda and Thai Yoga: Religious Therapeutics Theory and Practice"** at https://ln.run/EQpSH

3-Phase Marma Therapy: Detox, Balance, Rejuvenate

The 3-Phase Marma Therapy is a sophisticated sequence designed to holistically cleanse, balance, and revitalize the body through the strategic stimulation of Marma points. This therapeutic process begins with the detox phase, where targeted Marma points are activated to expel toxins and purify the system, setting a pristine foundation for subsequent healing.

In the balance phase, the focus shifts to regulating the body's three doshas – Vata, Pitta, and Kapha – ensuring they are in perfect harmony. This is achieved by manipulating specific Marma points that correspond to these elemental energies, thus stabilizing bodily functions and enhancing resistance to diseases.

The final phase, rejuvenate, centers on revitalizing the body's vital energies. Here, rejuvenation is facilitated through Marma points that boost organ function and promote cell regeneration. This culminates in restored vitality and a profound sense of well-being, rendering the therapy not only corrective but profoundly transformative.

Dosha-Specific Marma Sequences

In the realm of Ayurveda, understanding and balancing the three doshas—Vata, Pitta, and Kapha—is crucial for maintaining health. The Dosha-Specific Marma Sequences are meticulously designed to address these unique constitutions, employing specific Marma points that resonate with each dosha's energy centers.

For Vata, characterized by elements of air and ether, the sequence focuses on grounding and stabilizing the body. Marma points in the lower back and feet are emphasized, counteracting Vata's tendency towards dryness and anxiety. Pitta, with its fire element, benefits from cooling and soothing protocols. Points around the heart and small intestine are targeted to alleviate heat and promote calmness. Finally, Kapha, made up of earth and water, is stimulated through invigorating points in the chest and stomach to enhance metabolic processes and energize the body.

Each sequence is a thoughtful curation of specific touch techniques that not only aim to balance the doshas but also catalyze deep healing and rejuvenation. Employing these tailored approaches ensures holistic well-being, attuned to the subtle nuances of Ayurvedic wisdom.

Disease-Specific Treatment Sequences

The efficacy of Marma Chikitsa deepens with its application in disease-specific treatment sequences. These sequences are meticulously formulated to address specific health conditions, leveraging the power of Marma points to catalyze healing and restore bodily balance.
Conditions ranging from chronic pain syndromes, such as arthritis and migraines, to systemic ailments like hypertension and diabetes are treated through precise Marma protocols.
Each sequence is a bespoke amalgamation of Marma points, activated in a precise order to maximize healing impact. For instance, sequences for respiratory issues might focus on points across the chest and back, enhancing lung capacity and easing breath. Conversely, gastrointestinal disorders benefit from sequences targeting the abdomen to improve digestion and alleviate discomfort.
Practitioners combine detailed knowledge of Marma points with the individual's health profile, creating a personalized therapeutic approach. Regular application of these sequences promotes not only symptomatic relief but also a profound reharmonization of bodily functions, heralding a return to health and vitality.

Sequence for Energy Boosting and Mental Clarity

The Sequence for Energy Boosting and Mental Clarity is a specialized Marma protocol specifically crafted to invigorate the body's energy levels while sharpening mental acuity. This sequence begins with the stimulation of vital Marma points along the spinal column and head; areas traditionally associated with the activation of life force and cognitive function. The careful manipulation of these points encourages a surge of prana throughout the nervous system, effectively dispelling lethargy and boosting alertness.
To augment this effect, the protocol includes targeted maneuvers around the chest and arms, which enhance respiratory volume and circulation, critical elements in maintaining high energy levels and mental focus. This carefully choreographed sequence not only empowers one with immediate vibrancy but also sets the foundation for sustained mental clarity.
By integrating slow, deliberate breathwork with each point activation, practitioners guide the body into a state of balanced energy flow, optimizing conditions for peak cognitive performance and maintaining an energetic equilibrium throughout the day.

Reproductive Marma Sequence for Men and Women

The Reproductive Marma Sequence for Men and Women is a delicate interplay of Marma points designed to enhance reproductive health and vitality. This sequence begins by focusing on key points around the pelvic area, traditionally associated with reproductive functions, and gently extends to include the lower abdomen and lower spine. Each point is stimulated in a manner that supports hormonal balance and improves energy flow to reproductive organs.
Enhancement of fertility and mitigation of reproductive disorders are central goals of this protocol. For men, the sequence aims to promote vitality and regulate hormonal functions, whereas for women, emphasis is placed on regulating menstrual cycles and supporting overall uterine health. The sequence is designed to be nurturing, using smooth, gentle pressures to reassure and relax the body, encouraging a natural state of health.
Regular practice of this sequence can lead to significant improvements in reproductive health,

offering a natural aid for couples seeking fertility enhancements or overall reproductive wellness. Emotionally and physically, the sequence is structured to foster a deep sense of well-being and connection within one's own body.

Sleep Induction Marma Flow

The Sleep Induction Marma Flow is an exquisitely designed sequence that emphasizes the facilitation of deep, restorative sleep through the gentle stimulation of specific Marma points known to regulate sleep patterns and promote relaxation. It begins with the gentle activation of points around the head and neck; areas closely associated with mental relaxation and the reduction of stress. This helps calm the mind, setting a serene commencement to the sleep induction protocol.

The sequence progresses to include points along the spine and feet, well-regarded in Ayurvedic practice for their roles in grounding and soothing the nervous system. This methodical stimulation aids in diminishing physical tension, a common impediment to peaceful sleep. Subtle manipulations at these critical junctures encourage a natural descent into sleep, gently ushering the body into a state of tranquility.

By integrating rhythmic breathing techniques with each point activation, the flow culminates in a harmonious alignment of body and mind, making the transition into sleep seamless and swift. This protocol not only primes the individual for a night of deep sleep but also enhances overall sleep quality, crucial for health and vitality restoration.

Emotional Stability Sequence for Mood Regulation

Central to achieving emotional equilibrium, the Emotional Stability Sequence for Mood Regulation employs Marma therapy to manage mood swings and enhance emotional resilience. Targeting specific Marmas associated with emotional centers in the brain and heart, this sequence initiates by calming the nervous system, gradually reducing feelings of anxiety and depression.

The protocol incorporates gentle pressure on the head and heart regions; areas key to emotional processing. Practitioners focus on these critical points to release emotional blockages, facilitating a flow of balanced energy that supports stable moods. This approach not only helps in regulating stress responses but also promotes a deep sense of inner peace.

Integrating slow, focused breathing with each touch, the sequence engenders a meditative state, making it highly effective for those undergoing emotional distress. Over time, regular application of this sequence can transform emotional turbulence into serenity, fostering an enduring state of mental and emotional well-being.

High-Performance Athlete Recovery Protocol

The High-Performance Athlete Recovery Protocol is meticulously designed using Marma therapy techniques to enhance recovery and performance in athletes. Recognizing the immense physical demands placed on athletes, this sequence targets Marma points that facilitate rapid muscle recovery, reduce inflammation, and optimize energy distribution, which is crucial for high-intensity activities.

Initiating with Marma points along the legs and lower back, areas often subject to stress and injury in athletic endeavors, practitioners apply focused pressures to dissipate lactic acid buildup and accelerate tissue repair. The sequence transitions to stimulate Marmas around the shoulders and arms, crucial for relieving tension and promoting joint health to withstand rigorous training regimes.
Integrating vital points on the head and neck, this protocol additionally focuses on mental clarity and concentration, ensuring athletes remain sharp and focused. By restoring the body's natural balance, the sequence not only accelerates physical recovery but also enhances mental resilience, providing athletes with a holistic recovery tool essential for maintaining peak performance.

Marma for Immunity Strengthening

In the realm of Ayurvedic healing, the Marma for Immunity Strengthening stands as a pivotal protocol designed to fortify the body's natural defense mechanisms. This sequence meticulously targets Marma points associated with vital organs and the immune response, such as those along the chest, spine, and abdomen. By stimulating these specific areas, the protocol aims to enhance the body's capacity to ward off illnesses and maintain robust health.
The manipulation of these points is believed to activate and regulate the flow of prana, or life energy, which is crucial in stimulating the immune system. This not only helps prevent seasonal maladies but also enhances the body's resilience against more persistent health challenges. The sequence incorporates a combination of gentle pressures and rhythmic strokes to bolster lymphatic drainage and blood circulation, which are vital processes for immune efficiency. Regular application of this Marma sequence can lead to a noticeable improvement in overall vitality and a strengthened immune system, making it an essential practice for those seeking to enhance their body's natural protective mechanisms and achieve a balanced state of health.

Pre/Post-Operative Marma Protocol

The Pre- and Post-Operative Marma Protocol provides targeted support designed to optimize surgical outcomes and enhance recovery. This meticulously designed sequence engages Marma points to bolster the body's resilience both before and after surgery. Initially focusing on areas that stimulate vitality and strength, the protocol prepares the patient by promoting a balanced flow of energy, reducing pre-operative anxiety, and enhancing the body's natural defenses.
Following surgery, the focus shifts to accelerated healing and effective pain management. Key Marma points are stimulated to facilitate smoother recovery, reduce inflammation, and mitigate complications. This phase of the protocol utilizes gentle yet effective techniques to support tissue repair and detoxification, which are crucial in post-operative care. The application of Marma therapy here aims to reinvigorate the body and shorten recovery time.
Through both pre- and post-operative stages, practitioners offer a supportive touch that not only addresses physical recuperation but also aids in emotional stability, ensuring a holistic approach to surgical recovery. Regular sessions are recommended to maintain optimal benefits.

Sequence for Spiritual Awakening and Meditation

The Sequence for Spiritual Awakening and Meditation employs an exquisite combination of Marma point stimulation designed to heighten spiritual connectivity and enhance meditative depths. This session begins with focusing on the crown and third eye areas, pivotal centers for spiritual and intuition energies. Stimulating these specific Marmas is believed to unlock spiritual potential and foster a deeper connection to higher consciousness.

Continuing down to the heart and solar plexus, the sequence helps align personal energy with universal frequencies. This alignment is crucial for achieving a state of profound meditation and spiritual insight. By methodically engaging these critical energy centers, the practitioner can facilitate a flow of energy that nurtures the soul's vibrational needs, setting the foundation for advanced spiritual practices.

Incorporating soft, rhythmic pressures alongside controlled breathing, the session not only calms the mind but also prepares it to receive and interpret deeper spiritual messages. Regular practice of this sequence promises an enriched meditative experience and a significantly enhanced spiritual journey.

Chakra-Balancing Marma Sequence

The Chakra-Balancing Marma Sequence is intricately designed to harmonize the body's chakra centers, vital for maintaining spiritual and physical health. By focusing on key Marma points aligned with the seven major chakras, this sequence aims to remove blockages and restore the flow of energy throughout the body.

Initiation of the sequence involves applying gentle pressure to Marma points corresponding to the root chakra, gradually moving upward to the crown chakra. This methodical progression ensures each chakra is activated and balanced, promoting a sense of groundedness and connectivity with higher consciousness. Special attention is given to the heart and throat chakras, centers of love and communication, to foster emotional openness and clarity in expression.

Integrative techniques, including synchronized breathing and visualization, enhance the efficacy of the sequence, aiding in more profound relaxation and spiritual awareness. Regular practice can lead to profound changes in one's energetic health, facilitating a tranquil mind and a rejuvenated spirit.

Marma Flow for Joint Health and Flexibility

The Marma Flow for Joint Health and Flexibility is specially formulated to address issues of stiffness and restricted movement by targeting critical Marma points that influence joint health. The sequence begins with the stimulation of Marma points around key joints, knees, elbows, and shoulders to facilitate the removal of toxins that accumulate in joint areas, often causing pain and inflammation.

This protocol then incorporates sequences that enhance the flow of synovial fluid, essential for lubricating the joints and promoting smoother, pain-free movements. Techniques employed focus on re-establishing the balance of Vata, the dosha primarily responsible for movement and flexibility in the body. By harmonizing Vata, this sequence helps improve mobility and reduce joint discomfort.

The concluding part of the sequence emphasizes maintenance and prevention, integrating daily practices that help sustain joint health and prevent future issues. Regular application of this Marma routine promises enhanced flexibility, reduced joint pain, and a revitalized energy flow throughout the body, which is essential for overall wellness.

Skin Rejuvenation Marma Sequence

The Skin Rejuvenation Marma Sequence is an elixir for radiant, youthful skin, utilizing the profound principles of Ayurveda to revitalize and renew the body's largest organ. This sequence targets key Marma points across the face and body to stimulate blood circulation and enhance the delivery of nutrients to the skin cells, thereby promoting cellular regeneration and reducing signs of aging.

Practitioners employ gentle pressures combined with specialized oils that integrate herbal essences aligned with skin health, such as turmeric and saffron, known for their antioxidant and brightening properties. These sessions help in detoxifying the skin, minimizing pores, and smoothing fine lines, creating an overall effect of luminance and suppleness.

In addition to facial Marmas, the sequence includes points on the arms and legs to encourage overall body skin health. Regular treatments are recommended as part of a holistic approach to maintain the skin's elasticity, clarity, and vitality, thereby embodying a natural glow that resonates from within.

Beauty Marma Protocol (Facial and Scalp Focus)

The Beauty Marma Protocol (Facial and Scalp Focus) is exquisite in its essence, primarily aimed at enhancing facial radiance and scalp health through precise Marma point stimulation. This protocol integrates ancient wisdom with modern holistic techniques to invigorate the skin and hair follicles, promoting a youthful appearance and natural glow.

Initiating with gentle touches on the key Marma points across the face, the sequence boosts circulation, encouraging the removal of toxins and enhancing nutrient supply to skin cells. This not only diminishes signs of aging but also infuses the skin with a vibrant, healthy sheen. Simultaneously, the scalp treatment focuses on stimulating hair follicles to improve hair texture and stimulate growth, addressing issues like thinning and dryness.

The session ends with harmonizing techniques that align the inner energies, reflecting outward beauty. Regular application of this protocol can dramatically transform one's facial and scalp health, leading to a balanced, luminous complexion and robust, shiny hair.

Detox and Fasting Marma Plan

The Detox and Fasting Marma Plan is designed to complement the cleansing effects of fasting, using targeted Marma techniques to enhance elimination of toxins and invigorate the body's innate detoxification systems. This sequence begins by focusing on Marmas that influence the liver and kidneys, key organs responsible for the filtration and elimination of toxins.

With gentle pressures and specific oils known for their purifying properties, such as neem and guggulu, the plan works to stimulate these critical energy points, aiding in the breakdown and removal of toxin buildups. This not only supports the physical aspects of detoxification but also

elevates mental clarity and emotional peace, aligning with the holistic benefits of fasting.
As the fast continues, this Marma plan shifts to support metabolic functions and energy levels, ensuring that the body maintains vitality while in a state of reduced food intake. Regular application of this sequence during fasting periods promotes a deeper and more effective cleanse, restoring a sense of balance and health throughout the body.

Eye and Ear Health Marma Routine

The Eye and Ear Health Marma Routine is meticulously designed to enhance sensory health using precise Marma points relevant to ocular and auditory functions. The beginning of this sequence focuses on points around the eyes to improve vision acuity and alleviate strain from screen exposure, promoting relaxation and diffusion of accumulated eye tension.
Subsequently, the sequence addresses ear health by stimulating specific Marma points that help balance inner ear pressures and enhance auditory capabilities. This section is particularly beneficial for those experiencing tinnitus or general hearing inefficiencies, providing a soothing effect and facilitating clearer hearing.
By integrating techniques that encourage lymphatic drainage and increase local circulation, this routine helps in detoxifying the sensory organs. Regular practice can lead to improved sensory sharpness, potentially delaying the onset of degenerative sensory conditions. Emphasizing preventive care, this Marma routine offers a holistic approach to maintaining the vitality and functionality of the eyes and ears, which are integral to a balanced sensory experience.

Cardiovascular Toning Sequence

The Cardiovascular Toning Sequence is a specialized Marma protocol designed to enhance heart health and improve circulation throughout the body. Through strategic stimulation of critical Marma points, this sequence aims to fortify the cardiovascular system, aiding in the regulation of blood pressure and heart rhythms.
This therapeutic sequence begins by targeting Marmas situated around the chest and upper back, which are vital for supporting cardiac function. Gentle yet precise touches help to activate the body's natural healing mechanisms, promoting better blood flow and oxygenation to heart tissues. Techniques used not only focus on the physical aspects but also aim to release emotional stress that often impacts heart health.
As the sequence progresses, attention is given to Marmas that influence associated systems, such as the lungs and diaphragm, thereby enhancing overall respiratory capability and energy levels. Regular implementation of this Marma routine is recommended to maintain optimal cardiovascular health and vitality.

Children's Marma Development Protocol

The Children's Marma Development Protocol is specifically designed to support the evolving needs of children, promoting their physical and cognitive development through gentle stimulation of Marma points. This protocol employs specific sequences designed to strengthen the body's vital centers, fostering both robust health and mental alertness.
Beginning with gentle touches on key Marma points along the spine and limbs, the practice

promotes proper alignment, improves posture, and enhances neurological functions associated with learning and attention. Each session is tailored to the child's unique developmental stage, ensuring both safety and effectiveness. The inclusion of mild herbal oils, such as chamomile and lavender, aids in soothing and calming young minds, making it a perfect relaxation technique before bedtime.
Furthermore, this protocol not only aids in physical growth and emotional regulation but also enhances immune system capabilities, which are essential during these formative years. Regular engagement with the Children's Marma Development Protocol can lead to a harmonious balance in the child's energy systems, contributing significantly to holistic growth and overall well-being.

Elderly Care Sequence for Marma

The Elderly Care Sequence for Marma is meticulously tailored to address the specific needs of aging bodies, focusing on enhancing mobility, reducing pain, and promoting overall well-being. This protocol utilizes gentle Marma point stimulation to improve circulation and nerve function, crucial for elderly individuals who often experience reduced physical activity and vitality. Beginning with core Marma points along the spine and joints, the sequence eases stiffness and discomfort, which are common in the elderly. By targeting these crucial areas, the therapy helps to restore a sense of balance and flexibility, essential for maintaining independence and daily function. Additionally, special attention is given to Marma points that correlate with mental clarity and emotional stability, supporting cognitive functions and mood.
Concluding with Marma points that invigorate the heart and digestive system, the sequence aims to bolster these vital organs. Regular application of this Marma protocol can significantly enhance the quality of life for the elderly, ensuring a more active and joyful later life phase.

Women's Cycle Harmonizing Marma Plan

The Women's Cycle Harmonizing Marma Plan offers a refined approach to alleviating menstrual discomfort and enhancing reproductive health through targeted Marma therapy. This specialized sequence begins with the stimulation of key Marma points in the pelvic and abdominal areas, which are known to regulate hormonal balance and alleviate cramps, thereby promoting a smoother menstrual cycle.
Further into the sequence, techniques focus on Marmas that support ovarian and uterine health, fostering a nurturing environment for reproductive functions. The application of mild, soothing pressure helps reduce inflammation and discomfort, particularly during the premenstrual and menstrual phases. Herbal oils, such as rose and ylang-ylang, are used to enhance the effectiveness of the treatments, providing a calming and restorative experience.
To conclude, the plan incorporates stress-relieving Marma points that not only assist in emotional regulation during hormonal fluctuations but also promote overall well-being. Regular adherence to this protocol can lead to an enhanced sense of health and vitality, making it a cornerstone of women's holistic health management.

Summary

The chapter on 'Advanced Marma Protocols and Therapeutic Sequences' presents a dense exploration into Therapeutic Sequencing in Marma, aiming to maximize healing by ordering Marma point stimulation tailored to individual needs. This sequence begins with preparatory techniques to warm up the body, followed by detailed manipulation of Marma points to address specific health issues, such as detoxification and strengthening of organ systems, and concludes with techniques that stabilize the energy flow in the body. Each sequence is rigorously crafted considering the patient's health, medical history, and dominant dosha to ensure personalized and effective treatment.

Further segments describe various specialized sequences, such as the Full-Body Marma Reboot Protocol, which aims to rejuvenate the body's energy system from toe to head through coordinated Marma point activation, integrating rhythmic breath synchronization to deepen the therapeutic impact. The chapter also covers specific sequences for daily health maintenance, detoxification, dosha balance, disease treatment, boosting energy, reproductive health, sleep induction, mood regulation, and athletic recovery, each meticulously designed to harness the potential of Marma points in support of the intended therapeutic outcomes.

Moreover, specific sequences target enhancing immunity, preparing and recovering from surgical procedures, spiritual awakening, chakra balancing, joint health, skin rejuvenation, among others. Each protocol is carefully tailored to stimulate appropriate Marma points to address various physical, emotional, and spiritual needs, ensuring holistic well-being. The use of targeted Marma therapies serves not only as a remedy for specific ailments but also as a preventative measure to maintain overall health and vitality, underscoring the adaptability and depth of these protocols within the therapeutic landscape of Marma practice. The holistic approach of each sequence testifies to the comprehensive nature of Marma therapy, aiming to create sustained health benefits and a balanced energetic state.

References

[1] 'The foundation of Marma Therapy in Ayurvedic Medicine'. https://www.ayurveda-journal.com/foundation-marma-therapy

[2] 'Comprehensive Review of Marma Science'. https://www.healthjournal.org/marma-science-review

[3] 'Applying Ayurvedic Marma Point Therapy'. https://www.traditionalhealing.org/marma-point-therapy

Case Study: Integration of Holistic Marma Therapy in Modern Rehabilitative Care

In the bustling metropolitan city of Bengaluru, India, a pioneering wellness center integrates traditional Ayurvedic practices, focusing on Marma therapy, with contemporary rehabilitative medicine to enhance patient recovery processes. The case study revolves around Aarav, a 48-year-old IT professional who suffered from chronic lower back pain exacerbated by prolonged periods of sitting and minimal physical activity. Despite various medical treatments, including physiotherapy and pain medication, Aarav's condition showed minimal improvement, leading him to explore alternative therapies.

The wellness center, renowned for its holistic approach, designed a customized Marma therapy protocol for Aarav, categorizing his treatment into three phases: assessment, intervention, and maintenance. During the assessment phase, a detailed analysis of Aarav's physical health, lifestyle, and emotional state was conducted. The intervention involved a specific sequence of Marma point stimulation focusing on the spine, lower back, and legs to alleviate pain, improve circulation, and reduce muscular tension. This was complemented by dietary recommendations and yoga exercises aimed at enhancing the therapeutic effects of Marma therapy and promoting overall well-being.

The maintenance phase included regular follow-up sessions and adjustments to the therapy protocol based on Aarav's progress. Throughout the treatment, the practitioners maintained a meticulous record of his response to the therapy, noting significant improvements in pain reduction and mobility. Aarav reported not only physical relief but also an enhanced sense of mental clarity and emotional stability, attributing these changes to the integrated approach of Marma therapy within his rehabilitation.

This case study highlights the efficacy of Marma therapy in treating chronic conditions and its potential integration into modern healthcare regimes. It underscores the importance of a personalized, holistic approach to medical treatments, which considers not only the physical symptoms but also the emotional and psychological well-being of the patient, providing a comprehensive model for rehabilitative care.

Case Study: Enhancing Cardiovascular Health through Targeted Marma Therapy: A Clinical Approach

In an innovative clinical trial conducted at a specialized Ayurvedic healthcare facility in Pune, India, researchers investigated the efficacy of Marma therapy in managing cardiovascular diseases, with a primary focus on patients with hypertension and arrhythmias. The study included Geeta, a 55-year-old female patient diagnosed with hypertension, who had been on conventional medication with limited improvement in her overall health status.

The clinical team designed a Marma therapy protocol specifically tailored to address cardiovascular issues. This protocol aimed to stimulate key Marma points that influence heart functions and blood circulation. The treatment plan for Geeta included a detailed initial assessment of her cardiovascular health, a review of her personal health history, and an evaluation of her lifestyle habits. Based on this comprehensive evaluation, the therapy sessions were structured to focus primarily on Marma points around the chest, back, and arms.

Each session involved precision-targeted stimulation of these points to help regulate blood pressure and improve cardiac rhythm. Alongside Marma therapy, Geeta was guided through a series of lifestyle adjustments, including dietary changes and mild physical activities tailored to complement the Marma treatment and promote overall cardiovascular health.

Over a period of three months, Geeta's treatment was closely monitored, with regular evaluations to track progress and make necessary adjustments to the Marma protocol. Remarkably, she reported a significant reduction in her blood pressure levels and an improvement in her heart rate. The clinical trial not only demonstrated the potential of Marma therapy as a supplementary treatment for cardiovascular conditions but also highlighted the importance of a holistic approach in managing chronic diseases.

This case study serves as a pivotal example of how traditional therapies, such as Marma, can be scientifically adapted to modern medical practices, offering a complementary and integrative approach to cardiovascular healthcare.

Case Study: Revitalizing Mental Health with Marma Therapy: The Case of Prolonged Workplace Stress

The rapidly evolving corporate sector in Toronto, Canada, has seen a significant rise in cases of workplace stress, contributing to mental health issues such as anxiety and burnout. This case study focuses on Simran, a 35-year-old software developer, who experienced severe anxiety and decreased job performance due to high job demands and chronic stress. Traditional counseling and medication provided only temporary relief, prompting her to seek alternative treatments to complement her ongoing therapies.

A local holistic health clinic introduced Simran to Marma therapy, beginning her treatment with an in-depth assessment that considered her emotional, physical, and psychological health. The clinic's specialized practitioner designed a customized Marma sequence tailored to address Simran's specific symptoms of stress and anxiety, focusing on the head, neck, and shoulder regions, which are often affected by prolonged computer use and stressful work environments.

The treatment sessions, held twice a week, involved gentle stimulation of vital Marma points to release tension and enhance the flow of energy or prana. This stimulation was designed to calm the mind and reduce anxiety by activating the body's natural healing responses. Each session concluded with a guided meditation and recommendations for dietary modifications to support mental clarity and emotional stability.

The sequential Marma therapy sessions over three months significantly improved Simran's mental health, with noticeable reductions in anxiety levels and an enhanced sense of well-being. Follow-up assessments showed improvements in her emotional response to stress and increased resilience. Simran's case underscores the potential for Marma therapy to be effectively integrated into conventional treatments for mental health, offering a non-invasive approach that holistically addresses the causes and symptoms of workplace-related stress.

Case Study: Optimizing Diabetes Management through Marma Therapy

In the city of Kochi, India, a holistic health clinic specializing in traditional Ayurvedic treatments has been exploring the benefits of integrating Marma therapy into the management of chronic ailments, specifically type 2 diabetes. The case study centers on Anjali, a 62-year-old retired schoolteacher recently diagnosed with type 2 diabetes, which was increasingly challenging to manage despite regular medication and diet control. Her struggles included fluctuating glucose levels and frequent episodes of fatigue, prompting her family to seek alternative therapies to supplement her conventional treatment regimen.

The clinic's approach began with a comprehensive review of Anjali's health history, dietary habits, lifestyle, and medication regimen. After detailed consultations, a personalized Marma therapy protocol was developed, targeting points believed to optimize pancreatic function and improve insulin sensitivity. The sequences are particularly focused on the points related to metabolic functions and energy balance, in addition to regular Ayurvedic dietary counseling and stress reduction techniques using meditation and yoga.

Anjali underwent Marma therapy sessions bi-weekly. Each session involved the gentle stimulation of specific Marma points across her abdomen, lower back, and legs to enhance energetic flow and improve digestion, which is critical in the management of diabetes. Initial responses were promising, with Anjali reporting increased levels of energy and stability in her blood sugar levels.

Over six months, documented observations revealed significant improvements in Anjali's glycemic control. Her need for medications decreased under the supervision of her endocrinologist, highlighting the efficacy of Marma therapy in supporting conventional diabetic treatments. The case study highlights the potential of Marma therapy not only as a complementary treatment for enhancing physiological processes related to diabetes but also emphasizes the need for an integrated treatment approach that considers the patient's overall physical and emotional well-being.

Case Study: Elderly Well-being with Integrative Marma Therapy: A Case Study on Arthritis and Mobility Issues

In the scenic town of Coonoor, nestled in the Nilgiri Hills of southern India, a pioneering geriatric wellness program incorporates Ayurvedic Marma therapy to address mobility and pain management in elderly patients, specifically targeting arthritis, a common ailment among the elderly. The program's focal case study involves Sujata, an 82-year-old retired school principal suffering from osteoarthritis in her knees and lower back pain, limiting her mobility and significantly decreasing her quality of life.

The wellness program, held at a local Ayurvedic clinic renowned for its integrative approach to elder care, began with a thorough examination of Sujata's medical history, current health status, and an in-depth consultation to understand her pain points and mobility issues. The practitioners developed a tailored Marma therapy plan, initiating treatment with gentle stimulation of Marma points linked to joint health and pain relief. These included points on the legs, lower back, and key energy pathways that affect the joints.

Each session involved targeted Marma stimulation, combined with gentle herbal oil massages known for their anti-inflammatory properties, which helped ease joint stiffness and reduce swelling. Alongside physical therapy, Sujata was guided in customized, gentle yoga practices designed to complement the Marma therapy by strengthening muscles and improving joint flexibility.

Over several weeks, Sujata experienced notable improvements in her pain levels and range of motion. The therapy sessions were meticulously documented, providing valuable insights into the treatment's efficacy and areas for further improvement. Notably, Sujata's emotional well-being also improved, evidenced by her renewed interest in daily activities and enhanced social interactions, underscoring the holistic benefits of integrating Marma therapy into elder care.

This case study emphasizes the effectiveness of Marma therapy in managing elderly ailments, particularly osteoarthritis, highlighting its potential as a cornerstone in geriatric healthcare. The integrative approach adopted in Sujata's case opens avenues for broader applications, providing promising pathways for enhancing elder mobility and overall well-being through traditional Ayurvedic practices.

Case Study: Revitalizing Burnout with Comprehensive Marma Therapy: Leveraging Holistic Health Approaches

The increase in work-related stress in urban populations is an alarming issue that often culminates in burnout, severely impacting personal and professional lives. This case study inspects the holistic intervention provided by a renowned wellness center in Mumbai, India, which incorporates Marma therapy as a central component of its treatment regimen. The subject, Pranav, is a 40-year-old software engineer who approached the center suffering from severe burnout manifested by chronic fatigue, headaches, and a marked decrease in job performance.

Upon his initial consultation, Pranav was given a comprehensive physical and psychological evaluation to tailor a specific Marma therapy protocol suited to his individual needs. This evaluation revealed significant imbalances in his Prana (vital energy), majorly affecting his mental and neurological functions. The personalized therapy plan was set to deploy Marma therapy in conjunction with meditation, dietary modifications, and herbal supplementation. *

Pranav's therapy sessions were scheduled thrice weekly and involved stimulation of crucial Marma points across the body, particularly those affecting the nervous system and stress responses. Points such as Brahmarandhra (crown of the head) and Ajna (third eye) were targeted to alleviate mental stress, while Anahata (heart) was focused on to encourage emotional healing. The session included the application of specific oils like Brahmi oil, renowned for its efficacy in enhancing cognitive function and reducing stress.

Over the duration of three months, Pranav recorded a significant reduction in his symptoms of burnout. His cognitive function improved, as did his energy levels and overall job satisfaction. Follow-up sessions were scheduled to assess and sustain the improvements, ensuring a long-term resolution of his condition.

This case study highlights how integrative Marma therapy, when combined with other holistic practices, can effectively mitigate severe symptoms of burnout, offering a sustainable path to recovery and enhanced general well-being.

Case Study: Pioneering Postpartum Recovery with Marma Therapy: A Holistic Approach

In the suburban landscape of Chennai, India, a community healthcare initiative launched a pilot program aimed at supporting women through their postpartum recovery using traditional Ayurvedic methods, with a particular focus on Marma therapy. The case study centers on Meena, a 29-year-old first-time mother, who faced significant challenges with postpartum depression, physical fatigue, and hormonal imbalances after the birth of her daughter.

Understanding the complexities of postpartum recovery, the healthcare team initiated a comprehensive assessment of Meena’s physical, emotional, and psychological state. This assessment considered her birthing experience, her lifestyle, and her diet. Based on this evaluation, a customized Marma therapy plan was developed, targeting vital energy points known to promote hormonal balance, stress relief, and overall vitality. The therapeutic strategy included stimulation of specific Marma points along the spine to alleviate back pain, points on the head to address emotional and hormonal disturbances, and abdominal points to improve uterine health and digestion.

The therapy sessions were conducted weekly, each lasting for about forty-five minutes. Special attention was given to creating a supportive and relaxing environment to enhance Meena's comfort and receptivity to the treatment. Each session involved gentle stimulation of Marma points combined with soothing herbal oils that are conducive to healing and relaxation, such as lavender and chamomile. Additionally, guidance on nutrition, focusing on an Ayurvedic postpartum diet, was provided, aimed at restoring and revitalizing the body from within.

Positive outcomes were observed within the first few months as Meena reported significant improvements in her energy levels and a reduction in symptoms of depression. Hormonal tests indicated better regulation, and her sleep quality had improved markedly. The success of Meena's recovery through Marma therapy underscores the efficacy of incorporating traditional wellness practices in postpartum care. Additionally, this case study provides profound insights into the potential of Marma therapy, not only as a complementary medicine but also as a holistic approach to healing and recovery during a critical period in a woman’s life.

Case Study: Innovative Marma Therapy for Combatting Chronic Migraine in High-Pressure Work Environments

In the high-stakes environment of a New York City financial firm, David, a 38-year-old investment banker, struggled with chronic migraines that severely impacted his productivity and overall quality of life. Traditional medications provided only temporary relief and often came with undesirable side effects, prompting David to seek alternative treatments. This led him to explore the potential of Marma therapy, an ancient Ayurvedic practice purported to restore bodily balance and alleviate pain through targeted pressure on vital energy points.

The holistic health clinic that David approached offered a comprehensive Marma therapy program specially tailored to treat chronic migraines. The treatment protocol began with an in-depth consultation to understand the specific triggers and symptoms of his condition, as well as an evaluation of his lifestyle and stress levels, which are often overlooked in conventional treatments. The practitioner deduced that David's migraines were exacerbated by prolonged stress and irregular sleep patterns, common in high-pressure vocations.

The therapy sessions commenced with gentle stimulation of the Marma points on the head, neck, and shoulders—areas specifically affected during migraine episodes. This included the application of cooling oils to soothe David’s intense headaches. Each session also incorporated techniques aimed at balancing the 'Pitta' dosha, which in Ayurveda is often associated with metabolic and biochemical changes causing heat and inflammation in the body.

Over the course of several months, David experienced a significant reduction in the frequency and severity of his migraines. The holistic approach not only addressed the physical manifestations of migraines but also promoted better stress management and improved sleep patterns. Regular follow-ups and adjustments to the treatment ensured the therapy remained effective and aligned with his changing health dynamics.

This case study highlights the effectiveness of Marma therapy in managing chronic conditions, such as migraines, and demonstrates the benefits of incorporating holistic health practices into contemporary lifestyles. It highlights how personalized treatments can provide sustainable relief and promote an overall improvement in well-being, especially in high-stress environments.

Case Study: Revitalizing Sports Performance through Marma Therapy: A Case Study in Professional Athletics

In the competitive world of professional sports, maintaining peak physical performance and rapid recovery are critical. Thiago, a 30-year-old professional soccer player, faced recurring injuries and muscle fatigue, which hindered his performance and threatened his career longevity. Traditional treatments, including physical therapy and modern medicine, provided short-term relief but failed to address the underlying issues. This case study explores the integration of Marma therapy into Thiago's recovery and conditioning regimen to enhance his athletic performance and resilience.

The sports medicine clinic partnered with an Ayurvedic specialist to create a tailored Marma therapy protocol for Thiago. The treatment plan began with a comprehensive evaluation of his physical injuries, body mechanics, and psychological state to pinpoint energy imbalances and stress accumulation areas. Critical to this was understanding the role of Marma points in regulating the body's vital energy (prana) to enhance muscle recovery and reduce injury susceptibility.

The treatment sessions focused on stimulating key Marma points corresponding to major muscle groups and joints that Thiago frequently used during play. Special attention was given to Marma points along his legs, lower back, and shoulders. Each therapy session included manipulations to release blocked energy, improve circulation, and promote tissue healing. These were complemented by Ayurvedic oil applications, known for their anti-inflammatory and muscle-relaxing properties.

Over the therapy period, Thiago experienced noticeable improvements in muscle flexibility, a decrease in recovery time, and a reduced occurrence of injuries. The therapy also had a noticeable effect on his mental well-being, including greater stress resilience and improved focus during games. Duly, his performance metrics saw a consistent improvement.

This case study not only underscores the efficacy of Marma therapy as a pivotal addition to sports medicine but also showcases how traditional practices can be innovatively applied in modern high-demand settings. By holistically addressing the physical and mental aspects of athletic performance, Marma therapy provides a comprehensive model that can be applied across various sports disciplines to enhance athlete longevity and performance.

Case Study: Revitalizing Energy and Reducing Stress in Corporate Professionals Through Marma Therapy

In the high-pressure environment of Silicon Valley, California, a unique wellness initiative was launched at a leading tech company to combat employee burnout and improve overall wellness. The initiative included integrating Marma therapy, an ancient Ayurvedic practice, into their standard wellness programs. The case study focuses on Elena, a 37-year-old software engineer, who faced persistent fatigue and stress due to demanding project deadlines and chronic overwork.

Elena was initially skeptical about alternative therapies but decided to engage with the program as conventional methods, including counseling and stress management workshops, had provided only temporary relief. Her treatment began with a comprehensive assessment, focusing on her physical health, daily routine, and stress level analysis. Based on the findings, a tailored Marma therapy protocol was developed, primarily aimed at revitalizing energy and managing stress.

The sessions were carefully structured, starting with Marma points that facilitate relaxation and stress alleviation, specifically targeting her head, neck, and shoulders. This was followed by stimulation of the energy points associated with vitality and circulation, encompassing her arms and legs. Each session incorporated rhythmic breathing techniques, which combined with Marma point stimulation, worked to enhance prana flow and clear blockages in energy pathways.

Over a period of six months, Elena underwent bi-weekly sessions, with each session lasting about 45 minutes. She was closely monitored for changes in her stress indicators and energy levels. Remarkably, Elena reported a significant improvement in her overall energy and a decrease in stress-related symptoms. Her sleep quality improved, and she experienced heightened mental clarity and enhanced productivity at work.

This case study not only illustrates the effectiveness of Marma therapy in a modern corporate setting but also highlights the importance of integrating traditional holistic practices to promote employee health in highly stressful work environments. It serves as a model for other organizations aiming to enhance employee well-being through innovative, non-invasive, and holistic health interventions.

Review Questions

1. A 30-year-old female patient with a medical history of chronic stress and insomnia seeks alternative therapies to improve her sleep quality and overall emotional stability. After an initial evaluation, a practitioner decides to implement a Sleep Induction Marma Flow, focusing especially on Marma points around her head, neck, and feet. Which of the following is NOT an expected outcome of this therapy?

A) Enhanced mental relaxation and reduced stress
B) Immediate resolution of her insomnia
C) Reduction in physical tension across the body
D) Improved transition into deeper sleep phases

Answer: B

Explanation: The Sleep Induction Marma Flow targets specific Marma points known for regulating sleep patterns and promoting relaxation. While this therapy can effectively enhance mental relaxation, reduce physical tension, and improve the transition into deeper sleep phases, it is not expected to provide an immediate resolution to chronic insomnia. Addressing insomnia typically requires multiple sessions and may involve additional holistic interventions to address other underlying issues such as stress or dietary habits.

2. A professional athlete is recovering from a strenuous competitive season and experiencing lingering fatigue and muscle soreness. The practitioner initiates the High-Performance Athlete Recovery Protocol using Marma therapy. What is the primary focus of the treatment in the initial stages?
A) Enhancing mental clarity and concentration
B) Stimulating rapid muscle recovery and reducing inflammation
C) Targeting Marma points along the spine for improved energy flow
D) Balancing the doshas through whole-body treatments
Answer: B
Explanation: The High-Performance Athlete Recovery Protocol, when applied to athletes suffering from post-competition fatigue and soreness, primarily focuses on stimulating rapid muscle recovery and reducing inflammation. This involves targeting specific Marma points associated with muscle and tissue repair and relief from inflammation. While other focuses like enhancing mental clarity and balancing doshas are important, they are usually secondary in the initial recovery stages after intense physical activity.

3. A patient reports symptoms of generalized anxiety and frequent mood swings. The practitioner opts to use the Emotional Stability Sequence for Mood Regulation. By concentrating on the Marma points around the brain and heart, what is the expected therapeutic effect of this treatment?
A) Immediate cessation of anxiety attacks
B) Regulation of energy flow to enhance emotional stability
C) Sharp increase in cognitive functioning
D) Long-term treatment suppresses other emotional responses
Answer: B
Explanation: The Emotional Stability Sequence focuses on managing mood swings and enhancing emotional resilience by targeting specific Marma points associated with emotional processing in the brain and heart. The expected therapeutic outcome is the regulation of energy flow, which supports a more balanced emotional state. This helps in reducing anxiety and mood fluctuations. Unlike immediate cessation of anxiety attacks or suppression of emotions, this therapy aims for a gradual improvement in emotional regulation without significantly altering cognitive functions.

CHAPTER TEN: Integration with Yoga, Ayurveda, and Other Disciplines

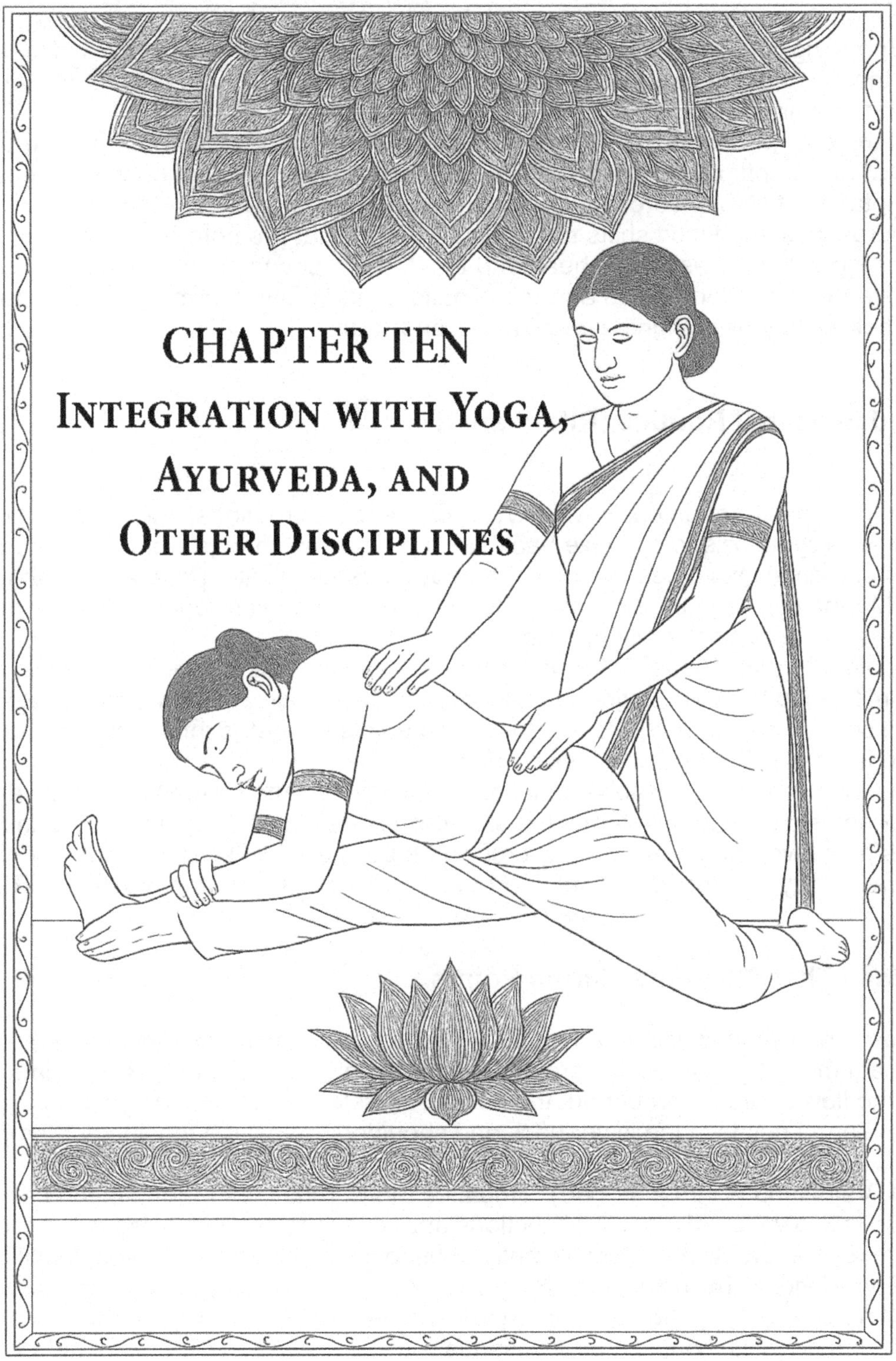

Marma in Ayurvedic Daily Routine (Dinacharya)

Marma therapy, an ancient Ayurvedic technique, is elegantly woven into the fabric of daily routines, termed Dinacharya, to promote sustained health and vitality. The practice begins at dawn, incorporating light stimulation of key Marma points to awaken the body's inner energy at the start of the day. This gentle activation supports the natural rhythms of the body, enhancing alertness and preparing the individual for the day's activities.

Throughout the day, Marma points related to digestion and metabolism are targeted before and after meals to aid in optimal digestion and energy assimilation. This not only enhances nutritional uptake but also ensures that energy levels remain steady.

As night approaches, the focus shifts to calming Marmas that promote relaxation and sleep. A routine involving soft touches on the head and feet Marma points encourages a deep, restorative sleep, crucial for healing and rejuvenation. Integrating Marma into Dinacharya thus supports a holistic balance, aligning body, mind, and spirit.

Marma and Seasonal Routine (Ritucharya)

Marma therapy aligns harmoniously with Ayurvedic seasonal routines, known as Ritucharya, crafting a unique symbiosis to optimize health as the seasons change. Each season, with its distinct environmental influences, impacts the body's doshas - Vata, Pitta, and Kapha. By integrating Marma point stimulation specific to the season, one can regulate these doshas, enhancing resilience against seasonal ailments.

During the cold, dry Vata season, Marma therapy focuses on points that increase warmth and circulation, mitigating the Vata aggravation that leads to dry skin and joint pain. Conversely, in the hot Pitta season, the emphasis shifts to cooling points to soothe inflammation and prevent Pitta-related issues like irritability and skin rashes.

As the monsoon ushers in the Kapha season, stimulating Marma points that enhance digestion, and metabolism is crucial to counteract the sluggishness and congestion typical of increased Kapha. This proactive approach not only fortifies the body against seasonal pathogens but also boosts overall vitality and mood, making Marma a pivotal element in the practice of Ritucharya.

Yoga Asanas That Stimulate Marma Points

Yoga asanas, when aligned with Marma therapy, open a profound dimension of healing and energy management. Specific poses are designed to apply pressure to Marma points, enhancing the flow of prana throughout the body. For instance, Balasana (Child's Pose) gently presses the Marma points in the lower back and shoulders, releasing tension and promoting calmness.

Additionally, Vajrasana (Diamond Pose) stimulates the Kurchashira Marma in the calves and thighs, which is known to aid digestive functions and relieve knee pain. Integrating such postures into regular practice can significantly boost one's vitality and address specific bodily concerns. Furthermore, the inclusion of Bhujangasana (Cobra Pose) targets the Marma points along the spine, invigorating the spinal energies and enhancing respiratory functions.

To maximize the benefits, coupling these asanas with synchronized breathing and mindful focus on the pressure points can lead to profound outcomes, making yoga a dynamic ensemble within Marma therapeutic practices. Regular engagement brings about a noticeable enhancement in one's physical and energy system integrity.

Pranayama and Marma Co-Activation

The convergence of Pranayama and Marma therapy offers a transformative healing approach, enriching both respiratory strength and energy flow. Classical Pranayama practices, such as Nadi Shodhana and Kapalabhati, are utilized to amplify the energy movements through key Marma channels. This co-activation not only enhances pulmonary capacity but also stabilizes the prana within the Nadis, the energy channels, fostering profound inner balance and vitality.
Incorporating Marma points such as Anahata (heart) and Vishuddha (throat) during Pranayama allows for a deeper engagement with the vital energies that govern respiratory and spiritual aspects. Stimulating these Marmas while regulating breathwork creates a feedback loop that intensifies the benefits, promoting clearer breathing pathways and enhancing meditative depth.
To tailor this practice for individual needs, adjustments are made based on one's doshic balance and current state of health. This personalized approach ensures that the dual benefits of enhanced lung function and energized Marma points effectively boost overall health, enabling an enriched sense of well-being.

Marma During Meditation Practices

Marma points serve as vital intersections of life force energy, making their integration into meditation practices a potent tool for enhancing spiritual clarity and physical relaxation. By concentrating on specific Marma points during meditation, practitioners can unlock deeper realms of consciousness and facilitate a more direct connection with their internal energies. This focused engagement promotes a profound sense of peace and alignment between the body and mind.
For example, the Adhipati Marma at the crown of the head is often targeted to enhance meditative depth and spiritual connection. Gentle pressure or visualization of energy at this point can help clarify thoughts and elevate the meditative experience. Similarly, stimulating the Hridaya Marma, located near the heart, during meditation accentuates emotional release and fosters a nurturing space for healing and self-reflection.
Integrating Marma in meditation not only amplifies the physical benefits, such as reducing stress and addressing bodily discomforts but also deepens the spiritual undertones of the practice. This holistic approach enriches the meditative journey, paving the way for a transformative spiritual and physical health experience.

Integration with Ayurveda's Panchakarma Detox

Marma therapy, integrated with Ayurveda’s revered Panchakarma detoxification process, provides a synergistic approach to holistic wellness. Panchakarma, known for its deep cleansing and rejuvenation capabilities, aligns inherently with Marma’s energy touchpoints to enhance therapeutic efficacy. During Panchakarma’s preparatory phase, known as Purvakarma, gentle stimulation of Marma points can amplify the body’s readiness for the detox, making the subsequent procedures both more effective and less taxing on the body.
Key Marma points such as Nabhi (around the navel), which influence the digestive fire, and Kshipra (on the hands and feet), which relate to detoxification, are particularly valuable. Stimulating these points can optimize the elimination of toxins during the primary Panchakarma

treatments like Vamana (therapeutic vomiting) and Virechana (purgation therapy).
In the rehabilitation phase or Pachatkarma, Marma therapy assists in revitalizing the body, restoring energy flow, and balancing the doshas. This integration not only enriches the detox process but also fortifies the body's defenses, enhancing overall vitality and well-being.

Nasya, Basti, and Shirodhara with Marma

Nasya, Basti, and Shirodhara are pivotal Ayurvedic therapies that holistically interact with Marma points to enhance therapeutic outcomes. Nasya involves administering herbal oils or powders through the nasal passages, directly stimulating Marma points within the sinus, throat, and head regions to clear blockages and improve respiratory and neurological functions.
Basti, an Ayurvedic enema, targets the Vasti Marma located in the lower back. By using specific oils and herbal concoctions, Basti influences the digestive and eliminative energies, harmonizing the Vata dosha and promoting detoxification. The synergy between Basti and Marma therapy can profoundly affect the Sakthi Marma (pelvic region), enhancing reproductive and digestive health.
Shirodhara, the gentle pouring of oil on the forehead, calms the mind and soothes the nerves. When integrated with Marma therapy, it targets the Adhipati Marma at the crown, facilitating deep mental relaxation and spiritual awakening, thus advancing a meditative state and emotional balance.

Ayurveda Diet Planning and Marma Activation

The fusion of Ayurvedic diet planning with Marma activation opens a nuanced pathway to personalized health and vitality. Ayurveda emphasizes the importance of tailoring dietary choices to one's unique constitutional type or dosha—Vata, Pitta, and Kapha. When these principles are integrated with Marma therapy, the stimulation of specific energy points can enhance digestive fire (Agni) and optimize nutrient assimilation.
For instance, stimulating the Kshipra Marma on the hands and feet during meals can invigorate the metabolic processes, while the Annavaha Srotas Marmas around the abdomen, when activated, can help in detoxifying and strengthening the gastrointestinal tract. This targeted approach not only boosts digestion but also aligns the body's energies, fostering a balance between physical health and emotional well-being.
Moreover, incorporating specific foods that resonate with the Marma points can amplify these effects. For example, incorporating ghee to soothe Pitta-related Marmas or ginger to activate Vata points ensures that the diet not only nourishes but also heals. This holistic convergence of diet and Marma therapy encapsulates the essence of Ayurvedic wisdom, promising a revitalized and harmonious state of health.

Jyotish Astrology and Marma Diagnostics

Jyotish Astrology, often termed Vedic Astrology, contributes a profound dimension to Marma Chikitsa by enabling diagnostic insights based on cosmic influences. Each astrological chart reveals planetary positions that can influence an individual's physical and energetic health. By correlating these celestial mappings with Marma points, therapists can pinpoint which energy centers may be blocked or weakened, thus customizing treatments to rectify these imbalances. Furthermore, specific transits and dashas (planetary periods) offer timing insights for when an individual is more susceptible to health issues or when treatment might be most effective. This timing, known as Muhurta in Jyotish, can be critically aligned with Marma therapy sessions to enhance efficacy; for example, targeting Kshipra Marma during a Jupiter transit may boost liver function and metabolic health.

Lastly, the integration extends to preventive wellness. By forecasting periods of potential health vulnerability, Jyotish Astrology can guide preemptive Marma treatments to fortify the body's resilience, harmonizing celestial energies with corporeal well-being, thus ensuring a holistic therapeutic approach that enhances longevity and vitality.

Integrating Mantra and Sound with Touch

The practice of integrating mantra and sound with touch in Marma Chikitsa opens a profound gateway to enhanced healing and consciousness. Mantras, when chanted during Marma therapy, vibrationally align the subtle energies at Marma points, magnifying their therapeutic potency. The resonance produced by specific sounds can help unblock or stimulate these energy points, facilitating deeper healing and emotional release.

For example, chanting 'Om' while gently touching the Sthapani Marma between the eyebrows can significantly enhance focus and calm the mind, promoting a higher state of meditation. Similarly, the use of bija mantras like 'Lam' or 'Vam' can be synchronized with touch at the Mooladhara and Swadhisthana Marmas to activate root and sacral energies, supporting grounding and emotional stability.

This fusion not only deepens the physical aspects of healing but also enriches the spiritual experience, fostering a unique blend of body-mind-spirit integration that is central to Ayurvedic medicine. Such holistic practices reinforce the foundation of Marma Chikitsa as a comprehensive modality in the healing arts.

Modern Physiotherapy and Marma Compatibility

The pioneering integration of Marma Chikitsa into modern physiotherapy brings an innovative dimension to holistic health practices. Physiotherapy, primarily focused on restoring movement and function, harmonizes well with Marma therapy, which targets vital energy points to optimize bodily functions and relieve pain. This synergy allows practitioners to enhance their therapeutic approaches, achieving more comprehensive treatment outcomes.

In practice, physiotherapists can adapt Marma techniques to alleviate musculoskeletal conditions by stimulating specific points that increase circulation and reduce muscle tension. For instance, stimulation of the Janu Marma around the knee can significantly aid in knee rehabilitation, blending the precision of physical therapy with the energetic healing of Marma.

Moreover, incorporating Marma therapy provides a dual benefit of addressing both the physical and subtle energy layers, offering a depth of healing that purely physical modalities might not reach. This integration promotes not only quicker recovery but also ensures a holistic balance, vital for long-term wellness and prevention of future injuries.

Acupuncture and Marma Combined Practices

The convergence of acupuncture and Marma Chikitsa represents a remarkable synthesis of two potent healing modalities, each with deep roots in the ancient medical practices of China and India, respectively. Acupuncture, known for its effectiveness in pain relief and addressing various systemic health issues through the stimulation of specific points along the body's meridians, parallels the Marma therapy of Ayurveda, which focuses on vital energy points to enhance health and vitality.

When these practices are integrated, they enhance each other's efficacy and broaden the therapeutic spectrum. For example, simultaneously targeting both acupuncture points and Marma points can lead to a more dynamic flow of energy or Qi (Chi) across the body, optimizing the healing process for conditions like chronic pain, digestive disorders, and emotional imbalances.

This integrative approach not only amplifies the individual strengths of each therapy but also introduces a novel pathway for holistic healing. Patients often report faster improvement in their symptoms, alongside a significant increase in their overall energy levels and well-being.

Reiki and Energy Medicine With Marma

The fusion of Reiki with Marma Chikitsa presents a transformative approach to holistic healing. Reiki, a Japanese technique known for its stress reduction and relaxation properties, channels universal energy through the palms. When integrated with Marma therapy, the energy flow specifically targets Marma points, intensifying the healing impact.

This combination allows practitioners to clear blockages in the subtle energy pathways, enhancing both physical and emotional well-being. For instance, channeling Reiki energy to Anahata Marma can profoundly impact heart health and emotional balance. The synergy elevates the energetic healing process, offering a deeper level of restoration and rejuvenation.

Furthermore, incorporating energy medicine modalities like Reiki with Marma therapy supports the body's natural healing processes. This holistic method amplifies innate vitality, promoting a harmonious balance within the bio-energetic fields. Ultimately, this integration not only aids in alleviating physical ailments but also enriches the spiritual journey, nurturing a profound connection between body and mind.

Siddha Varmam vs. Marma Techniques

Exploring the ancient healing sciences of Siddha Varmam and Marma Chikitsa reveals both similarities and distinct differences. Originating from different cultural baselines within India, both techniques emphasize the manipulation of vital energy points in the body to promote healing and vitality. Siddha Varmam, integral to Siddha medicine primarily practiced in Tamil Nadu, focuses on varmam points that are seen as junctures where life energy resides or passes through.

Conversely, Marma Chikitsa, a facet of Ayurvedic practice prevalent across broader South Asia, involves 107 Marma points which, when stimulated, are believed to directly influence bodily organs and systems, facilitating healing. While both modalities aim at energy manipulation, Siddha Varmam often incorporates martial arts techniques and is somewhat more physically intensive compared to the generally gentle touch of Marma therapy.

Understanding both allows practitioners to adopt a more integrated approach to healing that respects both the therapeutic intensity and the subtle energy nuances each tradition offers, cultivating a comprehensive modality that enhances overall well-being.

Marma and Thai Yoga Therapy Comparison

Exploring the intricate relationship between Marma Chikitsa and Thai Yoga Therapy unveils a fascinating intersection of therapeutic modalities designed to balance energy pathways within the body. Both practices, while originating from different cultural traditions—Marma from ancient India and Thai Yoga from Thailand—focus on energy points that are crucial for healing and vitality restoration.

In Marma Chikitsa, the application involves gentle touches on specific Marma points, linked to various bodily organs and vital systems, which are believed to enhance healing and promote energy flow. Comparatively, Thai Yoga Therapy incorporates a more dynamic interaction with the body through assisted stretches and massages, targeting similar points known as 'Sen' lines, which also aim to improve energy flow and alleviate physical ailments.

While both modalities share a common goal of restoring energy balance, their methodologies differ notably. Marma therapy is generally subtler, emphasizing the energetic impact of gentle touches, whereas Thai Yoga is physically more engaging, employing comprehensive body movements to stimulate energy flow. This comparison not only highlights their uniqueness but also their complementary nature in holistic healing practices.

Integration with Naturopathy and Homeopathy

The integration of Marma Chikitsa with naturopathy and homeopathy creates a holistic trifecta that targets the physical, emotional, and energy systems, promoting comprehensive healing. Naturopathy, grounded in the principle of facilitating the body's inherent ability to heal, encompasses a wide range of natural therapies including herbs, nutrition, and lifestyle modifications. When synergized with Marma Chikitsa, it enhances vital energy flow and balances the doshas, effectively amplifying the body's natural healing processes.

Homeopathy, by contrast, employs a principle of 'like cures like', using minute doses of natural substances to stimulate a healing response. Integrating Marma points activation with homeopathic remedies can lead to a deeper, more nuanced treatment response. This approach not only quickens recovery but also targets root causes of illness, harmonizing body energies and boosting overall vitality.

This distinctive blend of Marma Chikitsa, naturopathy, and homeopathy offers a nuanced dimension to traditional treatments. It enriches the therapeutic landscape by providing a comprehensive, energetically aware protocol that aligns and balances multiple aspects of health, from biochemical pathways to energetic fields.

Biofield and Aura Healing With Marma

Biofield and aura healing are intrinsic components of holistic health, emphasizing the manipulation of the body's energy fields to promote wellness. Marma Chikitsa, with its roots deeply embedded in Ayurvedic traditions, intersects remarkably with these practices by focusing

on vital energy points. Harnessing Marma points for biofield and aura healing facilitates a profound rebalancing mechanism, restoring equilibrium to the body's intrinsic energy fields.
The treatment process involves gentle stimulation of specific Marma points, which correlate with energy centers that influence the aura and biofield. This activation triggers natural healing processes within the body, aligning physical health with emotional and spiritual well-being. The impact is a holistic rejuvenation, noticeable not just physically but resonating through the vibrational fields surrounding everyone.
Practitioners who blend Marma therapy with biofield and aura healing often report enhanced therapy outcomes, witnessing accelerated healing and deeper emotional releases. This synthesis not only amplifies healing potential but also propels the patient towards a more integrated state of health, where energy flows uninterrupted, supporting both body and spirit comprehensively.

Chronotherapy: Marma Activation by Time of Day

Chronotherapy, the practice of synchronizing healing interventions with the body's natural rhythms, finds a unique ally in Marma Chikitsa by integrating time-specific Marma point activation. This alignment with the circadian cycles enhances the efficacy of interventions, tapping into the body's peak energy flows at various times of the day to maximize healing and vitality restoration.
Morning hours, revered for their Vata-pacifying qualities, are ideal for activating Marma points that stimulate mental clarity and physical mobilization. Conversely, evening treatments focus on Kapha-related Marma points, promoting relaxation and detoxification. This time-specific approach ensures that Marma therapy is not only aligned with Ayurvedic principles but also with the physiological needs dictated by the time of day.
Incorporating chronotherapy into Marma Chikitsa empowers practitioners to craft personalized treatment schedules that align vital energy flow with daily biorhythms, facilitating deeper healing and more sustained energy levels throughout the day. This synchronization enhances both immediate relief and long-term wellness, embodying a holistic approach to health.

Healing Environments: Space Energy and Marma

The concept of healing environments merges the architectural and energetic organization of spaces with Marma Chikitsa to create areas that optimize wellbeing. This approach incorporates the principles of Vastu Shastra—the traditional Indian science of architecture and space—to align the physical layout with the energetic grid of Marma points, intensifying the healing potential of a space.
In such environments, everything from room orientation to furniture arrangement is meticulously planned to enhance the flow of prana, or life force. For example, treatment rooms might be oriented to receive morning sunlight, believed to activate specific Marma points that invigorate and cleanse the body energetically. The placement of water features or plants could also be strategically chosen to bolster certain energy fields within the room.
Integrating these elements into the design of wellness centers and spas not only enhances the effectiveness of Marma therapies performed within them but also ensures that every aspect of the client's experience is rooted in the principles of energy alignment. The result is a synergistic blend of environmental design and traditional healing arts, promoting an atmosphere that inherently supports recovery and vitality restoration.

Integration in Wellness Retreats and Spas

Integrating Marma Chikitsa into wellness retreats and spas brings a profound dimension to holistic healing practices, meticulously harmonizing ancient wisdom with modern health paradigms. As guests step away from the stresses of daily life, the introduction of Marma therapy enhances their encounter with serenity and wellness. These spaces are sanctuaries where subtle energies are nurtured and where Marma's therapeutic touch amplifies the healing journey.

In this setting, practitioners can employ a combination of tailored Marma protocols alongside spa treatments such as aromatic massage oils and herb-infused steam, each designed to actuate Marma points that rebalance and revitalize the body's energy pathways. The inclusion of serene music and muted lighting further complements the Marma experience, inviting deeper relaxation and receptivity to the healing effects.

Such integration offers guests not only immediate relief from physical discomfort but also long-lasting improvements in mental clarity and emotional stability. By seamlessly blending the ambiance and treatments, wellness retreats and spas provide an ecosystem that supports comprehensive well-being.

Ayurveda Psychology and Marma Mind Therapy

An exploration of Ayurveda psychology interwoven with Marma Mind Therapy reveals a profound approach to psychological health based on the deep wellspring of Ayurvedic wisdom. This symbiosis articulates not only the treatment of psychological ailments but also the promotion of mental and emotional wellness. Marma points, when specifically targeted, can modulate mental states, therefore offering therapeutic interventions directly influencing mental health.

Marma Mind Therapy incorporates techniques where Marma points associated with psychological attributes are gently stimulated to release emotional blockages and foster mental clarity. This practice is rooted in the understanding that mental wellness is intrinsically linked to the flow of prana (life energy) within the body. Optimizing this flow enhances cognitive functions and emotional resilience, leading to a better stress response and heightened coping strategies.

Ayurveda Psychology, in conjunction with Marma Therapy, not only revitalizes the mind but also harmonizes the spirit, unlocking pathways to profound inner peace and mental stability.

Together, these disciplines craft a holistic paradigm that deeply nourishes and aligns the mind-body continuum, establishing a foundation for lasting psychological well-being.

Aromatherapy and Marma

Aromatherapy, employing essential oils derived from herbs, flowers, and roots, converges gracefully with Marma Chikitsa to enhance healing and vitality across sensory and energy planes. The activation of Marma points through specific aromatic compounds can significantly amplify the therapeutic effects, serving both physical alleviation and aromatic pleasure. This synergy not only heightens the sensory experience but also deepens the therapeutic impact, fostering a pronounced balance within the body's energy systems.

For instance, the application of lavender oil on Marma points could soothe the nervous system, while peppermint might invigorate energy flows at other strategic points. These therapies intertwine seamlessly, each aroma tailored to stimulate corresponding Marma channels that govern emotional and physiological responses, thereby encouraging a comprehensive sense of well-being.

Furthermore, incorporating seasonal aromatherapy with Marma therapy adapts body energies to environmental shifts. Springtime might accentuate floral scents to detoxify channels, while winter calls for warming oils to fortify the system. In this refined dance between scents and touch, every nuance is aimed at harmonizing the life force, thereby restoring vitality and enhancing wellness holistically.

Marma With Crystals and Yantras

Marma therapy, when integrated with crystals and yantras, transcends conventional energy healing, offering a multidimensional approach to revitalizing the body's energy system. Crystals, known for their ability to store and transmit energy, are strategically placed on or around Marma points to amplify the healing vibrations and fine-tune the body's resonance. Clear quartz may enhance clarity and remove energy blockages, while rose quartz can soothe the heart Marma, promoting emotional release.

Yantras, geometric representations of mantras, play a complementary role by anchoring divine energies. When used during Marma therapy, they infuse the treatment space with specific frequencies that correspond to different aspects of consciousness and physiological health. This sacred geometry helps in focusing the healing energies, enhancing the efficacy of the Marma practice.

Together, crystals and yantras create a healing synergy that deeply nurtures the pranic body, facilitating profound transformations in health. This integrative approach not only aligns the physical and energetic entities but also reignites the body's innate healing capabilities.

Breathwork and Trauma Release Marma Combo

The integration of breathwork with Marma Chikitsa in trauma release scenarios presents a groundbreaking therapeutic approach. This combination leverages the profound effects of directed breathing to enhance the activation of Marma points, vital centers in the body where concentrated life energy resides. Through specific breathing techniques, prana—life force—is dynamically circulated, impacting the emotional and physiological systems that store trauma. When trauma is energetically lodged in the body, the application of Marma therapy, in concert with rhythmic breathwork, accelerates the release of these deep-seated emotional blockages. The symbiotic action supports the body's innate healing processes, promoting a release that is both gentle and profound, restoring a sense of balance and peace.

Moreover, this combination augments the healing by stimulating the parasympathetic nervous system, crucial for relaxation and recovery. Practitioners carefully curate breath patterns that resonate with specific Marma points, facilitating a targeted therapeutic effect that is tailored to individual needs, ensuring a holistic restoration of well-being.

Summary

The chapter 'Integration with Yoga, Ayurveda, and Other Disciplines' discusses the seamless incorporation of Marma therapy, a traditional Ayurvedic technique, into various holistic practices, enhancing overall well-being. It covers daily and seasonal routines, specific yoga asanas, Pranayama, meditation, and more intricate integrations with Ayurvedic cleansing therapies and other holistic modalities. Marma points, vital life force intersections, are stimulated in accordance with daily routines, known as Dinacharya, to enhance vital energy from dawn to dusk, optimizing functions like digestion, metabolism, relaxation, and sleep. The seasonal routine, Ritucharya, adapts Marma therapy to seasonal changes, addressing the balance of body doshas — Vata, Pitta, and Kapha — to enhance resilience. Yoga asanas tailored to stimulate specific Marma points enhance energy flow and address bodily concerns, integrating postures like Balasana and Bhujangasana with targeted pressure on these points. Pranayama techniques co-activate Marma points, enriching respiratory strength and energy flow, aligning spiritual and physical domains harmoniously. Furthermore, the integration with Ayurveda's detoxification processes such as Panchakarma leverages Marma points to boost detox efficacy. Marma therapy also extends to other areas like modern physiotherapy, where it aids in musculoskeletal conditions, and traditional therapies like acupuncture, enhancing each other's therapeutic effects. Moreover, energies are combined in practices like Reiki, enhancing healing impacts through Marma points. The chapter emphasizes not just physical healing but also psychological and spiritual wellness, revealing the profound depth and versatility of Marma therapy across various therapeutic and wellness disciplines.

References

[1] Lad, V. (2002). Textbook of Ayurveda. https://www.amazon.com/Textbook-Ayurveda-Fundamental-Principles/dp/1883725070

[2] Frawley, D. (2000). Ayurvedic Healing: A Comprehensive Guide. https://www.amazon.com/Ayurvedic-Healing-Comprehensive-David-Frawley/dp/0914955977

[3] Jouanny, J. (1990). Essentials of Homeopathic Therapeutics. https://www.amazon.com/Essentials-Homeopathic-Therapeutics-Jacques-Jouanny/dp/9990157048

[4] Mishra, L. (2004). Scientific Basis for Ayurvedic Therapies. https://www.crcpress.com/Scientific-Basis-for-Ayurvedic-Therapies/Mishra/p/book/9780849313660

[5] Svoboda, R. E. (1999). Prakriti: Your Ayurvedic Constitution. https://www.amazon.com/Prakriti-Ayurvedic-Constitution-Robert-Svoboda/dp/0965620832

Case Study: Integrating Marma Therapy into Modern Lifestyle Wellness Programs

The case study revolves around the integration of Marma therapy into a comprehensive lifestyle wellness program at a modern holistic health center. The program aims to address the physical, emotional, and energetic needs of a diverse group of clients using a blend of traditional Ayurvedic practices and modern wellness techniques.

To begin with, the center introduced Marma therapy sessions, focusing on personalizing treatments to align with individual health profiles and specific concerns. One example is Emily, a 42-year-old software developer, who experiences chronic back pain and stress from her intense work schedule. During her initial consultation, the practitioner assessed her doshic balance and discovered a predominance of Vata, which often leads to dryness, pain, and anxiety.

As a key part of her treatment, Emily underwent Marma therapy, where the practitioner gently stimulated key Marma points known to alleviate pain and reduce stress. These included the Kurchashira Marma on the legs to help ease leg and back pain, and the Anahata Marma on the chest to calm anxiety and improve emotional resilience. These sessions were combined with guided meditation, using specific mantras to deepen the relaxation response and aid in emotional processing.

Furthermore, the program included dietary recommendations based on Ayurvedic principles, to nurture Emily's doshic balance. Foods that are warm, moist, and grounding were suggested to counteract the dry and erratic nature of Vata. The practitioner also recommended lifestyle adjustments, such as regular sleep hours and warm oil massages using specific oils like sesame to pacify Vata.

This integrated approach not only addressed Emily's immediate physical symptoms but also enhanced her overall emotional and energetic well-being. By the end of the eight-week program, she reported significant reductions in her pain levels, improved sleep quality, and a better capacity to manage stress. This case exemplifies how Marma therapy, when integrated with other holistic practices and tailored to individual needs, can profoundly impact health and wellness.

Case Study: Enhancing Athlete Recovery and Performance with Marma Therapy

This in-depth case study explores the application of Marma therapy in enhancing athletic performance and recovery, focusing on a high-performance sports academy that integrates Ayurvedic practices to support its athletes. The case centers on a professional tennis player, Alex, aged 28, who seeks to improve his recovery times and overall performance through holistic practices. Initially, Alex struggles with recurrent shoulder and knee injuries, which adversely impact his training schedule and performance consistency.

The academy's wellness team, including a sports physiotherapist and an Ayurvedic practitioner, collaborates to design a customized Marma therapy regimen tailored to Alex's specific needs. The program's first phase involves identifying Marma points that correspond to his injury areas and overall energy balance requirements. Vital points such as the Ani Marma, located in the shoulder, and the Janu Marma in the knee, are targeted to alleviate pain and enhance joint mobility. The therapy sessions are meticulously scheduled post-training to optimize recovery and pre-event to enhance performance, utilizing gentle stimulation and specific herbal oils known for their anti-inflammatory properties.

Parallel to Marma therapy, Alex is coached on integrating yoga stretches that focus on the same Marma regions, promoting self-care between therapy sessions. His routine includes poses like Gomukhasana for shoulder flexibility and Virabhadrasana to strengthen the knee joint, reinforcing Marma benefits throughout his training regimen.

Moreover, the program integrates dietary adjustments aligned with his doshic constitution, predominantly Pitta, focusing on cooling and energy-sustaining foods to support intense physical activity and recovery. The holistic regimen culminates in notable improvements over six months: Alex reports a significant reduction in pain, enhanced flexibility, and a marked increase in stamina and performance. Regular Marma therapy, complemented by targeted yoga practices and dietary adjustments, exemplifies a comprehensive approach to athlete care, demonstrating Marma's potential in professional sports settings.

Case Study: Revitalizing Elderly Care with Marma Therapy

The increasing interest in holistic elder care solutions brings forward a unique case study of integrating Marma therapy to enhance the quality of life for the elderly at the Serenity Retirement Home. The program aims to address the common physical ailments and emotional struggles faced by older adults, using Marma therapy not only as a tool for physical health but also as a means for emotional and spiritual healing.

The case centers on Margaret, an 82-year-old widow, who has been experiencing chronic arthritis pain and bouts of depression. Following her initial holistic health assessment, it was noted that her symptoms were exacerbated by a sedentary lifestyle and isolation. The custom-tailored Marma therapy plan included stimulation of specific Marma points associated with joint health and mood enhancement. Key points such as the Janu Marma for her knees and Manibandha Marma for her wrists were targeted to alleviate joint discomfort. Additionally, to uplift her spirits and balance her mental state, the Hridaya Marma around the heart and the Brahmarandhra Marma at the crown of the head were also treated, offering both emotional relief and a sense of spiritual connection.

Beyond individual therapy sessions, the retirement home organized group sessions focusing on gentle Marma stimulation, which encouraged social interaction among residents. During these sessions, practitioners focused on the Anahata (heart) Marma to foster emotional openness and the Svadhisthana (sacral) Marma which is linked to vitality and dynamic energy flow, enhancing communal engagement and overall mood.

Moreover, the integration of Marma therapy was accompanied by senior-friendly yoga classes and meditation sessions. These group activities were designed not only to physically stimulate the Marma points but also to support mental health and community bonding. The comprehensive approach resulted in noticeable improvements in residents' mobility and emotional well-being. Margaret remarked significant reductions in her pain levels and showed more enthusiasm in her daily interactions. Her progress underscores how Marma therapy, when used alongside other complementary practices and within a community setting, can transform elder care by providing a holistic, integrative health solution.

Case Study: Holistic Management of Chronic Migraines Using Marma Therapy

This extensive case study examines the effectiveness of integrating Marma therapy into the treatment plan for chronic migraine sufferers. The focus is on Anita, a 35-year-old graphic designer, who has been dealing with severe migraines for over a decade. Her condition often results in days lost from work and significant disturbances in her daily life. Initial consultations reveal a history of ineffective conventional treatments and a growing interest in alternative therapies.

Anita's treatment began with a detailed assessment of her lifestyle, dietary habits, and previous health records. The Ayurvedic practitioner identified key imbalances in her Pitta dosha, which were believed to be contributing to her migraine attacks. A personalized Marma therapy regimen was designed to specifically target the Marma points known to influence head and neck regions, orchestrate pain relief, and restore doshic balance.

The Marma points such as Sthapani (forehead), Adhipati (crown), and Krikatika (base of the skull) were focused on extensively during sessions. Initial treatments involved gentle stimulation using aromatic oils like sandalwood and mint, known for their cooling properties, which help soothe Pitta. Each session lasted for about 45 minutes, during which Anita experienced gradual relief from the pulsating pain typical of her migraines.

Parallel to Marma therapy, Anita was advised on dietary changes to reduce Pitta exacerbation, including avoiding hot and spicy foods and increasing intake of cooling fruits and vegetables. Inclusion of yoga and meditation helped her manage stress, a significant trigger for her migraines. This combination of treatments aimed to not only relieve the current pain but also reduce the occurrence of future episodes.

After six months of consistent treatment, Anita reported a dramatic reduction in the frequency and intensity of her migraines. The holistic approach, including lifestyle adjustments alongside regular Marma therapy, provided a sustainable method of managing her condition, markedly improving her quality of life. The case highlights the potential of Marma therapy as a pivotal part of integrative health strategies for chronic conditions like migraines. Anita's ongoing commitment to the prescribed lifestyle changes and periodic Marma sessions continues to help maintain her health improvements.

Case Study: Cultivating Wellness Through Marma and Ritucharya: Case Study on Seasonal Adjustment

The intricate alignment of Marma therapy with the Ayurvedic concept of Ritucharya (seasonal routine) offers unique insights into how traditional practices can be entwined to foster holistic health attuned to nature's cycle. This case pertains to Sarah, a 34-year-old teacher experiencing seasonal affective disorder (SAD) and related digestive discomforts, which typically aggravate during the transition from autumn to winter—a period associated with Vata dominance according to Ayurveda. Observing her escalating symptoms, her Ayurvedic practitioner suggests a captivating blend of Marma therapy specific to the season's requirements along with dietary and lifestyle adjustments in line with Ritucharya.

Initial sessions focus on enhancing Sarah's Agni (digestive fire), through stimulation of Marma points like Nabhi (umbilicus area) and Kshipra (base of the thumb and big toe), which are significant in regulating metabolic processes and grounding Vata's airy qualities. Given the cooling and drying nature of the Vata season, the practitioner also introduces sesame oil applications on Sarah's body before sessions to counteract Vata's cold and rough attributes. Season-specific herbal recommendations like ginger tea and warm, mushy foods are suggested to support internal warmth and easy digestibility.

To align with the tranquility of the season and address Sarah's SAD, evening Marma therapy sessions incorporate soothing pressure on the head's Marma points such as Adhipati (crown) and Sthapani (forehead) to calm her nervous system. A ritual inclusion of meditative practices focusing on Anahata (heart) and Manipura (solar plexus) Marma, fosters emotional stability and internal warmth, essential during her challenging months.

Furthermore, Sarah is educated about the influence of lunar cycles on human biorhythms in the context of Vata management, enhancing her engagement with the treatment. After incorporating these tailored therapeutic practices over the course of the season, Sarah reports not only a significant reduction in her physical symptoms but also a noticeable improvement in her emotional resilience and overall energy levels. Her case exemplifies the profound capabilities of integrating Marma therapy with Ritucharya to effectively address seasonal health variations.

Case Study: Integrative Marma Therapy for Postpartum Recovery

The following in-depth case study examines the application of Marma therapy as a vital component in an integrative postpartum recovery program. The subject, Lisa, a 30-year-old first-time mother, experienced significant physical and emotional strain following an arduous labor, leading to postpartum fatigue and anxiety. Traditional postpartum care seemed inefficient in addressing her holistic needs, prompting the integration of Marma therapy into her recovery regimen.

Initially, Lisa's postpartum challenges included severe muscle aches, frequent headaches, and emotional instability, often culminating in anxiety attacks. During her initial evaluation, a specialized practitioner identified imbalances primarily in her Vata and Pitta doshas, which were aggravated due to sleep deprivation and the physical strain of childbirth. A tailored Marma therapy plan was developed, focusing on points that would address both her physical pain and emotional unrest.

Key Marma points such as the Gandusha Marma around the jaw and neck were stimulated to alleviate her headaches and neck stiffness. Similarly, the Hridaya Marma, located near the heart, was targeted to help stabilize her emotional state and reduce anxiety. Sessions were conducted in a quiet, comfortable setting, ensuring Lisa felt relaxed and receptive to the treatment. Soft, calming music and diffused lavender scent created a soothing environment conducive to healing.

Complementarily, Lisa received guidance on postpartum nutrition, focusing on warm, easy-to-digest foods that would help balance her doshas and promote better sleep. Gentle yoga poses and pranayama (breathwork) specifically chosen for postpartum care were also integrated into her daily routine to support her physical healing and mental well-being.

After six weeks of integrated care, Lisa reported significant improvements: a reduction in headaches, more stable mood patterns, and enhanced overall vitality. Her experience highlights the effectiveness of Marma therapy as part of a comprehensive postpartum recovery plan, addressing the multifaceted challenges new mothers may face and underlining the importance of holistic health approaches in postpartum care.

Case Study: Marma Therapy Integration into Corporate Stress Management Programs

The continuous evolution of workplace wellness programs has begun to integrate more holistic approaches to employee health, with Marma therapy emerging as a key component in tackling chronic stress and related ailments. This case study explores the implementation of Marma therapy within a large corporate environment, specifically focusing on a group of mid-level managers at a technology firm who reported high stress levels, poor sleep quality, and recurrent headaches.

The program was initiated with an introductory workshop where an Ayurvedic practitioner explained the principles of Marma therapy and its potential benefits for stress reduction and overall wellness. Following the workshop, interested employees were offered a 12-week program involving weekly Marma therapy sessions tailored to address stress-related symptoms by targeting specific Marma points known for their calming effects, such as the Adhipati Marma on the crown of the head, and Anahata Marma around the heart area.

Participants were also educated on self-care techniques to stimulate Marma points at home, particularly those affecting sleep and relaxation. Techniques included gentle tapping and the application of mild pressure on the Sthapani Marma between the eyebrows, which is traditionally associated with emotional balance and tranquility.

Over the course of the program, the practitioners closely monitored the participants' progress through regular feedback and stress assessments. Adjustments to the therapy were made based on individual responses and changes in symptoms. By the end of the program, participants noted a marked improvement in their stress levels and general health. Many reported better sleep patterns and a significant reduction in headache frequency and intensity.

Moreover, the corporation noted a decrease in employee absenteeism and an improvement in workplace morale. The success of the program prompted the firm to integrate Marma therapy sessions permanently into their annual health initiatives, reflecting a broader trend towards adopting integrative health strategies in corporate wellness programs.

Case Study: Reviving Traditional Healing in Urban Settings: A Marma Therapy Initiative

The surge of interest in alternative medicine brought forth by an increased awareness of self-care and wellbeing practices in urban populations catalyzed the inception of a novel Marma therapy initiative in a bustling metropolis. The initiative, dubbed 'Urban Revive', aimed at integrating ancient Ayurvedic Marma techniques with contemporary wellness needs, focusing on addressing stress, lifestyle diseases, and general malaise prevalent in urban settings.

'Urban Revive' collaborated with local Ayurvedic practitioners and wellness experts to establish a center that was accessible yet serene, balancing the hectic outer city life with a tranquil healing space. Among the highlighted cases was that of John, a 38-year-old IT professional plagued by chronic stress, insomnia, and early signs of hypertension. His lifestyle was typical of many city dwellers - sedentary and high-pressure, with limited attention to personal health regimes.

John's treatment protocol began with a comprehensive assessment of his doshic imbalances, primarily identifying an aggravated Vata, which was manifesting as anxiety and sleep disorders. The chosen treatment regimen involved targeted stimulation of the Marma points such as the Brahmarandhra and Anahata, aiming to relieve mental tension and promote cardiac wellness. Each session was augmented by the soothing sounds of calming music and aromatic herbal oils tailored to soothe Vata dosha.

Parallel to Marma therapy, John participated in workshops designed to teach participants about managing stress through mindfulness and Ayurvedic nutrition. These workshops incorporated practical tips on integrating Marma self-massage techniques into daily routines, aimed at fostering independence in maintaining health and preventing disease.

Upon concluding a six-month series of bi-weekly Marma sessions, John reported a significant improvement in his sleep patterns and a noticeable reduction in his stress levels. His blood pressure also stabilized, which he attributed to the holistic treatment regimen. The success of John's case strongly advocated for the relevance of Marma therapy in modern urban health management, showcasing how traditional practices can be revitalized to complement and enhance contemporary lifestyle.

Case Study: Combining Marma Therapy with Advanced Rehabilitative Techniques for Stroke Recovery

This comprehensive case study examines the integration of Marma therapy with modern rehabilitative techniques in the management and recovery of stroke patients. The case centers around Michael, a 60-year-old retired bank manager, who suffered an ischemic stroke, leading to right-sided paralysis and speech difficulties.

Following the initial medical interventions, Michael's recovery plateau was significant, with modest improvements in mobility and communication. His daughter, familiar with holistic approaches, sought out an innovative recovery plan incorporating Marma therapy alongside his conventional stroke rehabilitation program. The goal was to enhance his neuroplasticity and holistic recovery through an integrated approach.

A specialized neuro-rehabilitation team, including a physiotherapist and an Ayurvedic practitioner trained in Marma therapy, designed a personalized treatment protocol. Their plan targeted Marma points that potentially stimulate neural activity and enhance circulation, particularly those along the head, spine, and extremities associated with motor function and speech articulation.

Therapy sessions began with gentle manipulation of the Brahmarandhra Marma at the crown and the Sthapani Marma on the forehead to address cognitive functions and communication faculties. This was complemented by physiotherapeutic exercises aimed at strengthening physical mobility. The Marma points such as the Kshipra Marma on the hands and Gulpha Marma on the ankles were also targeted to improve fine motor skills and overall limb responsiveness.

Additionally, Michael's regimen included nutritional guidance based on Ayurvedic principles to support nerve health and reduce Vata aggravation, recognized as a contributing factor in neural instability post-stroke. The dietary adjustments focused on grounding and nourishing foods to help rebuild strength and vitality.

Over several months, Michael exhibited notable improvements. His speech clarity increased, and motor skills improved significantly, as evidenced by his ability to perform finer tasks like writing and self-feeding. The integrated approach not only accelerated his physical rehabilitation but also enhanced his mental and emotional resilience, demonstrating the potential of combining Marma therapy with conventional rehabilitative techniques in stroke recovery.

Case Study: Optimizing Mental Health and Emotional Resilience Through Marma Therapy

This extensive case study explores the effectiveness of Marma therapy integrated into a mental health and wellness program aimed at individuals suffering from chronic stress, anxiety, and mild to moderate depressive disorders. The focal point of this study is Brenda, a 40-year-old school administrator, dealing with stress-induced anxiety and recurrent depressive episodes, exacerbated by the challenging dynamics of her professional environment.

The intervention began with a thorough holistic assessment conducted by an Ayurvedic practitioner, specializing in psychological wellness, who mapped out Brenda's doshic imbalances, focusing particularly on her elevated Vata and aggravated Pitta, which often manifest as anxiety and irritability, respectively. A customized therapeutic plan was tailored to address these imbalances through the stimulation of specific Marma points associated with emotional and mental regulation.

Key focus areas included the Hridaya Marma to promote emotional balance, the Ajna Marma to enhance mental clarity, and the Sthapani Marma to relieve stress headaches. Each session involved gentle, methodical stimulation of these points using soothing herbal oils like Brahmi and Jatamansi, known for their efficacy in calming the mind and nurturing the nervous system.

Parallel to the Marma therapy, Brenda was counseled on incorporating meditative practices into her routine. Guided sessions focusing on mindfulness and centered breathing techniques were provided to deepen her stress management strategies. Additionally, dietary recommendations were customized to include nourishing meals rich in grounding and cooling properties, such as sweet juicy fruits and cooling vegetables like cucumbers, to mitigate Pitta and balance Vata.

Over the course of six months, Brenda experienced a pronounced decrease in her anxiety levels and noted substantial improvements in her overall mood. Regular Marma therapy sessions augmented her ability to manage stress and cultivated greater emotional resilience. This integrative approach not only alleviated Brenda’s clinical symptoms but also significantly enhanced her quality of life, demonstrating the profound impact of Marma therapy when effectively incorporated into mental health treatment programs.

Review Questions

1. A 32-year-old female yoga instructor, who has been teaching various yoga asanas that stimulate Marma points, feels a significant increase in her vitality. She incorporates Balasana regularly in her sessions due to the common shoulder and back tension her students face. Which Marma point is most likely being stimulated in Balasana for releasing tension?
A) Vajrasana
B) Anahata
C) Sthapani
D) Adhipati
Answer: D
Explanation: Balasana, known as Child's Pose, is used in yoga to create a calming effect on the nervous system and to release tension in the back and shoulder areas. The pose involves resting the forehead on the ground, which gently stimulates the Adhipati Marma point located at the crown of the head. This stimulation is known to help in calming the mind, reducing stress, and alleviating physical tension in the upper part of the body, thereby enhancing relaxation and rejuvenation.

2. A 45-year-old male patient undergoes Pranayama sessions to improve his respiratory health. His therapist incorporates Marma therapy by focusing on two specific points during his breathing exercises. If the aim is to enrich respiratory and spiritual health, which Marma points are likely being targeted?
A) Anahata and Vishuddha
B) Vishuddha and Sthapani
C) Anahata and Sthapani
D) Kurchashira and Kshipra
Answer: A
Explanation: During Pranayama sessions focused on enhancing both respiratory and spiritual health, the Anahata (heart) and Vishuddha (throat) Marma points are typically targeted. Stimulating the Anahata point affects the cardiac region and emotional well-being, supporting deeper emotional release and respiratory improvements. The Vishuddha point, located at the throat, directly influences the respiratory tract and communication abilities, thereby fostering better breath control and spiritual communication.

3. A 39-year-old female, who frequently experiences joint pain and digestive issues during the Vata season, consults an Ayurvedic practitioner. The practitioner decides to use Marma therapy to alleviate her symptoms. Which Marma points are most appropriate to stimulate to increase warmth and circulation thus addressing her Vata aggravation?
A) Nabhi and Kshipra
B) Kurchashira and Hridaya
C) Kurchashira and Nabhi
D) Adhipati and Hridaya
Answer: C
Explanation: In Marma therapy, Kurchashira and Nabhi points are pivotal during the Vata season, which is characterized by cold and dry conditions. Stimulating the Kurchashira Marma, found in the calves and thighs, enhances circulation and warmth, thus mitigating joint pain associated with Vata aggravation. The Nabhi Marma, located around the navel, is crucial for stimulating digestive fire which helps in combating the digestive issues that often worsen during colder months. Targeting these points effectively reduces the symptoms by balancing the Vata dosha.

CHAPTER ELEVEN: Regional Practices – Marma Across Asia

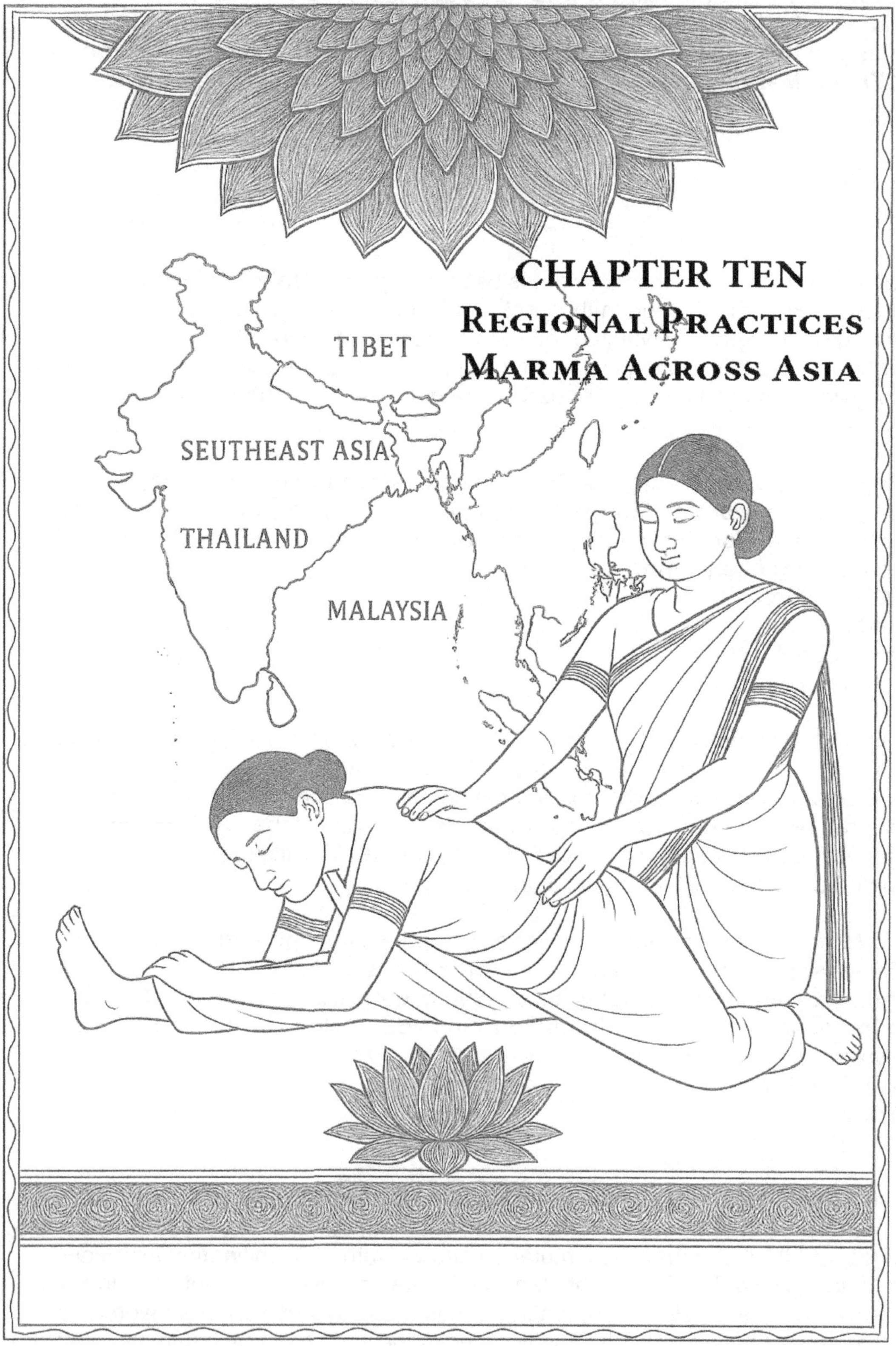

Kalari Marma in Kerala, India

In the lush landscapes of Kerala, India, the ancient martial art of Kalaripayattu intertwines seamlessly with Marma Chikitsa, forming a distinctive tradition known as Kalari Marma. This holistic approach not only emphasizes physical prowess but also integrates the profound knowledge of vital energy points—marmas—to heal and invigorate the body.
Practitioners of Kalari Marma possess a deep understanding of the human anatomy, focusing on 107 marma points that are considered gateways to body and mind rejuvenation. During training or healing sessions, these points are stimulated through precise strikes or gentle touches, promoting the flow of prana, or life force, thereby enhancing vitality and strength.
The practice is revered not only for its combat techniques but also for its therapeutic efficacy. It addresses a range of ailments from muscle injuries to emotional imbalances, making it a revered component of traditional wellness in Kerala. Kalari Marma showcases the intricate bond between martial prowess and energy healing, embodying a legacy of health and discipline.

Siddha Varmam in Tamil Nadu

In the heart of Tamil Nadu, the ancient Siddha medicine tradition thrives, encapsulating the profound practice of Varmam. Unlike other regional therapies, Siddha Varmam is deeply entrenched in siddhar wisdom, focusing on 'varma points' which are considered pivotal energy junctures capable of unlocking profound healing and rebalancing the body's energies.
Masters of Siddha Varmam are known as varmam asans, who possess an intricate understanding of these points, utilizing them to both heal and harm - a knowledge traditionally guarded with fervent secrecy. These healing sessions frequently accompany holistic siddha treatments like herbal medicines and rigorous lifestyle adjustments, aiming to achieve a symbiotic restoration of physical and spiritual health.
This remarkable system of healing is not merely medical but is intertwined with Tamil culture, reflecting in martial arts, dance, and spiritual practices. Through public demonstrations and teachings in cultural festivals, Siddha Varmam remains a vibrant, living tradition that continues to fascinate and heal across generations.

Marma in Sri Lankan Ayurveda

In the verdant realm of Sri Lanka, the ancient wisdom of Ayurveda permeates deeply, with Marma Chikitsa emerging as a pivotal aspect of traditional healing practices. Unique to Sri Lankan Ayurveda is the integration of local herbal lore and Buddhist philosophies, which enrich the understanding and application of Marma therapy. This confluence creates a distinctive healing modality focused on revitalizing both the physical and spiritual planes of existence.
Practitioners, often monks or traditional healers, are adept at identifying and manipulating specific Marma points that correlate with the Ayurvedic principles of Vata, Pitta, and Kapha. Their skilled touch, coupled with chants and meditative techniques, is believed to release blockages and restore the body's inherent balance. The lush island's biodiversity provides a rich arsenal of herbal preparations that are topically applied during Marma sessions, enhancing the therapeutic effect.
Marma therapy in Sri Lanka also extends into preventive care, educating individuals on daily routines and self-care Marma practices. This holistic approach not only addresses acute

ailments but also promotes long-term health resilience, making it a revered component of Sri Lankan Ayurveda.

Nepalese Marma Traditions and Monastic Healing

In the shadow of the Himalayas, Nepal's Marma traditions flow deeply through its monastic communities, serving as both spiritual and physical therapy. Monks, who are custodians of this esoteric knowledge, apply Marma techniques to cultivate healing and spiritual enlightenment. These practices are often intertwined with Buddhist teachings, enhancing the holistic nature of the healing process.

The techniques used in Nepalese Marma involve precise manipulations of vital points to stimulate the body's innate healing abilities. This is often complemented by herbal remedies sourced from the abundant local flora, which are believed to possess potent energetic properties that amplify the effects of Marma therapy. The monks' deep understanding of the interconnection between body and spirit guides their application, ensuring a treatment that addresses both physical ailments and spiritual well-being.

Nepal's Marma practices are not merely medical interventions but are considered a way of life that harmonizes the energies of the body with the rhythms of nature. Through public festivals and private sessions within monastery walls, these sacred practices are preserved and passed down through generations, embodying a rich legacy of holistic health and spiritual integrity.

Tibetan Kunye Therapy and Marma Points

In the serene expanse of Tibet, the traditional practice of Kunye therapy merges seamlessly with the principles of Marma Chikitsa, creating a unique and holistic form of healing known locally as 'Kunye Marma'. This method combines gentle massage techniques, utilizing not only the hands but also traditional tools like stones and sticks to stimulate specific Marma points across the body.

Kunye therapy emphasizes the balance of the body's elemental energies—earth, water, fire, air, and space. By targeting these energies through Marma points, practitioners facilitate a deep healing process that addresses both physical ailments and emotional disturbances. The inclusion of aromatic oils and warming herbs in the treatment enhances the therapeutic impact, promoting relaxation and energy flow.

These sessions often take place in monastic settings, surrounded by the tranquil landscapes of Tibet, which adds to the therapeutic ambiance. The holistic approach of Kunye Marma respects the body's wisdom and innate capacity to heal, embodying the spirit of Tibetan medicinal practices.

Thai Massage and Sen Lines vs. Marma

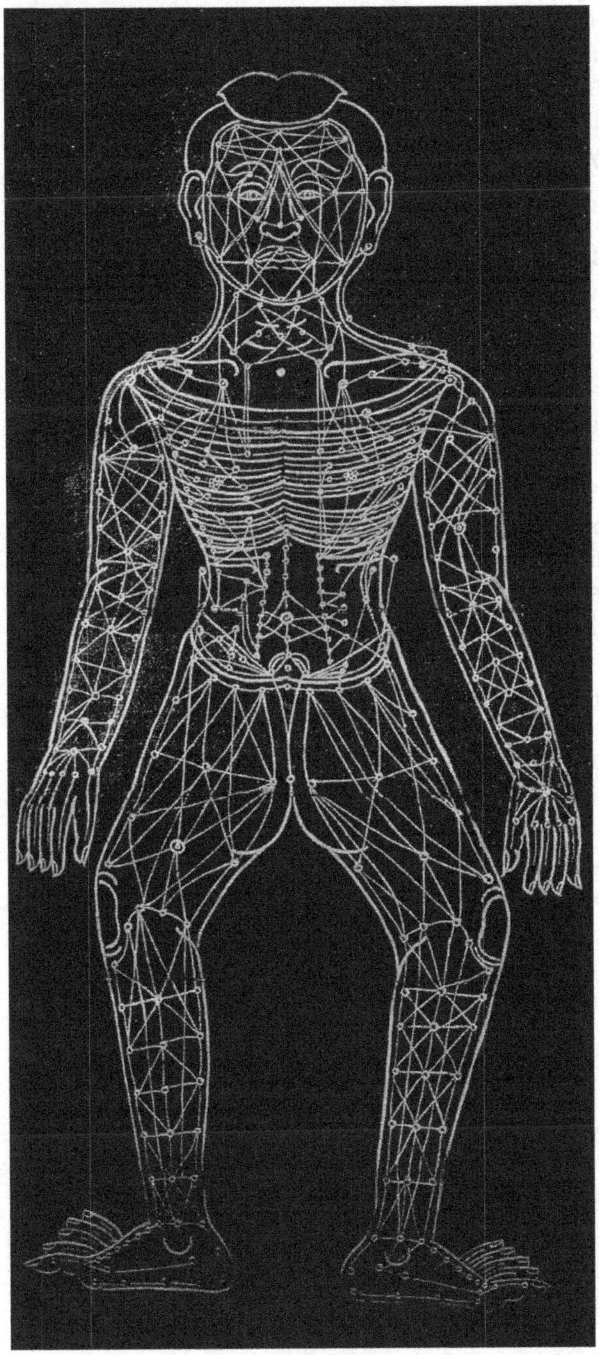

In the tranquil heart of Thailand, Traditional Thai Medical Massage, or '*Ryksaa Thang Nuad Phaen Boran Thai*', transcends mere physical therapy, intertwining deeply with spiritual and healing traditions. Central to this practice are the 'Sen Lines', pathways of flowing life energy akin to Nadis in Ayurveda. While Marma points in Ayurveda specifically target junctures of vital life forces, Thai Massage stimulates these Sen Lines, promoting an unblocking of energy that enhances holistic wellness.

The dance-like rhythm of a Thai Massage, with its stretching and calm syncopation, contrasts

with the more static pressure applied on Marma points. Despite the differences, both practices share a profound respect for the body's hidden energies and potential for self-healing. Thai therapists use their hands, elbows, and sometimes even feet to engage with these lines, suggesting a dynamic, whole-body approach to healing.
This juxtaposition highlights not just a cultural exchange but also a deep, mutual understanding that spans across borders - from the Indian subcontinent to the heart of Southeast Asia. Both modalities thrive on a philosophy of balance, energy, and the subtle science of life itself.

Balinese Healing Touch and Marma Analogs

In the verdant landscapes of Bali, the traditional art of healing transcends mere physical touch, weaving ancient local practices with Marma Chikitsa to form a unique therapeutic experience known as Balinese Healing Touch. This method leverages not only the island's ancient wisdom but also parallels the holistic principles found in Marma therapy, focusing intensely on vital energy points that rejuvenate both body and spirit.
Bali's healers, revered in their communities, incorporate gentle finger pressure, soothing strokes, and harmonious movements that closely mirror the Marma techniques, aimed at unblocking energy pathways and fostering deep relaxation. This synchronization of therapies offers a profound healing experience, bolstered by the island's serene environment and the spiritual ambiance that permeates its culture.
The amalgamation of Balinese modalities with Marma analogs represents a rich tapestry of cultural healing wisdom. As a vital part of holistic tourism, these practices not only draw visitors worldwide but also preserve the deep-rooted traditions that define Balinese spiritual and medicinal practices.

Chinese Meridian Theory vs. Marma Channels

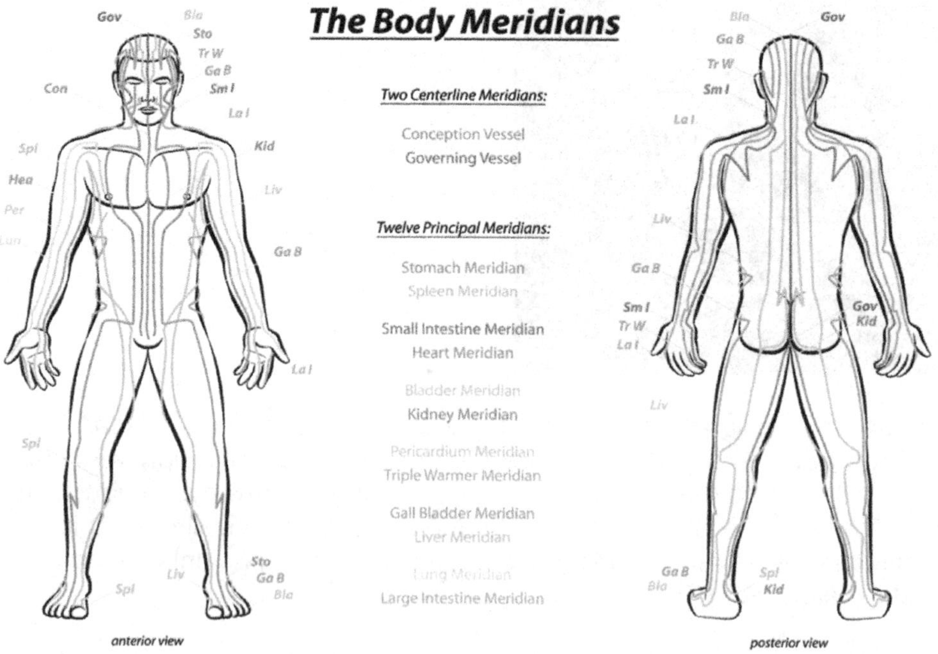

In the intricate world of healing, both Chinese Meridian Theory and Marma Channels from Ayurveda serve as fundamental systems for understanding bioenergetic pathways. Chinese Meridian Theory revolves around the flow of 'Qi' or vital energy through specific pathways, integral to practices like acupuncture and Qigong. These meridians, counting twelve primary and numerous secondary paths, are believed to influence physical and emotional health by regulating internal balance.

Contrastingly, Marma Channels center on 107 vital points which, when stimulated, unlock profound therapeutic benefits aligning with the Ayurvedic elements of air, fire, water, earth, and space. These points, encompassing both physical and ethereal aspects, are strategic gates where flesh, veins, arteries, tendons, bones, and joints converge, influencing energy flow and organ function.

Despite their distinct origins and philosophies, the comparison reveals a shared core belief: the body as a map of invisible paths crucial to health. Understanding these nuances not only respects their cultural heritage but also underscores a global interconnectivity in holistic healing.

Japanese Shiatsu and Marma

In the serene ambiance of Japan, the traditional practice of Shiatsu presents a fascinating parallel to Marma Chikitsa. Shiatsu, meaning 'finger pressure,' involves rhythmic sequences of pressure applied to specific points across the body, much like the stimulation of Marma points in Ayurvedic medicine. These pressure points in Shiatsu are believed to align closely with the pathways of energy, or 'Ki', akin to the 'Prana' in Marma therapy.

The technique, deeply rooted in the principles of traditional Chinese medicine, also reflects the holistic spirit found in Marma. Both therapies underscore the belief in the body's innate ability to heal itself. Shiatsu practitioners use palms, fingers, and even elbows to restore balance and enhance the body's natural healing capabilities, echoing the Marma practice of using pressure to release energy blocks.

This integration of body, mind, and spirit in Japanese Shiatsu enriches the understanding and application of Marma across Asia. Both modalities, nurturing the subtle dance of life energies, offer a profound pathway to health and vitality, bridging traditional wisdom with contemporary practices.

Bhutanese Energy Healing and Marma

In the mystical landscape of Bhutan, traditional energy healing practices intertwine with the principles of Marma Chikitsa, converging into a holistic healing technique deeply embedded in local spirituality and medicinal wisdom. Bhutanese "*Serkhap*" (Golden Needle Therapy) is a unique and indigenous medical practice within Bhutan's traditional healing system, known as "*gSo-ba Rig-pa*. "It integrates spiritual, physical, and energetic principles rooted in Buddhist philosophy and Tibetan medicine. Below is an overview of Serkhap therapy, its spiritual foundations, techniques, integration with other modalities, and supporting references.

Known for their serene monastic life and profound connection with nature, Bhutanese healers employ an intimate understanding of energy channels that closely mirror the Marma points recognized in Ayurveda. These healers, often monks or spiritual practitioners, use subtle touches and pressure on specific points to release blockages and restore energy flow. This method is not only therapeutic but also deeply spiritual, providing both physical relief and spiritual harmony. Integrating chants and meditative practices enhances the effectiveness of the treatments, aligning the patient's body and spirit with the rhythmic energies of the universe.

The practice is revered in local communities and remains a vital part of Bhutan's cultural heritage, promoting health and spiritual well-being while maintaining a sacred link to ancient healing traditions. This unique therapeutic approach stands as a testament to the enduring power of integrated bodily and energetic health practices across Asian cultures.

Mongolian Bone Setting and Pressure Points

Mongolia, with its vast steppes and nomadic heritage, harbors unique traditional practices, among which bone setting and pressure point therapy stand prominent. These techniques, deeply embedded in the rugged lifestyle of its people, offer a pragmatic yet profound approach to healing. Bone setting, known locally as 'Zetkik,' involves manual adjustment of the skeletal structure, while focused pressure is applied to specific points, similar in concept to Marma points, to alleviate pain and restore bodily functions.

The practice is not just a medical intervention but a cultural rite, passed down through generations of Mongolian herders and warriors, emphasizing resilience and holistic wellness. The healers, often elderly and respected members of the community, possess an intimate knowledge of the human anatomy, guided equally by tradition and intuitive experience.

This therapeutic symbiosis between bone setting and pressure point manipulation reflects a broader Asiatic narrative where physical and energetic healing intertwines. Mongolian methods, though less known globally, represent a rich motif in the tapestry of regional Marma practices, highlighting both diversity and interconnectedness in Asian healing traditions.

Indigenous Malaysian Practices and Marma

In the lush greenery of Malaysia, a quietly practiced form of Marma Chikitsa merges with indigenous healing methodologies, manifesting in unique therapeutic approaches. Rooted deeply in Malaysian culture, these practices reflect a profound understanding of natural remedies and body energy points like those in Ayurveda. Local healers, often regarded as repositories of communal knowledge, apply their skills with intuitive precision, focusing on vital points to align and rejuvenate the body's energy flow.

This integration extends to the use of local herbs and rituals that enhance the therapeutic effects, embodying a holistic approach to healing. The application of pressure, coupled with herbal poultices, is common, mirroring the Marma principle of unlocking energy pathways to promote healing and wellness. Village elders and traditional healers often pass these techniques down through generations, preserving a rich heritage of natural health care.

The confluence of traditional Malaysian and Marma practices continues to support local health while contributing to a larger tapestry of Asiatic healing arts. This synergy not only enriches the cultural narrative but also underlines the universality of using body points in traditional medicine across Asia.

Vietnamese Marma-Like Therapies

Vietnamese traditional medicine, with its rich tapestry dating back to indigenous roots, presents a unique approach parallel to Marma Chikitsa. Known as 'Cẩm nang,' these local practices involve the stimulation of specific body points to harmonize and revitalize the body's energy flow, echoing the fundamental concepts found in Ayurvedic Marma therapy.

These therapeutic techniques are often intertwined with local folklore and spiritual beliefs, attributing healing powers not just to physical touch but also to the energy infusions from the natural surroundings. Practitioners, usually elder community healers, apply manual pressures and sometimes integrate herbal applications to enhance the therapeutic effects.

The resemblance these methods hold to Marma is profound, showcasing a shared belief in the crucial role of energy channels in health and healing across different cultures. Despite the geographical and cultural distances, both practices aim at mastering the hidden flows of life energy, providing a compelling example of the universal application of energy-based healing systems.

Thus, Vietnamese Marma-like therapies enrich the dialogue on cross-cultural health practices, highlighting enduring communal knowledge and its integration with universal healing principles.

Korea's Traditional Chuna and Marma Overlap

In the culturally rich landscape of Korea, the traditional Chuna therapy offers intriguing similarities with Marma Chikitsa. Chuna, a form of manual manipulation used in Korean medicine, focuses on correcting bodily imbalances through targeted adjustments, akin to the Marma technique of activating vital energy points to enhance healing.

Chuna practitioners, much like Marma therapists, believe in the intrinsic healing power of the body and utilize strategic touches to realign the spine, joints, and musculoskeletal structures. This not only alleviates physical ailments but also stimulates the energy flow, enhancing overall vitality—a core principle in both Chuna and Marma practices.

The integration of these methods within Korea's medical framework illustrates a significant cultural exchange. Both systems embody a holistic approach, viewing the patient's wellness through a combined lens of physical alignment and energetic health. As a result, the overlap between Chuna and Marma not only enriches Korean therapeutic offerings but also bridges traditional Asian health practices, underscoring a shared heritage of healing wisdom.

Cultural Rituals of Marma in Asia

Across the diverse landscapes of Asia, cultural rituals involving Marma Chikitsa form a fascinating tapestry of ancient healing wisdom. These ceremonies are deeply interwoven with local traditions, folk beliefs, and communal spirituality, reflecting the holistic view of health and healing prevalent in Asian civilizations.

In many Asian cultures, Marma therapy is not solely a curative practice but a part of significant life events such as births, marriages, and even harvest festivals. For instance, in rural India, specific Marma points are gently stimulated during wedding ceremonies to ensure vitality and harmonious energy flow between couples. Similarly, during planting or harvest times, community healers perform Marma rituals to invoke blessings for abundance and communal well-being.

These practices are often accompanied by ancient chants and specific herbal applications, creating a ceremonial atmosphere that enhances the therapeutic effects. Thus, Marma not only cures physical ailments but also supports spiritual and communal health, maintaining a balance that has been revered through generations.

Healing Ceremonies Involving Marma in Sri Lanka

In Sri Lanka, healing ceremonies involving Marma take a distinctively vibrant form, deeply rooted in ancient spiritual and medicinal traditions. These ceremonies, often presided over by Ayurvedic experts and spiritual leaders, are integral to Sri Lankan cultural and health practices. They beautifully blend the mysticism of religious rituals with the empirical wisdom of Marma therapy, providing a holistic approach to health that resonates deeply with the local populace.

One notable practice involves elaborate rituals during full moon nights, believed to enhance the energetic potency of Marma treatments. Participants, adorned in traditional attire, gather in sacred spaces, where healers perform precise Marma manipulations amid chants and drum rhythms, aligning spiritual energies with bodily ones. This practice not only aims at physical healing but also spiritual cleansing and emotional well-being.

Furthermore, these ceremonies often commemorate seasonal festivals and life milestones, tying the community together under the auspices of wellness and shared heritage. Through these communal gatherings, Marma therapy transcends its role as mere physical treatment, embodying a pivotal element of Sri Lankan societal and spiritual life.

Martial Arts and Marma in Kalari and Silat

Marma Chikitsa intertwines deeply with the martial traditions of Asia, particularly in the distinct practices of Kalari in Kerala, India, and Silat across Malaysia and Indonesia. Kalari, one of the oldest fighting systems in existence, integrates Marma points into its training, enabling practitioners to both heal and inflict pain with precision. This martial art emphasizes the synchronization of body, mind, and energy flow, utilizing knowledge of Marma points to enhance strength and spiritual energy.

Silat, although diverse in its forms, shares a similar trait where fighters use knowledge of vital points to subdue adversaries. This approach is not merely about combat efficiency but is also therapeutic, as the correct stimulation of these points can also heal injuries and rebalance the body's energy.

This profound integration of Marma within these martial arts underscores a holistic approach to the warrior's path, where healing and combat are inextricable, reflecting a deep respect for life's dualities. Thus, Marma Chikitsa serves as both a warrior's tool and a healer's balm.

Traditional Healing Songs and Prayers

In the realms of Marma Chikitsa across Asia, traditional healing songs and prayers are integral, weaving a spiritual dimension into the therapeutic practices. These auditory elements are believed to amplify the healing energies during Marma sessions. Local healers often recite ancient mantras or sing sacred songs, which resonate with the vibrational frequencies of the body's marma points, facilitating deeper healing and energetic balance.

In cultures where oral traditions predominate, these songs and prayers are passed down through generations, encapsulating the ancestral wisdom of Marma therapy. The specific intonations and rhythms are tailored to invoke natural elements which are associated with the body's energy centers, enhancing the therapeutic impact of the physical manipulations conducted by the practitioners.
Moreover, these healing songs often accompany important communal and spiritual events, thereby enriching the cultural tapestry of Marma practices. They serve not only as therapeutic tools but also as a bridge connecting the community through shared spiritual and healing experiences, reinforcing the holistic nature of Marma Chikitsa.

Esoteric Schools of Marma Knowledge

Within the vast expanses of Asia, esoteric schools of Marma Knowledge remain closely guarded, enigmatic sources of profound healing wisdom. These schools, often veiled in secrecy, operate on the periphery of mainstream Ayurvedic practices, and hold the keys to ancient techniques that delve deep into human energy systems. Entrusted to a select few, the teachings focus on mastering the intricate energy channels and vital points that govern physiological and spiritual health.
The curriculum in these schools bypasses conventional learning; instead, it emphasizes direct transmission of knowledge from master to pupil, a method preserving the purity and power of their practices. Each school maintains its unique set of philosophies and techniques, tailored according to their geographical and cultural contexts, which enrich the diversity within the Marma tradition. The rituals, often suffused with spiritual undertones, serve as both therapeutic and transformative experiences for the initiated.
Viewed with a blend of reverence and mystique, these schools not only perpetuate ancient knowledge but also explore new dimensions of healing, continuously evolving while staying rooted in tradition. Their practices, while elusive to the public eye, contribute significantly to the cultural heritage and medicinal landscape of Asia, bridging ancient wisdom with contemporary needs.

Secret Manuscripts and Lineages

The realm of Marma Chikitsa, rich in its diversity and depth across Asia, is intricately linked to secret manuscripts and lineages that have safeguarded its esoteric teachings for centuries. These texts, often written in ancient scripts and stored in monastic libraries or private collections, comprise detailed methodologies for mastering Marma points and energy channels. These lineages, typically familial or tied to specific spiritual schools, are charged with the preservation and passing on of knowledge. The process of learning and mastery involves rigorous discipline and a deep spiritual commitment, typically under the guidance of a guru or master. Rare glimpses into these manuscripts reveal a complex system of healing that transcends mere physical touch, delving into the realms of energy manipulation and spiritual healing.
Ultimately, these manuscripts and the lineages that protect them are not merely historical artifacts but living streams of knowledge. They offer a continuous link to the past, ensuring the survival and purity of Marma Chikitsa across generations, adapting subtly with each new custodian of their secrets.

Common Themes Across Asian Practices

Across the diverse landscapes of Asia, Marma Chikitsa reveals shared thematic threads woven into the fabric of regional healing traditions. Despite variations in methodology and cultural expressions, a common commitment to holistic well-being and the integration of spiritual elements with physical healing pervades these practices.

Central to these is the understanding of the body as an interconnected system where energy flows through specified points. Whether it is through the rhythmic pressures of Thai massage or the precise touch in Japanese Shiatsu, the manipulation of these energy paths is aimed at restoring balance and enhancing life force.

Moreover, the reverence for knowledge passed through generations—be it via secret manuscripts in China or esoteric schools in Tibet—highlights a deep respect for ancestral wisdom. This shared heritage fosters a collective identity among practitioners, transcending national boundaries and creating a pan-Asian tapestry of therapeutic knowledge.

Thus, Marma Chikitsa not only offers physical alleviation but also serves as a spiritual bridge, connecting individuals to both their cultural roots and universal energies.

Comparative Tables: Techniques and Points

The comparative tables of Marma Chikitsa techniques and points across Asia offer a unique vista into this ancient healing art. These tables juxtapose diverse methodologies from various cultures, showcasing differences and similarities in approach and application. One might see, for example, how the precise finger pressures in Japanese Shiatsu align with or diverge from the deep palm presses employed in Thai massage, both manipulating vital Marma points but with nuanced techniques influenced by their cultural ethers.

Furthermore, these tables not only catalog different techniques but also outline the specific Marma points targeted within each regional practice. This allows for a deeper understanding of how local geography and culture influence the interpretation and prioritization of energy points. For instance, the focus on abdominal Marma points in Balinese healing touch contrasts with the emphasis on spinal points in Tibetan Kunye Therapy.

Thus, these comparative insights serve not merely as academic knowledge but also as practical guides for practitioners and enthusiasts seeking to explore Marma Chikitsa's rich diversity. They enhance the practitioner's ability to integrate these techniques, fostering a more holistic approach to healing that respects and utilizes the vast tapestry of Asian medical traditions.

Healing Centers in Asia Using Marma

Across Asia, specialized healing centers have emerged as bastions of Marma Chikitsa, dedicated to the practice and preservation of this ancient healing art. These centers, often nestled in regions rich in Ayurvedic tradition, provide a sanctuary not only for pain relief and disease reversal but for the profound revitalization of vitality through energy healing. From the lush landscapes of Kerala to the vibrant streets of Kathmandu, these institutions have become pivotal in fostering holistic well-being.

Each center, while adhering to the core principles of Marma therapy, incorporates local healing practices and herbs, creating a unique blend of traditional and regional treatments. The

therapists, often trained in age-old lineages, wield deep knowledge of energy pathways and Marma points, skilled in tailoring their approach to individual needs.
Furthermore, some of these centers are involved in educational initiatives, aiming to train new generations of practitioners. They hold workshops and courses, spreading awareness and understanding of Marma Chikitsa's benefits. These centers not only serve as healing hubs but also as cultural preservation sites, maintaining and revitalizing ancient wisdom in modern times.

Government Recognition and Regulation

The role of government in recognizing and regulating Marma Chikitsa varies significantly across Asia, reflecting diverse medical paradigms and cultural valorizations of traditional practices. In countries like India, where Ayurvedic therapies like Marma are deeply intertwined with national heritage, there is substantial formal recognition. Institutions govern standards, certifying practitioners and overseeing educational frameworks to maintain the integrity and efficacy of these ancient treatments.
Conversely, in regions where Marma practices blend subtly into broader traditional healing systems without distinct nomenclature, such as in Vietnam or Korea, governmental oversight is less pronounced. Here, Marma-like therapies may fall under general traditional medicine regulations without specific mention, relying more on communal trust and historical continuity than on formal licensure.
This varied landscape of recognition and regulation not only influences the practice and proliferation of Marma Chikitsa but also impacts its integration into public health policies. Governmental attitudes can either pave the way for its advancement or hinder its formal acceptance, significantly affecting how these ancient knowledge systems survive in contemporary medical environments.

Summary

The chapter 'Regional Practices – Marma Across Asia' explores the intricate tapestry of Marma-related healing traditions across various Asian regions, highlighting how these practices are deeply interwoven with regional cultures, martial arts, and spiritual beliefs. In Kerala, India, Kalari Marma integrates the martial art of Kalaripayattu with Marma Chikitsa, emphasizing the stimulation of vital points for both therapeutic and combat purposes. Tamil Nadu's Siddha Varmam leverages 'varma points' in conjunction with Siddha medicine, enhancing physical and spiritual health through guarded knowledge passed down by varmam asans. Sri Lankan Ayurveda uniquely combines local herbal knowledge with Buddhist philosophies to enhance Marma therapy's effectiveness, focusing on preventive care and holistic wellness. Nepal's Marma practices in monastic settings use herbal and physical therapies to promote spiritual and physical healing, reflecting the Buddhist influence. Tibetan Kunye Therapy incorporates Marma principles using traditional tools to balance elemental energies, while Thai Massage and Marma share a focus on energy pathways albeit through different methodologies. Balinese healing also parallels Marma techniques, focusing on energy point stimulation to foster health. The practices in Vietnam and Korea, although not explicitly labeled as Marma, show parallels in their focus on vital points and energy flow. Cultural rituals across Asia also integrate Marma Chikitsa into communal and spiritual life, showcasing its role beyond mere physical healing. Healing centers across the region serve as custodians of this knowledge, facilitating the spread and preservation of Marma techniques. This wide array of practices not only illustrates the adaptability and integration of Marma into various cultural fabrics but also underscores a common belief in the importance of energy balance, holistic health, and the body's innate healing capabilities.

References

[1] Zarrilli, Phillip B. 'A South Indian Martial Art and the Yoga and Ayurvedic Paradigms.'. https://www.jstor.org/stable/10.7722/j.ctt14brv6x.12

[2] Thompson, T. & Leberman, S. (2005). 'Siddha Varmam – A Traditional Indian Medicine Technique.'. https://www.ncbi.nlm.nih.gov/pmc/articles/PMC5423738/

[3] White, David Gordon. 'Marma Science and its applications in Sri Lankan Ayurveda.'. https://www.sciencedirect.com/science/article/pii/S222541101630027X

[4] Shroff, F. (2014). 'The Cultural Context of Therapeutic Choice: Tibetan Kunye Massage Practice in Nepal.'. https://books.google.co.uk/books?id=dFacBAAAQBAJ

[5] Zysk, K.G. 'The Science of Resuscitation: Traditional Thai Massage and Marma Therapy of India.'. https://www.jstor.org/stable/41371453

[6] Connor, L. (1995). 'The Power of Touch: Balinese Healing Techniques with Marma Points.'. https://www.sciencedirect.com/science/article/abs/pii/S0926669096000325

Case Study: Integrating Marma Chikitsa into Modern Clinics: A Case Study from Kerala, India

In the serene landscapes of Kerala, a revolutionary approach to traditional healing has emerged within a modern clinical setting, spearheading a new paradigm in healthcare that integrates Marma Chikitsa with contemporary medical practices. This case study delves into a clinic in Thrissur, which has begun incorporating Marma therapy alongside allopathic treatments, creating a holistic health environment that caters to both physical and energetic health dimensions.

The clinic, founded by Dr. Ananya Rajesh, a dual specialist in Ayurvedic and allopathic medicine, focuses on patients suffering from chronic pain and neuromuscular disorders. Dr. Rajesh observed that while allopathic medicine offered immediate pain relief and surgical options, it often failed to address the underlying energy imbalances seen in her patients. To tackle this issue, she introduced Marma Chikitsa, which she had mastered under the tutelage of renowned Ayurvedic healers in Kerala.

In one illustrative case, a 45-year-old male presented with chronic lower back pain, a common ailment with usually prescriptive treatments such as painkillers and physiotherapy. Instead of following the conventional path, Dr. Rajesh employed a hybrid treatment regimen. Initial allopathic assessments ensured no structural damage that required surgical intervention, followed by a series of Marma therapy sessions aimed at revitalizing the Marma points associated with spinal and muscular health. The patient experienced notable relief not only physically but also reported increased vitality and a reduction in stress levels.

Reflection on this integrative approach shows promising results for patient recovery times and overall health improvement. The synchronization of Marma Chikitsa with allopathic care provides a template that could reshape modern medical practices by reintroducing ancient wisdom in a new light. This holistic model does not just heal physically but also balances the body's energies, potentially reducing dependence on pharmacological interventions and making preventive health a tangible goal for modern society.

This case study suggests that the blending of Indian traditional and modern medical practices could serve as a beacon for global health systems exploring integrative health solutions, highlighting the potential of cultural wisdom in contemporary medical frameworks.

Case Study: Revitalizing Community Wellness Through Marma Chikitsa in Rural Sri Lanka

In the tranquil village of Digana, located in the central province of Sri Lanka, a transformative approach to community health revival showcases the profound impact of integrating Marma Chikitsa into local healthcare practices. This case study explores the initiative launched by Ayurvedic practitioner Dr. Lakmini Wijeratne, who introduced a community-based Marma therapy program aimed at enhancing overall wellness and reducing the prevalence of chronic ailments among the villagers.

Dr. Wijeratne, who was trained in both traditional Sri Lankan Ayurveda and Western medical science, observed that many rural communities lacked access to comprehensive healthcare, primarily relying on intermittent medical clinics and traditional home remedies. Noticing the high incidence of stress-related illnesses and chronic pain disorders among the villagers, she proposed a tailored Marma therapy program that would address both physical and emotional health needs.

The program involved training local healers in the identification and stimulation of key Marma points, crucial for managing health issues prevalent in rural settings, such as arthritis, digestive problems, and anxiety. Alongside hands-on training, Dr. Wijeratne organized workshops with visual aids and practical demonstrations to educate the community about the benefits of Marma Chikitsa, including its preventive aspects and its role in promoting a balanced lifestyle.

The initiative's impact was multifaceted; it not only alleviated physical symptoms in patients but also enhanced their understanding of body-energy dynamics, leading to healthier lifestyle choices. For instance, a community survey conducted six months after the program's inception showed a significant reduction in the use of over-the-counter painkillers and a noticeable improvement in mental health parameters among the participants.

Throughout the program, challenges such as initial skepticism and the adaptation of Marma practices to suit local needs were addressed through continuous education and alignment with local cultural practices. This community-based model demonstrated that by empowering local practitioners and integrating ancient wisdom like Marma Chikitsa into routine care, rural populations could achieve remarkable improvements in both health outcomes and quality of life.

Case Study: Cultural Adaptation and Preservation of Marma Therapy in Urban Nepal

In the bustling urban landscape of Kathmandu, Nepal, a unique initiative has been taken by the Jivanmukti Cultural Center to preserve and adapt the ancient practice of Marma Chikitsa to suit the needs of a rapidly modernizing society. This case study explores how the center integrates traditional Marma healing techniques with contemporary health modalities to cater to the diverse population of the city, highlighting cultural preservation alongside modern therapeutic needs.

The center, founded by Dr. Aarav Bhattarai, a renowned practitioner of Nepalese traditional medicine, begun its quest with a dual objective: to offer effective health solutions through Marma Therapy and to educate the urban populace about the rich heritage of Nepalese holistic practices. Dr. Bhattarai, along with a team of multidisciplinary experts including Ayurvedic physicians, physiotherapists, and yoga instructors, devised a comprehensive wellness program that includes workshops, treatment sessions, and public seminars focusing on the principles and applications of Marma Chikitsa.

One illustrative example involved a 38-year-old software developer suffering from chronic stress and insomnia, conditions prevalent among professionals in the city. Traditionally treated with medication and counseling, Dr. Bhattarai's team instead utilized a tailored Marma therapy protocol focusing on vital points that enhance mental clarity and relieve stress. The therapy was complemented by guided yoga practices and dietary adjustments based on Ayurvedic principles.

The results were profound. The patient reported significant improvements in sleep quality and overall well-being within weeks. The success story was systematically documented and shared in one of the center's seminars, leading to heightened interest and participation in Marma therapy programs.

Reflecting on this integration, the Jivanmukti Cultural Center has not only provided a therapeutic modality that bridges the gap between ancient wisdom and contemporary health challenges but also fostered a renewed appreciation for Nepalese cultural heritage. By adapting Marma Chikitsa to modern lifestyles, the center ensures the survival and relevance of this ancient practice in urban settings, while also contributing to the global dialogue on integrative health practices.

Case Study: Reviving Traditional Marma Practices in Remote Tibetan Villages

In the remote mountainous regions of Tibet, the ancient practice of Marma Chikitsa, integrated into the monastic healing system, presents a riveting model of how traditional knowledge can be revitalized and adapted to serve contemporary health needs. This case study revolves around a pioneering project initiated by Dr. Tenzin Choedrak, a renowned Tibetan monk-physician, who sought to reinvigorate this age-old healing modality, ensuring its transmission to future generations while also addressing the pressing health issues faced by local communities.

Dr. Choedrak, trained both in Tibetan medicine and modern medical techniques, recognized the potential of Marma therapy to complement modern healthcare, especially in areas where medical resources are scarce. He embarked on a mission to train local healthcare providers, including monks and village healers, in the art of Marma Chikitsa, focusing particularly on the integration of herbal medicine and energy healing techniques.

The training program was set in place with support from both local leaders and international health organizations. It included detailed workshops on identification and manipulation of Marma points, tailored to address common ailments such as arthritis, digestive issues, and respiratory conditions prevalent in the high-altitude environment of Tibet. Dr. Choedrak's program emphasized sustainable practices, such as the use of local herbs and incorporation of ritualistic techniques that align with the cultural and spiritual nuances of Tibetan life.

An illustrative example of the program's success is the case of an elderly woman suffering from chronic arthritis. Traditional pain management strategies had failed to relieve her symptoms. Under Dr. Choedrak's guidance, local healers employed a combination of Marma manipulation and specially prepared herbal concoctions. Within weeks, the woman reported significant improvements, demonstrating the effectiveness of this integrated approach.

This case study highlights the program's multifaceted impact, not only in enhancing the health and wellbeing of individuals but also in revitalizing a crucial aspect of Tibetan cultural heritage. By marrying traditional Marma practices with modern healthcare strategies, the project showcases a sustainable model of healthcare that preserves ancient wisdom while advancing medical practice in remote regions.

Case Study: Enhancing Athletic Performance through Marma Chikitsa: A Case Study in Malaysian Sports

In the competitive world of sports in Malaysia, a groundbreaking initiative has been launched integrating Marma Chikitsa into athletic training to enhance performance and recovery. This case study revolves around the Malaysian National Sports Academy's recent adoption of these ancient practices, tailored to meet the rigorous demands of professional athletes.

The academy, known for its commitment to holistic training methods, initiated a pilot program under the guidance of Dr. Amirul Mukminin, an expert in both sports medicine and traditional Malaysian healing techniques. The project aimed to incorporate Marma therapy into routine training regimens, with a focus on improving energy flow, enhancing muscular flexibility, and reducing injury recovery time.

One significant aspect of the implementation was the customized approach taken for different sports. For instance, badminton players received Marma therapy focused on wrist and ankle joints to prevent common injuries and boost agility, while track athletes focused on back and leg Marma points to enhance sprinting capability. Each regimen was meticulously designed to align with the athlete's specific physical demands and competitive challenges.

An early assessment showed promising results. A notable case was of a long-distance runner who had been struggling with recurring hamstring injuries. Traditional treatments had offered only short-term relief. Through regular Marma sessions, targeting specific points that correlate with muscle healing and pain relief, the runner reported not only a faster recovery time but also improved endurance during races.

Reflecting on the initial success of the program, Dr. Mukminin highlighted the importance of an integrative approach in sports training. He noted that Marma Chikitsa does not just address physical ailments but also promotes mental clarity and emotional stability, which are crucial for high-level performance. The academy plans to continue this program and conduct further research on its efficacy, positioning Marma therapy as a core component of athletic training in Malaysia's sports framework.

This case study underscores the potential of traditional healing practices in enhancing modern athletic performance, offering insights into how ancient wisdom can be effectively integrated into contemporary health and wellness practices.

Case Study: Expanding Marma Chikitsa in Pediatric Care in Bhutan

In the serene landscape of Bhutan, an innovative healthcare initiative is changing the way pediatric care is approached by integrating Marma Chikitsa into routine pediatric treatments. This case study elaborates on the pioneering efforts by the Jigme Dorji National Pediatric Center in Thimphu, which has adopted Marma therapy as a complementary modality in the treatment of common childhood ailments such as asthma, digestion issues, and sleep disturbances.

The center, under the leadership of Dr. Pema Yangchen, a pediatrician trained in both conventional medicine and traditional Bhutanese healing practices, recognized the gentle nature of Marma Chikitsa as particularly suitable for children, whose bodies are sensitive and still developing. The initiative began with a pilot project involving 50 children suffering from chronic asthma, a condition prevalent in the cold, damp climate of Bhutan.

Dr. Yangchen, together with a team of Ayurvedic specialists, developed a specialized protocol where specific Marma points related to respiratory health were stimulated using mild pressure and herbal oils suited for children. The treatment sessions were designed to be short and non-invasive, making them more acceptable to young patients and their parents. After three months of incorporating Marma therapy into their routine care, the children showed remarkable improvement in their symptom control and overall vitality.

The success of the asthma protocol led to wider application in other chronic conditions. Children with digestive troubles and sleep disturbances were treated with customized Marma protocols targeting points that enhance gastrointestinal health and promote relaxation. Parents reported improvements such as better appetite, reduced gastric discomfort, and more regular sleep patterns after their children underwent Marma treatments.

This case study not only highlights the versatility of Marma Chikitsa in treating a range of pediatric conditions but also illustrates how traditional practices can be seamlessly integrated into modern medical care. The initiative has spurred further research into pediatric Marma protocols and is increasingly viewed as a model for holistic pediatric care in traditional medicine settings.

Case Study: Navigating Through Marma Chikitsa in Orthodox Medicine: A Modern Therapeutic Fusion in Vietnam

In the evolving landscape of health care in Hanoi, Vietnam, a unique initiative bridges the gap between traditional Vietnamese healing practices resembling Marma Chikitsa and orthodox medical treatments. This case study explores the pioneering integration undertaken by the Hanoi Holistic Health Center (HHHC), which aims to amalgamate these age-old practices within the framework of conventional medicine to address the increasing prevalence of lifestyle diseases affecting modern society.

Dr. Minh Vu, a practitioner of both Western medicine and traditional Vietnamese healing, spearheaded a program to incorporate Marma-like therapeutic methods into the treatment regimens for patients with chronic conditions such as hypertension and diabetes. He noticed the limitations of typical pharmacological interventions, often laden with side-effects, and proposed a more sustainable approach blending Marma Chikitsa's holistic benefits with medical science.

A notably successful case involved a 52-year-old male patient diagnosed with hypertension, traditionally managed with beta-blockers. Observing the patient's reluctance towards lifelong medication due to side-effects, Dr. Vu opted for an integrative treatment plan. Initial consultations and thorough medical assessments were followed by strategic stimulation of specific Marma (pressure) points that correspond to cardiovascular stability. These sessions were supplemented by lifestyle counseling and dietary adjustments rooted in naturopathy.

This patient's journey through the blended treatment saw a remarkable improvement not only in blood pressure readings but also in overall vitality and stress reduction, which traditional medication alone had not achieved. The integrative approach also led to a reduction in the patient's dependency on pharmaceuticals.

This case shows that Marma Chikitsa, when implemented with careful consideration of modern diagnostic tools and medical understanding, can offer a novel pathway to managing chronic conditions that enrich the traditional therapeutic focus on vitality and balance. It also underscores the role of innovative health paradigms in bridging cultural medical wisdom and scientific methodologies, fostering a more comprehensive treatment outlook which respects both patient preference and contemporary medical standards.

Case Study: Holistic Health Incorporation in Sports: Marma Chikitsa for a Professional Football Team in Japan

In the world of professional sports, particularly within the high-intensity realm of football in Japan, the Sapporo City Football Club (SCFC) has embarked on an innovative journey to integrate Marma Chikitsa into their training and rehabilitation programs. This case study explores the pioneering adoption of these ancient Ayurvedic practices aimed at enhancing player performance, recovery rates, and overall team vitality.

Initially met with skepticism, the integration began with the hiring of Dr. Aiko Yamamura, a renowned sports therapist with a background in both modern sports medicine and traditional Indian healing techniques. Dr. Yamamura introduced Marma Chikitsa in a phased approach, starting with educational sessions for the coaching staff and medical team, and followed by non-invasive treatments for players reporting chronic injuries.

One significant example involves a midfielder, Kenji Sato, who had struggled with recurrent knee injuries, hindering his performance. Traditional treatments kept him off the field for prolonged periods during the season. Dr. Yamamura implemented a targeted Marma protocol focusing on specific Marma points around the knee and lower back, accompanied by custom herbal oils known to facilitate musculoskeletal healing.

The results, documented over the course of the season, showed a remarkable improvement in

Sato's recovery time and reduction in the reoccurrence of his knee issues. Furthermore, generalized implementation across the team led to decreased overall injury rates and improved stamina and mental focus during games. Players also reported enhanced sleep quality and lower anxiety levels, attributed to the holistic nature of Marma Chikitsa that balances the body's energies.

Reflecting on this integrative health strategy, the SCFC has set a precedent in sports medicine. By incorporating a multi-disciplinary approach, they not only addressed the physical aspects of sports injuries but also enhanced the athletes' emotional and psychological resilience. This case study sheds light on the potential of Marma Chikitsa in sports, providing a blend of ancient wisdom and modern science to foster a healthy, sustainable athlete lifestyle in highly competitive environments.

Case Study: The Integration of Marma Chikitsa in Mental Health Programs in Bhutan

In the serene and spiritual landscape of Bhutan, a pioneering mental health program incorporates Marma Chikitsa to treat psychological ailments, showcasing a novel approach to holistic mental health. This case study focuses on the Bhutan National Mental Health Initiative (BNMHI), which has embarked on integrating traditional Bhutanese healing practices, specifically Marma Chikitsa, alongside modern psychological therapies.

The BNMHI, spearheaded by Dr. Sonam Tshering, a psychiatrist with extensive training in both Western psychiatric methods and traditional Bhutanese therapies, aims to address the rising issues of depression and anxiety among the youth. Recognizing the limitations of conventional medication, which often provides only symptomatic relief and carries the risk of side effects, Dr. Tshering and his team sought to explore the benefits of Marma Chikitsa, known for its efficacy in restoring emotional balance through energy point stimulation.

The integration involved structured training sessions for mental health professionals in identifying and stimulating Marma points that are specifically effective for emotional regulation. The therapeutic protocols developed combined Marma therapy with cognitive-behavioral techniques to create a multifaceted treatment approach. In one notable instance, a 30-year-old female patient suffering from severe anxiety and insomnia experienced significant improvement after undergoing a tailored treatment plan, which included Marma point stimulation and mindfulness exercises.

The continued success stories have led to wider acceptance of this integrative approach within the community. Benefits reported by patients include not just alleviation of symptoms but also enhanced coping mechanisms, increased self-awareness, and greater overall well-being. These outcomes are documented and analyzed to refine treatment protocols continually.

This case study illustrates the potential of Marma Chikitsa to transform mental health treatment paradigms by providing a more comprehensive, culturally appropriate, and side-effect-free approach to emotional healing. The BNMHI's efforts may serve as a model for other nations looking to integrate traditional healing arts with modern medical practices, potentially revolutionizing the global approach to mental wellness.

Case Study: Reinvigorating Marma Chikitsa in Geriatric Care: A Case Study from Kyoto, Japan

In the culturally rich city of Kyoto, Japan, an innovative approach to geriatric healthcare integrates Marma Chikitsa into conventional elderly care, offering a unique perspective on managing aging-related health issues. This case study explores the Harmony Elderly Wellness Center that has adopted Marma therapy as part of its comprehensive care program for the elderly, focusing particularly on those suffering from chronic pain and cognitive decline.

The center, led by Dr. Hiroshi Tanaka, a geriatric specialist with a profound interest in integrative medicine, recognizes the potential of Marma therapy to complement traditional treatments and improve the quality of life for older adults. The program initiated at the center includes a combination of Marma therapy, conventional medication, and cognitive behavioral therapies tailored to individual patient needs.

One notable case involves an 82-year-old female patient with osteoarthritis and mild cognitive impairment. Traditional treatments had limited success in managing her pain and mobility issues. Under Dr. Tanaka's guidance, a Marma therapy protocol was designed to focus on key points believed to enhance joint health and mental clarity. The treatment sessions involved gentle manipulation of specific Marma points combined with aromatherapy using traditional herbs known for their anti-inflammatory properties.

Over several weeks, the patient exhibited significant improvements in joint mobility and a reduction in pain levels. Additionally, her family reported that she showed greater engagement and clarity during conversations, suggesting cognitive benefits from the therapy. This holistic approach not only addressed physical symptoms but also supported cognitive function, proving crucial for the patient's overall well-being.

The case reaffirms the potential of Marma Chikitsa as a vital tool in geriatric care, emphasizing the importance of an integrative approach that addresses the complex health needs of the elderly. The success at Harmony Elderly Wellness Center has prompted discussions about expanding Marma therapy programs, aiming to set benchmarks for elderly care that can be emulated globally, thereby reshaping how aging populations are cared for in diverse healthcare settings.

Review Questions

1. A 32-year-old male practitioner of Kalaripayattu from Kerala, India reports experiencing muscle stiffness and minor injuries frequently. Based on the regional practice of Kalari Marma, what would be the most appropriate therapeutic approach to address his ailments?

A) Focused therapeutic massages at non-specific random points
B) Stimulation of specific marma points known to benefit muscle recovery
C) Avoidance of physical therapy and reliance on oral medications only
D) Application of cold packs and refraining from further physical activity

Answer: B

Explanation: In Kalari Marma, a traditional practice from Kerala, therapy includes the stimulation of specific marma points integral to treating muscle stiffness and injuries. This approach, which is deeply rooted in Kalaripayattu, utilizes the understanding of 107 marma points across the human body. These points, when properly stimulated, help in enhancing the flow of prana (life force) which facilitates faster recovery and revitalization. This choice stands out because it integrates the cultural and traditional medical wisdom unique to Kerala.

2. While attending a cultural festival in Tamil Nadu, you observe a demonstration by a varmam asan who explains the use of varma points for both healing and martial applications. How does this practice differ fundamentally from conventional massage therapies?
A) It primarily focuses on superficial skin stimulation
B) It involves deep pressure techniques on muscle tissue only
C) It combines knowledge of energy pathways and both healing/harming techniques
D) It is strictly a non-contact form of therapy
Answer: C
Explanation: Siddha Varmam, as practiced in Tamil Nadu, uniquely integrates the deep and esoteric knowledge of varma points which are crucial energy junctures on the body. Unlike conventional massages that may focus more on muscle and tissue manipulation for relaxation or superficial stimulation, Siddha Varmam uses these points strategically for therapeutic benefits and, in martial contexts, can be applied to harm. This dual application showcases a profound understanding of the body's energy pathways, aligning with the holistic approach of traditional Siddha medicine.

3. A Sri Lankan monk specializing in Marma Chikitsa plans to treat a patient suffering from chronic stress and emotional imbalances. Which aspects of the therapy should be emphasized to align with local therapeutic practices and philosophical underpinnings?
A) Use of topical treatments only with no emphasis on spiritual practices
B) Heavy reliance on synthetic medications as per modern standards
C) Incorporation of chants and local herbal preparations alongside manipulation of marma points
D) Sole focus on physical massage without energy or spiritual considerations
Answer: C
Explanation: In Sri Lankan Ayurveda, the approach to healing is profoundly holistic, merging local herbal knowledge with philosophical and spiritual elements intrinsic to their culture. Marma Chikitsa in this region is not just about physical touch but also encompasses spiritual healing through chants and meditative techniques. The use of local herbs enhances the therapeutic effectiveness. This integration helps in addressing not just the physical symptoms like stress but also aims at emotional and spiritual balance, reflecting the cultural depth of the therapy.

CHAPTER TWELVE: Teaching, Research, and the Global Future of Marma Chikitsa

CHAPTER TWELVE

TEACHING,
RESEARCH,
AND
THE GLOBAL FUTURE
OF MARMA CHIKITSA

The Need for Standardized Marma Education

The proliferation of Marma Chikitsa across Asia, while enriching, has led to a pressing need for standardized education within the discipline. As the therapy gains popularity, a structured educational approach becomes critical to ensuring its efficacy and authenticity. This standardization involves defining core curricula, developing uniform teaching methodologies, and establishing baseline competencies that practitioners must achieve.
Currently, the teaching of Marma Chikitsa varies widely, reflecting local customs and individual interpretations of ancient texts. Standardized education would not only elevate the practice by ensuring consistency but also facilitate its integration into broader medical systems. Educators and practitioners could reliably measure and augment the therapy's effectiveness, based on a unified knowledge base.
Furthermore, the establishment of formal educational standards would bolster international credibility and aid in the dissemination of Marma Chikitsa to new geographic and professional areas. It would define clear pathways for learner progression from novice to expert, ensuring the longevity and vitality of the practice on a global scale.

Certification Programs and Accreditation

As Marma Chikitsa expands globally, creating standardized certification programs and accreditation processes becomes paramount. This initiative aims to fortify the credibility of practitioners and institutes, ensuring a uniform level of proficiency and knowledge across all operators within this traditional discipline.
Certification programs provide benchmarks for practitioner competence, encompassing both theoretical knowledge and practical skills. This formal recognition not only uplifts the profession but also reassures patients of the therapeutic integrity and safety of treatments received.
Accreditation of institutions, on the other hand, ensures that educational bodies adhere to globally recognized standards in curriculum development, faculty qualifications, and training facilities. This comprehensive approach assures quality control and fosters public trust in Marma Chikitsa as a legitimate medical practice.
Moreover, well-structured accreditation helps bridge the gap between traditional healing arts and modern healthcare systems, promoting integrative health solutions. Establishing robust certification and accreditation frameworks also paves the way for the inclusion of Marma Chikitsa into mainstream healthcare policies worldwide, enhancing its accessibility and acceptance.

Development of a Global Marma Curriculum

The expansion of Marma Chikitsa across diverse regions necessitates the creation of a global curriculum that encapsulates the essence and complexities of this ancient practice while ensuring its relevance across cultural boundaries. A unified curriculum would serve as a cornerstone for interdisciplinary learning and practice, leveraging accumulated knowledge from various healing traditions to establish a comprehensive educational framework.
This global curriculum would be structured around core principles of Marma therapy, enriched with modern scientific research and regional healing practices. It would integrate traditional Ayurvedic teachings with contemporary health sciences, ensuring a well-rounded pedagogical

approach. Through such integration, practitioners worldwide could apply Marma Chikitsa effectively within their local contexts, ensuring both cultural adaptability and technical proficiency.
Further, a globally standardized curriculum would facilitate reciprocal recognition of qualifications among countries, enhancing professional mobility and global collaboration in Marma practice. It aims to sculpt practitioners who are not only skilled in technique but also versed in the ethical, cultural, and scientific dimensions of healthcare, preparing them to be pioneers in both local and global health landscapes.

The Role of Online Courses in Marma Education

In the expanding world of Marma Chikitsa, online courses play a pivotal role by bridging geographical divides and making this ancient practice accessible to a global audience. These digital platforms offer flexible learning environments that cater to students across different time zones, accommodating various lifestyles and commitments. Through well-designed online modules, learners can delve into the intricate knowledge of Marma points, energy pathways, and therapeutic techniques at their own pace.
Moreover, online education in Marma Chikitsa not only democratizes learning but also ensures a standardized dissemination of knowledge, crucial for maintaining the efficacy and integrity of the practice. Interactive elements like webinars, virtual workshops, and real-time discussions facilitate a dynamic learning experience, engaging students more deeply than traditional textbook methods.
Emerging technologies such as virtual reality could enhance these courses further, enabling students to experience hands-on practice sessions in a simulated environment. This integration of technology promises to enrich the learning experience significantly, paving the way for a new era in the education of Marma Chikitsa.

Workshops and Seminars: Expanding Knowledge Globally

The dissemination of Marma Chikitsa through global workshops and seminars is pivotal in fostering a worldwide comprehension and application of this ancient healing art. These interactive sessions serve as vital platforms for both novice and seasoned practitioners to engage directly with experts, enhancing their practical skills and deepening their theoretical understanding. Furthermore, these gatherings facilitate a diverse exchange of ideas, merging traditional wisdom with contemporary practices.
In regions where Marma Chikitsa is less known, workshops and seminars play a crucial role in introducing and embedding these practices within local healthcare paradigms. They act as catalysts for cultural exchange and adaptation, allowing Marma Chikitsa to be tailored to meet specific regional health needs while respecting local medicinal traditions. This adaptability is central to the global spread and sustainability of Marma practices.
Finally, as centers of learning and innovation, such events also spark collaborations that bridge various health disciplines. Integrating Marma Chikitsa into the broader medical community not only enriches holistic health approaches but also paves the way for more interdisciplinary healthcare solutions, impacting global health outcomes positively.

Teaching Marma Chikitsa in Universities

Integrating Marma Chikitsa into university curricula marks a pivotal step towards formalizing this ancient healing art within academic institutions. By introducing Marma Chikitsa as a course of study, universities can provide a structured, scholarly environment that fosters both theoretical understanding and practical proficiency. This educational approach not only prepares a new generation of practitioners but also enhances research opportunities in the field.
Furthermore, university-based programs could collaborate with medical schools to offer interdisciplinary training, blending Ayurvedic wisdom with modern medical techniques. Such initiatives would expand the therapeutic landscape, offering students a holistic view of health that bridges eastern and western modalities.
Lastly, the presence of Marma Chikitsa in higher education would stimulate global academic interest and recognition, attracting international students and scholars. This global exchange enriches the educational experience, promoting a deeper, culturally nuanced understanding of Marma practices that could inform and transform contemporary approaches to health and wellness.

Partnerships Between Marma Institutions and Healthcare Facilities

The integration of Marma Chikitsa into mainstream healthcare through partnerships with institutions is a transformative stride towards holistic health. Such collaborations aim to blend traditional Marma practices with contemporary medical treatments, ensuring a comprehensive approach to patient care. Institutions dedicated to Marma can provide invaluable expertise and resources that enhance the therapeutic offerings of modern medical facilities, creating a symbiotic relationship that benefits both providers and recipients of care.
Moreover, these partnerships facilitate the sharing of knowledge and methodologies, fostering innovation in both fields. As healthcare facilities begin to recognize the value of integrating Marma Chikitsa, these alliances can lead to the development of new treatment protocols that harness the strengths of both traditional and modern practices, potentially setting new standards in healthcare excellence.
Finally, institutional collaborations open doors for rigorous clinical research, providing the empirical evidence needed to further validate Marma Chikitsa's efficacy and embed it more deeply within global health systems. This not only enhances patient outcomes but also elevates the credibility of Marma therapy in the eyes of the medical community and the public at large.

Promoting Research in Marma Chikitsa

Elevating Marma Chikitsa to a globally recognized therapeutic approach demands a structured emphasis on scientific research. Developing rigorous methodologies to investigate Marma's efficacy will boast its integration into the evidence-based medical community. Initiatives must prioritize clinical studies that ascertain therapeutic outcomes, contributing to its legitimacy and broader acceptance.
Fostering partnerships with academic and healthcare institutions can streamline the process of conducting large-scale research, harnessing their resources and expertise. These collaborations would aid in crafting comprehensive studies that not only explore the physiological impacts but also the holistic benefits Marma Chikitsa offers, potentially

revolutionizing pain management and disease treatment practices worldwide.
Moreover, establishing dedicated research centers could serve as beacons for ongoing Marma studies, attracting global talent and funding. These centers would function as hubs for innovation, pushing the boundaries of conventional medicine and opening new horizons for holistic health solutions.
Ultimately, promoting research in Marma Chikitsa is vital for its evolution from ancient wisdom to modern-day miracle, ensuring its sustainability and relevance in the future of global healthcare.

Funding and Grants for Marma Studies

Securing funding and grants is crucial for advancing Marma Chikitsa, particularly as it endeavors to gain recognition and validation within the global scientific and medical communities. Financial support allows for comprehensive research, which is necessary to integrate this ancient practice into contemporary medicine effectively. It enables the execution of extensive clinical trials, development of standardized protocols, and publication of findings in acclaimed journals.
Governments, private foundations, and international health organizations can play significant roles by allocating funds specifically for Marma studies. Such backing not only aids in scientific exploration but also in the dissemination of knowledge through conferences and symposia. Encouraging public and private sectors to invest in Marma research could spur significant breakthroughs in holistic health practices.
Moreover, establishing dedicated funds to support students and scholars in Marma Chikitsa can foster an environment of innovation and learning. Scholarships and research grants help attract a new generation of practitioners and scholars, ensuring the growth and sustainability of Marma Chikitsa for future applications in global health solutions.

Clinical Trials and Evidence-Based Approaches

Undertaking clinical trials is essential for substantiating the efficacy of Marma Chikitsa within the global medical framework. These trials should adhere to international standards for research to ensure their credibility and replicability. Rigorous, well-designed clinical studies will help bridge the gap between traditional practices and contemporary scientific validation, offering solid evidence of its benefits and mechanisms.
Implementing evidence-based approaches involves integrating results from these trials into clinical practice, thereby enhancing patient trust and acceptance of Marma Chikitsa. It necessitates collaboration among researchers, practitioners, and healthcare professionals to translate research findings into practical, effective treatment protocols that can be universally adopted.
Finally, the outcomes from these trials will not only elevate Marma Chikitsa's profile in academic and healthcare sectors but also pave the way for its inclusion in guidelines and policymaking worldwide. This integrated approach promises to uphold the rigor of scientific inquiry while honoring the holistic essence of Marma Chikitsa.

Publications and Journals Dedicated to Marma Research

The proliferation of dedicated publications and journals in Marma Chikitsa serves as a cornerstone for advancing this ancient practice into the limelight of global healthcare discourse. These specialized platforms not only disseminate peer-reviewed research, increasing the scientific community's awareness and understanding of Marma therapy but also elevate its credibility and scholarly significance.

Journals focused on Marma Chikitsa provide a critical linkage between traditional knowledge and modern scientific inquiry. They offer a repository for case studies, clinical trials, and longitudinal research, contributing substantively to the body of evidence that supports the efficacy of Marma practices. Moreover, these publications are instrumental in defining and refining methodologies, setting benchmarks for future research and practice in the field.

Furthermore, the existence of these journals encourages scholars and practitioners to contribute to the growing body of Marma knowledge. This not only fosters a vibrant academic community but also ensures continuous improvement and innovation within the discipline, maintaining its relevance in changing medical landscapes.

Patient Outcome Studies and Longitudinal Research

Longitudinal research and patient outcome studies are pivotal in substantiating the long-term effectiveness and safety of Marma Chikitsa. By tracking patient progress over extended periods, these studies can illuminate trends, outcomes, and potential areas for refinement in Marma practice. This type of rigorous empirical evaluation is critical for Marma Chikitsa's integration into the wider health care systems globally.

Moreover, outcome studies provide valuable data that can influence policy decisions, treatment protocols, and patient care standards. They help in identifying efficacy patterns, enhancing treatment approaches, and optimizing patient health over time. This information is crucial for healthcare professionals and researchers aiming to create a more effective, integrative approach to medicine.

Continuing to invest in these research strategies will ensure that Marma Chikitsa is not only preserved as a traditional therapy but also evolves as a scientifically validated health solution. Ultimately, this commitment to longitudinal research will drive better health outcomes and foster wider acceptance of Marma therapy within the medical community.

Integrating Marma Therapy into Conventional Medicine

The journey to integrate Marma Therapy into conventional medicine challenges the boundaries between traditional and modern therapeutic practices. Establishing a collaborative mindset among healthcare professionals is paramount. Training and educating medical practitioners on the principles and benefits of Marma Chikitsa can cultivate a new era of interdisciplinary treatment strategies, merging holistic healing with contemporary medical protocols.

Crucial to this integration is the development of evidence-based models that demonstrate Marma's effectiveness and safety within conventional medical settings. Pilot programs in hospitals and health centers could serve as proving grounds for these models, combining Marma techniques with medical treatments to enhance patient recovery and well-being. Such initiatives would serve as case studies demonstrating the practical benefits of integrated care

approaches.
Ultimately, for Marma to be embraced by the mainstream medical community, it must adhere to the rigorous demands of scientific validation. This involves not only continuous clinical evaluation but also an adaptation of Marma practices to meet the stringent requirements of contemporary medical practice. Achieving this could dramatically shift the therapeutic landscape, enhancing patient care through the synthesis of ancient wisdom and modern science.

Global Legislation and Policy Framework for Marma Practice

The establishment of a global legislative and policy framework is crucial for the recognition and standardization of Marma Chikitsa as a legitimate form of medical practice. Such frameworks must navigate varied medical and legal environments, ensuring that Marma Chikitsa is both respected and regulated appropriately across different countries. This necessitates collaborative efforts with healthcare authorities, legal experts, and international bodies to create universally acceptable regulations that honor both the traditional and scientific aspects of Marma Chikitsa. Key objectives include protecting practitioner rights, ensuring quality and safety standards, and promoting ethical practices. Clear guidelines and licensing requirements would help prevent malpractices and ensure the provision of high-quality care. Establishing these norms will also facilitate international exchange of knowledge and practitioners, further advancing the global presence of Marma Chikitsa.
Moreover, harmonization of these laws will support the integration of Marma Chikitsa into mainstream healthcare systems, making it more accessible to patients worldwide. As this field grows, continual adaptation and revision of policies will be necessary to reflect the evolving understanding and application of Marma Chikitsa.

Setting Global Standards for Marma Practice

As Marma Chikitsa transcends regional boundaries and integrates into global healthcare, establishing universal standards becomes imperative. These standards would define the qualifications necessary for practitioners, the procedures followed during therapy, and the ethical guidelines that ensure patient safety and respect for cultural variances.
Adopting a standardized approach facilitates consistency in practice and simplifies the evaluation of outcomes across different demographic segments. This would bolster the credibility of Marma Chikitsa, fostering trust and wider acceptance within the international medical community. Additionally, uniform standards would assist regulatory bodies in monitoring and accrediting practitioners and therapy centers, ensuring a high level of care.
Ultimately, global standards would support the integration of Marma Chikitsa into existing health systems and enhance collaborative research efforts. They would serve as the bedrock for building robust educational programs that aspire to cultivate skilled practitioners dedicated to this ancient healing art, enriching its application and ensuring its preservation for future generations.

Ethical Considerations in the Practice and Teaching of Marma

The ethical landscape of Marma Chikitsa hinges significantly on the principles of integrity, respect, and commitment to patient welfare. As practitioners navigate the confluence of ancient wisdom and modern medical practices, upholding ethical standards is paramount. This includes ensuring informed consent, maintaining patient confidentiality, and delivering treatments with cultural sensitivity and awareness.

Moreover, ethical teaching in Marma Chikitsa requires a structured curriculum that imbues students with a deep understanding of their responsibilities. Educators must emphasize the importance of ethical behavior in both classroom settings and clinical practice, preparing students to confront ethical dilemmas professionally. This attention to ethics fortifies the therapist's role as a guardian of traditional knowledge, while respecting the boundaries and expectations of contemporary healthcare.

As Marma Chikitsa progresses globally, consistent ethical guidelines across different regions will become crucial. Establishing these standards will not only safeguard the therapeutic integrity but also enhance public trust in Marma practices. Ultimately, these ethical frameworks will serve as a beacon, guiding practitioners in delivering compassionate and competent care.

Innovations in Marma Therapy Tools and Techniques

The landscape of Marma Chikitsa is evolving with groundbreaking innovations in tools and techniques that propose enhanced efficacy and patient comfort. Advances in biotechnology have paved the way for biofeedback devices that can measure the body's responses to Marma therapy, providing practitioners with real-time data to tailor treatments more precisely.

Additionally, modern engineering has introduced ergonomic tools designed to facilitate the precise application of pressure on Marma points. These tools not only increase the precision but also ensure uniformity and safety during the therapy sessions. Innovations such as these support practitioners in delivering more effective treatments and open new pathways for clinical research.

The integration of virtual reality and augmented reality technologies into Marma therapy training presents yet another exciting development. Through immersive simulations, practitioners can hone their skills and understand complex concepts in a controlled and enriched environment. Such technological advancements are set to redefine traditional practices, making Marma Chikitsa more accessible and effective for future generations.

The Future of Technology in Marma Practice

As Marma Chikitsa strides forward, the interplay between technology and traditional healing techniques is set to revolutionize this age-old practice. The integration of advanced diagnostic tools, such as bioenergetic scanning systems, will enhance the precision of Marma point identification, facilitating targeted and effective treatments.

Moreover, the adoption of wearable technology and mobile applications is poised to monitor patient reactions and progress in real-time. Such technologies not only streamline the monitoring process but also empower patients to engage actively in their healing journey. This interactive approach supports a more personalized Marma therapy experience, adapting treatments to individual needs and responses.

Looking ahead, the development of AI-driven algorithms promises to predict patient outcomes, optimize therapy plans, and even simulate Marma treatments through virtual reality. As these technologies mature, they will undoubtedly expand the boundaries of Marma Chikitsa, making it more accessible and effective on a global scale. Bridging the ancient with the avant-garde, the future of Marma therapy is brightly innovative.

Artificial Intelligence and Machine Learning in Marma Studies

The integration of Artificial Intelligence (AI) and Machine Learning (ML) in Marma Chikitsa heralds a transformative era in this traditional practice. By harnessing AI's analytical power, researchers can decode complex patterns in patient data, enhancing diagnosis, treatment personalization, and outcome prediction. ML algorithms are particularly potent in recognizing subtle nuances in the vast datasets collected during therapy sessions, enabling precision medicine tailored to individual physiological responses.

Moreover, AI-powered systems can continuously learn and adapt from each interaction, constantly refining treatment methodologies based on real-time feedback. This facilitates a dynamically evolving practice that is both rooted in ancient wisdom and at the forefront of technological innovation. AI's capability to simulate various therapy outcomes also allows for safer clinical trials, minimizing risks before direct patient application.

The synergy between AI and Marma Chikitsa not only elevates patient care but also propels Marma into the global scientific community, ensuring its relevance and sustainability. By forecasting trends and potential breakthroughs, AI contributes to ongoing research efforts, setting the stage for next-generation therapies that hold the promise of revolutionizing holistic healing.

International Marma Chikitsa Conferences and Symposia

The proliferation of International Marma Chikitsa Conferences and Symposia exemplifies the burgeoning global interest in this ancient healing practice. Such gatherings convene experts, practitioners, and researchers from various corners of the globe, creating a vibrant forum for sharing insights, innovations, and breakthroughs in Marma therapy. These events not only deepen the understanding of Marma Chikitsa but also foster international collaborations that could propel the practice to new heights.

Central to these conferences is the dissemination of cutting-edge research and clinical findings, which are pivotal for establishing evidence-based practices and enhancing therapeutic efficacy. Workshops and expert panels facilitate hands-on learning and real-time discussions on pressing issues such as integration into conventional healthcare systems and navigating global regulatory landscapes.

Moreover, these symposia serve as critical networking platforms, cultivating a community of practice that spans cultures and continents. The exchange of knowledge here helps to tailor Marma Chikitsa effectively to diverse populations, ensuring its relevance and sustainability in a global context.

Building a Global Community of Marma Practitioners

The global expansion of Marma Chikitsa hinges on nurturing a unified community of skilled practitioners. This initiative aims to weave a tapestry of practitioners enriched by diverse cultural insights and bound by a commitment to health restoration. Establishing interconnected networks across borders encourages the sharing of seminal practices and novel advancements, thus elevating the collective expertise.

Key to this community is the role of digital platforms which facilitate seamless exchanges of knowledge and collaboration on a grand scale. Social media groups, online forums, and virtual conferences make it possible for practitioners to connect, share case studies, and discuss treatment strategies irrespective of geographical limitations. This digital approach not only broadens the scope of practice but also democratizes access to specialized knowledge and training.

Moreover, creating a global community also focuses on mutual respect and learning. Recognizing and incorporating the traditional healing practices of diverse cultures enriches the Marma Chikitsa curriculum, fostering a more holistic and inclusive approach. This synergy ensures the survival and thrives the rich heritage of Marma Chikitsa, promoting a more profound global healing dialogue.

Cultural Sensitivity and Adaptation in Global Practice

As Marma Chikitsa expands across diverse cultural landscapes, the need for cultural sensitivity and adaptation becomes paramount. Marma practitioners must understand the nuanced cultural beliefs and practices that influence health perceptions and treatment acceptability in different regions. This understanding can guide the adaptation of Marma techniques to align with local customs, enhancing both the acceptance and effectiveness of treatments.

Training modules specifically designed to address cultural diversity are essential. These modules should teach practitioners how to navigate cultural nuances sensitively, ensuring that Marma Chikitsa does not just transplant an age-old practice into a foreign context, but rather integrates it meaningfully. Ethnographic studies could support this by providing deeper insights into cultural health narratives that shape patient expectations and responses to Marma therapy.

Ultimately, the global practice of Marma Chikitsa should champion cultural empathy and adaptability, paving the way for a truly holistic approach to health that respects and utilizes cultural diversity as a strength in healing practices.

Marma Chikitsa as a Tool for Social Change and Wellness

Marma Chikitsa transcends its primary role as a healing technique, emerging as a potent force for social change and wellness. By focusing on holistic well-being, this ancient practice catalyzes community-level health improvements, extending its benefits beyond the individual to influence entire populations. Effective application within diverse communities demonstrates the adaptability and universal relevance of Marma Chikitsa, making it a bridge between traditional wisdom and contemporary needs.

Furthermore, as societies grapple with increasing health disparities, Marma Chikitsa offers an accessible and affordable solution that can be integrated into various social programs. Its principles can underpin public health initiatives aimed at preventing disease and promoting vitality among underserved populations, thereby addressing social justice in healthcare access. Lastly, the wellness paradigm advocated by Marma Chikitsa encourages a sustainable lifestyle, emphasizing preventive care and self-awareness. As a tool for social change, it fosters a cultural shift towards health autonomy, empowering individuals with knowledge and techniques to maintain their well-being, thus reducing societal health burden.

Vision for the Next 50 Years in Marma Chikitsa

As we stand at the threshold of a new era for Marma Chikitsa, the next 50 years promise transformative shifts guided by technological integration and global collaboration. The forthcoming decades will likely see Marma Chikitsa ascend to an unparalleled prominence in both traditional and modern healthcare frameworks worldwide, bridging ancient practices with cutting-edge medical innovation.

Strategic international partnerships will be pivotal, forging a nexus between Marma practitioners and healthcare systems across the globe. This integration will facilitate a cross-cultural exchange of knowledge, enhance treatment models and broaden the scope of research methodologies. With an emphasis on sustainability, Marma Chikitsa will adapt to environmental changes and evolving health landscapes, maintaining its relevance and efficacy.

Visionary initiatives will focus on inclusivity, ensuring that Marma Chikitsa's benefits reach diverse populations. Increased accessibility and the spread of standardized training programs will democratize the practice, making it a cornerstone of global wellness and healthcare. As an advocate for holistic health, Marma Chikitsa will lead the charge towards a more balanced, health-centric world.

Summary

The chapter explores the evolution and global expansion of Marma Chikitsa, an ancient Ayurvedic practice, focusing on the need for standardized education, certification, and a global curriculum to ensure its efficacy, authenticity, and integration into modern healthcare systems. It begins by highlighting the diversity in teaching and practice of Marma Chikitsa across different regions, necessitating standardized education through clearly defined curricula and teaching methodologies, thereby ensuring consistent training and competency among practitioners. The development of certification programs and accreditation processes is discussed as crucial for establishing professionalism and trust in Marma Chikitsa, aligning it with global health standards and facilitating its recognition as a legitimate medical practice. The chapter also underscores the importance of a global curriculum that incorporates traditional knowledge and modern scientific research, aiming to make the practice culturally adaptable and globally relevant. Furthermore, it emphasizes the role of online courses in democratizing access to Marma Chikitsa education, allowing for widespread dissemination and standardization. Workshops and seminars are identified as platforms for practical training and international exchange of ideas, enriching practitioners' knowledge and skills. Moreover, integrating Marma Chikitsa into university curricula is suggested to foster academic recognition and research, whereas partnerships between Marma institutions and healthcare facilities are seen as pivotal for blending traditional and modern medical practices. The chapter also addresses the need for robust research, adequate funding, global legislative frameworks, and ethical considerations to enhance the practice's credibility and integration into conventional medicine. Innovations in tools and techniques, including the use of technology and AI, are predicted to revolutionize Marma

Chikitsa, making it more effective and accessible globally. Ultimately, the chapter calls for building a global community of practitioners and maintaining cultural sensitivity, projecting Marma Chikitsa not only as a therapeutic tool but also a means for social change and wellness in the coming decades.

References

[1] Birch, J., & Felt, R. L. (2013). Understanding Acupuncture. Churchill Livingstone.. https://www.elsevier.com/books/understanding-acupuncture/birch/978-0-443-05627-9

[2] Gogte, V. M. (2000). Ayurvedic Pharmacology and Therapeutic Uses of Medicinal Plants (Dravyagunavignyan). Bharatiya Vidya Bhavan.. https://books.google.com/books?id=B8eIPQAACAAJ

[3] Sharma, H., & Clark, C. (2012). Contemporary Ayurveda: Medicine and Research in Maharishi Ayur-Veda. Churchill Livingstone.. https://www.elsevier.com/books/contemporary-ayurveda-medicine-and-research-in-maharishi-ayur-veda/sharma/978-0-443-05594-4

[4] Subbarayappa, B. V. (1997). The Roots of Ancient Medicine: An Historical Outline. Journal of Biosciences, 22(2), 135-143.. https://link.springer.com/article/10.1007/BF02703361

[5] World Health Organization. (2002). WHO Traditional Medicine Strategy 2002–2005.. https://apps.who.int/iris/handle/10665/67163

Case Study: Standardizing Marma Chikitsa Curriculum Across Diverse Cultural Contexts

In an era of globalization, as Marma Chikitsa, an ancient Indian healing practice, begins to permeate across different continents, the need for a universally cohesive yet culturally adaptable educational framework becomes apparent. The fictional case of the Transnational Institute of Marma Studies (TIMS) serves as an illustrative example of the complexities involved in creating such a curriculum that transcends geographical and cultural boundaries while maintaining the authenticity of Marma Chikitsa.

TIMS, established in 2023, sought to standardize the Marma Chikitsa curriculum used in their centers spread across Asia, Europe, and North America. Their primary challenge was to integrate the traditional Indian principles of Marma therapy with the diverse cultural healthcare beliefs predominant in each country they operate in. For instance, while European centers focused more on the alignment with modern medical practices, the Asian counterparts emphasized adherence to traditional holistic approaches.

To address this, TIMS convened a global conference with leading educators, practitioners, and cultural anthropologists from its various centers. The discussions aimed to pinpoint core elements of Marma Chikitsa that were universally essential such as the identification of Marma points and the therapeutic techniques. They also debated on customizable aspects of the curriculum that could be adapted to respect cultural sensitivities and regional medical norms. Significant was their effort to include modules that dealt with local herbs, alternative healing modalities, and language-specific educational materials.

Throughout two years of rigorous collaboration and several iterative adjustments in teaching methods and curriculum design, TIMS managed to roll out a standardized global curriculum. The curriculum was well-received due to its balanced approach that preserved the integral essence of Marma Chikitsa and embraced local practices, thereby enhancing both student engagement and therapeutic effectiveness across regions.

Case Study: Integrative Approaches to Marma Chikitsa in Western Hospitals

The fictional case of Bethany Hospital in the United States presents an intriguing example of how Marma Chikitsa can be integrated into the conventional medical system in a Western setting, thereby highlighting challenges and solutions in melding traditional Indian healing practices with modern Western medicine. In 2025, Bethany Hospital introduced a pilot program aimed at incorporating Marma Chikitsa into their pain management and rehabilitation services. This initiative was part of a larger strategy to embrace integrative health solutions that combine the best of Western medicine and traditional holistic approaches.

The hospital faced several significant challenges at the outset. Firstly, there was skepticism among medical staff who were unfamiliar with Marma Chikitsa's principles and its efficacy. To address this, the hospital organized extensive training sessions conducted by expert practitioners from India, supplemented by a series of workshops that focused on the scientific and clinical aspects of Marma therapy. Additionally, the hospital had to navigate regulatory hurdles related to the accreditation of non-conventional medical practices within hospital settings.

To measure the success and acceptance of this integrative approach, Bethany Hospital set up a detailed evaluation system. They conducted pre- and post-treatment surveys with patients and staff, collected data on patient recovery times, and compared the outcomes with traditional pain management treatments. The findings revealed noticeable improvements in patient recovery rates and significant reductions in the usage of pharmacological interventions.

The success of the pilot program led to the establishment of a dedicated Marma Chikitsa wing at the hospital by 2028. This wing worked on a collaborative model where Marma practitioners and Western-trained doctors worked side by side. This case illustrates not only the potential for integrating Marma Chikitsa into mainstream Western healthcare but also the importance of education, regulatory adaptation, and rigorous evaluation in achieving successful integration.

Case Study: Advancing Global Marma Chikitsa Education through Digital Platforms

With the rising globalization of Marma Chikitsa, a traditional Indian healing practice, access to standardized training and education in this field has become paramount. The fictional case of the Global Institute of Marma Therapy (GIMT) highlights the challenges and solutions in creating and distributing a digital learning platform tailored to both aspiring practitioners worldwide and existing practitioners seeking further certification.

Established in 2024, GIMT developed a comprehensive online platform designed to offer courses ranging from beginner to advanced levels, all structured around the core principles of Marma Chikitsa. A major hurdle they encountered was ensuring the platform's accessibility to users in remote or underserved regions, where internet connectivity could be unreliable. Additionally, GIMT faced the challenge of maintaining the integrity and authenticity of the teachings while adapting the content to a format that was engaging and effective for online learners.

To address these issues, GIMT collaborated with technology experts to develop low-bandwidth versions of courses and mobile-friendly materials. They also incorporated interactive elements such as virtual reality simulations of Marma point locations and therapy techniques to enhance the learning experience. Furthermore, GIMT established a tier-based certification system endorsed by known international bodies of traditional medicine, ensuring that their courses met global educational standards.

The impact of GIMT's online platform was significant. By 2026, the platform had attracted students from over 40 countries, many of whom were able to initiate local practices or integrate Marma Chikitsa into existing health services. Feedback from a continuous quality improvement program indicated high satisfaction with the practical applications of the courses and a deeper understanding of the cultural and scientific aspects of Marma therapy.

GIMT's case illustrates the potent role digital education platforms can play in transcending geographic boundaries, making traditional practices like Marma Chikitsa accessible and applicable in a global context. This approach not only democratizes learning but also enhances the scalability of traditional knowledge preservation worldwide.

Case Study: Implementing Marma Chikitsa in Community Health Initiatives

In the evolving landscape of global healthcare, integrating traditional practices like Marma Chikitsa into community health programs presents unique challenges and opportunities. The fictional case of Harmony Health Initiative (HHI), a community-based health program in Southeast Asia, showcases the complexities and benefits of incorporating Marma Chikitsa into community health services.

In 2026, HHI launched a pilot project aimed at reducing the incidence of chronic pain and enhancing overall wellness in rural areas through Marma Chikitsa. The project faced significant initial hurdles, including cultural hesitations about non-conventional medical practices and a lack of trained Marma practitioners in the region. In response, HHI collaborated with local health authorities and Marma education institutions to facilitate workshops and training programs, aiming to cultivate a skilled workforce from the local population.

The HHI also had to consider logistical aspects, such as the procurement of resources and the adaptation of Marma techniques to suit local cultural contexts. They developed a model where local healers were trained in basic Marma techniques, supplemented with modern medical knowledge. This combination promoted a holistic approach, encouraging community acceptance and engagement.

To assess the impact of the Marma Chikitsa interventions, HHI established a comprehensive evaluation framework. Community health workers collected data on patient outcomes, which included improvements in pain management, mobility, and general well-being. The data demonstrated significant health benefits, leading to an expansion of the program across other communities.

Through this case study, HHI's experience highlights the importance of community involvement in health care interventions, the need for adaptable health solutions across different cultural settings, and the potential of traditional practices like Marma Chikitsa to complement modern medical techniques in addressing comprehensive health needs.

Case Study: Establishing a Global Marma Research Network

In the realm of traditional medicine, ensuring the legitimacy and efficacy of treatments is crucial for wider acceptance in the global healthcare community. This case study examines the establishment of the International Marma Research Network (IMRN) in 2025, a consortium aimed at promoting high-quality research and evidence-based practices in Marma Chikitsa.

IMRN was founded through collaborative efforts between universities, healthcare institutions, and traditional medicine practitioners from India, Europe, and North America. One of the foremost challenges faced by the IMRN was creating standardized research protocols that could be applied across different research environments while respecting the diverse traditional knowledges and methods associated with Marma Chikitsa. This difficulty was compounded by varying regulations concerning traditional medicine in different countries, which affected how research could be conducted and how findings could be implemented in practice.

To tackle these challenges, IMRN organized several global workshops and seminars to discuss and establish common research methodologies. These gatherings included stakeholders from various backgrounds, including medical researchers, Marma practitioners, and policymakers. One significant outcome was the development of a comprehensive digital database for sharing research data and case studies amongst researchers, which supported transparency and facilitated the replication of studies.

Moreover, IMRN focused on building capacities for conducting clinical trials that meet international standards. They developed a training program for researchers and practitioners to ensure that studies on Marma Chikitsa were designed robustly, conducted ethically, and reported accurately. The network also pursued partnerships with pharmaceutical companies and medical technology firms to support the development of innovative Marma therapy tools and techniques.

Despite these strides, the IMRN continuously grapples with maintaining a balance between modern research practices and the traditional ethos that underpins Marma Chikitsa. They strive to produce research that not only enhances the scientific understanding of Marma therapies but also promotes its integration into mainstream healthcare systems globally.

Case Study: Establishing Marma Chikitsa Centers in Non-Traditional Markets

The global spread of Marma Chikitsa faces unique challenges, particularly when introduced in non-traditional markets, such as Scandinavia, where public and academic familiarity with Ayurvedic principles is minimal. A fictional Northern European wellness company, 'Nordic Harmony', ventured to establish Marma Chikitsa centers across Sweden, Norway, and Finland in 2027 with the goal of integrating this ancient practice into Scandinavian wellness culture.

Nordic Harmony's initiative began with a research phase, identifying key cultural barriers and consumer wellness trends in Scandinavia. The findings revealed a strong regional focus on evidence-based medical practices and a high value placed on mental health and stress reduction, areas where Marma Chikitsa could potentially offer significant benefits. However, the unfamiliarity of Marma Chikitsa in the region posed a considerable challenge in terms of acceptance and clientele building.

To mitigate this, Nordic Harmony launched an extensive educational campaign, collaborating with local healthcare providers and engaging in community wellness events to raise awareness. They offered free introductory sessions and published collaborative research with Scandinavian health institutes illustrating Marma Chikitsa's efficacy in stress relief and mental wellness. Recognizing the importance of credible endorsements in health-related matters, Nordic Harmony also sought accreditation from notable health organizations in each country.

The strategy included tailoring the Marma therapy offerings to align with local health practices, such as integrating light therapy during the dark winter months, a popular method in Scandinavia for fighting seasonal affective disorder. By 2029, the efforts began to show results; client intake numbers improved as Marma Chikitsa's stress reduction benefits became more recognized. Mini-case studies from patients who experienced significant improvements in their mental and physical health were documented and shared, further establishing credibility.

This case exemplifies the complex interplay between traditional healing practices and modern health systems, underlining the importance of strategic cultural adaptation and evidence-based practice to successfully integrate Marma Chikitsa into non-traditional markets.

Case Study: Leveraging International Partnerships to Standardize Marma Chikitsa Education

The fictional Alliance for Global Marma Education (AGME) illustrates the pivotal role of international partnerships in standardizing and spreading Marma Chikitsa education globally. Established in 2027, AGME comprises a coalition of educational institutions from India, Thailand, the United States, and the United Kingdom, each bringing a unique perspective and expertise related to holistic and integrative health practices.

AGME's primary mission was to create a standardized educational framework that could be adaptable to various global regions while preserving the integrity and effectiveness of Marma Chikitsa. One of the initial challenges was the varying levels of acceptance and familiarity with Marma Chikitsa in different countries. For instance, in Thailand, there was a profound respect and acceptance for traditional therapies like Marma, whereas in the US and the UK, there was a significant need for integration into existing healthcare education models and a push for evidence-based practice to gain wider acceptance.

To tackle these challenges, AGME initiated a series of collaborative research projects aimed at scientifically validating the efficacy of Marma Chikitsa. This involved experimental designs that could be replicated across different research facilities internationally, employing a multidisciplinary approach that combined modern scientific techniques with traditional knowledge. Furthermore, AGME facilitated student and faculty exchange programs among the coalition institutions, which were instrumental in fostering a deeper mutual understanding and appreciation of the global diversity in healthcare practices.

By 2029, AGME successfully rolled out a global curriculum that included core modules on Marma point techniques, elective courses focusing on regional treatment practices, and a robust component on clinical research methods. Through continuous feedback loops involving online forums and annual symposiums, AGME refined the curriculum iteratively to better meet the educational needs across different contexts, thereby ensuring its global relevance and applicability.

Case Study: Revolutionizing Rural Healthcare with Marma Chikitsa Mobile Clinics

The fictional case of the Mobile Marma Health Initiative (MMHI) vividly illustrates the impact of mobile clinics on rural healthcare accessibility and education in Marma Chikitsa. Launched in 2025, MMHI aimed to bridge the healthcare gap in remote areas of India where access to traditional and modern medical facilities was limited. Each mobile clinic was equipped with the necessary tools and staffed by trained practitioners who could deliver Marma Chikitsa, along with basic healthcare services, directly to these underserved communities.

The initiative initially faced several challenges, including geographical barriers, cultural hesitancy towards non-conventional medical practices, and logistical issues related to the maintenance and operation of mobile clinics. To overcome these obstacles, MMHI conducted community engagement sessions to educate locals about the benefits of Marma Chikitsa, emphasizing its non-invasiveness and historical relevance in Indian culture. Additionally, the program worked closely with local governments and other healthcare organizations to integrate into existing health systems, ensuring a collaborative and supportive approach to rural health.

As MMHI clinics began to operate, they kept detailed records of patient interactions, treatments provided, and follow-up outcomes. This data not only facilitated the ongoing assessment and adaptation of the service model but also served as valuable research material to analyze the effectiveness of mobile Marma therapy interventions. Over three years, MMHI observed a significant improvement in community health metrics, such as reduced prevalence of chronic pain and improved mobility among the elderly population. The clinics also played a crucial role during the public health emergencies by providing immediate care and disseminating health information.

This case not only underscores the adaptability and effectiveness of Marma Chikitsa in mobile healthcare settings but also showcases how innovative service delivery models can profoundly impact public health. By leveraging mobility, MMHI was able to democratize access to specialized care, making Marma Chikitsa a viable option for rural health enhancement. The success of MMHI has sparked interest in replicating this model in other parts of the world, tailoring the approach to meet diverse healthcare and cultural needs.

Case Study: Fostering Marma Chikitsa through Healthcare Policy Integration in Emerging Economies

In the fictional scenario, the government of the emerging economy of Rupland decided to integrate Marma Chikitsa, a traditional healing practice from India, into its national healthcare system in 2027. This initiative was propelled by a growing recognition of the benefits of integrative health approaches and bolstered by a surge in public interest following successful implementation stories from neighboring countries. Rupland's Ministry of Health envisioned that incorporating Marma Chikitsa could address several pressing healthcare challenges, particularly in rural areas lacking in conventional medical facilities.

The first major challenge was the lack of a standardized Marma Chikitsa curriculum and insufficient trained practitioners in Rupland. To counter this, the government collaborated with the Global Institute of Traditional Medicine (GITM) to develop an education and certification program specifically tailored for local cultural contexts and health needs. This program was designed to enable quick scalability, focusing on training healthcare workers already operating in the community, elevating their skill set with Marma techniques.

To facilitate this integration, the Rupland government proposed amendments to existing healthcare policies, which included recognizing Marma Chikitsa as a certified medical practice and establishing funding for training centers and clinical research. Legislative changes were met with mixed reactions; while there was support from various traditional medicine proponents, skepticism remained among conventional medical practitioners who questioned the efficacy of Marma Chikitsa based on scientific evidence.

As part of the policy integration, pilot projects were launched in select rural districts where access to conventional healthcare was critically limited. These projects not only provided essential healthcare services but also served as living labs for practicing and refining Marma Chikitsa applications, gathering data on patient outcomes and practitioner experiences. This grassroots level implementation helped in aligning Marma Chikitsa with localized health services, enhancing its acceptance and effectiveness in Rupland's broader medical framework.

Case Study: Global Collaboration for Standardizing Marma Chikitsa Practitioner Training

In the growing global arena of traditional therapeutic practices, the pressing need for standardized training and universally recognized certifications in Marma Chikitsa has become evident. Here, we explore the case of the International Council for Marma Therapy Standards (ICMTS), established in 2030, which plays a crucial role in this endeavor.

ICMTS was formed through a coalition of traditional medicine institutions from India, China, and the United States, recognizing the need for a hybrid model of education that balances traditional knowledge with modern pedagogical approaches. The core challenge faced by ICMTS was harmonizing the diverse training methodologies and substantive content across different cultures without diluting the essence of Marma Chikitsa.

To achieve its goals, ICMTS initiated a multi-phased project involving the development of a unified practitioner training framework. The first phase focused on extensive research to understand the existing landscape of Marma Chikitsa education worldwide, engaging with a wide range of stakeholders including seasoned practitioners, academicians, and students. The second phase involved a series of international workshops and symposiums designed to draft a preliminary standard that included key competencies, ethical guidelines, and examination protocols.

Despite initial resistance due to the perception of undermining regional practices, ICMTS proceeded by incorporating feedback mechanisms and pilot testing phases in varied locales. This approach facilitated adaptation, highlighted region-specific needs, and incorporated supplementary modules such as local herbology and integration with other complementary traditional practices like acupuncture or chiropractic adjustments.

By 2033, ICMTS successfully launched a global certification program for Marma practitioners, endorsed by international healthcare bodies. This not only standardized training but also helped bridge the gap between traditional and modern medical practices, enhancing the legitimacy and global reach of Marma Chikitsa.

Review Questions

1. A university decides to incorporate Marma Chikitsa into their curriculum as an official course of study. The dean of the medical faculty is exploring various approaches to ensure a comprehensive and structured education model. What should be the initial focus to integrate Marma teachings effectively in the university setting?

A) A. Developing a core curriculum that includes both theoretical and practical components
B) B. Immediately starting practical Marma healing sessions for students
C) C. Focusing solely on the historical and philosophical aspects of Marma Chikitsa
D) D. Partnering with local Marma practitioners for guest lectures only

Answer: A

Explanation: Integrating Marma Chikitsa into a university curriculum effectively requires a balanced approach that includes both theoretical knowledge and practical skills. Starting with the development of a core curriculum ensures that students receive a structured and comprehensive education that covers all fundamental aspects of Marma therapy. This should ideally include the study of its history, theoretical underpinnings, and practical applications in clinical settings to ensure students are well-prepared for professional practice. While guest lectures and practical sessions are important, they should complement a well-defined core curriculum.

2. Marma Chikitsa is gaining traction across global medical communities, necessitating structured certification to establish professional standards. What would be the most critical outcome of implementing standardized certification programs for Marma practitioners?

A) A. Decreasing the need for traditional medical treatments
B) B. Ensuring uniform levels of practitioner competence and patient safety
C) C. Eliminating other forms of traditional therapies
D) D. Only enhancing the reputation of Marma Chikitsa practitioners

Answer: B

Explanation: Implementing standardized certification programs for Marma practitioners primarily ensures that there is a uniform level of competence among practitioners and enhances patient safety. Certification establishes a reliable benchmark for the skills and knowledge expected of competent practitioners, which in turn reassures patients regarding the integrity and safety of their treatments. This step is crucial for integrating Marma Chikitsa into broader medical practices globally, where consistent and reliable therapeutic practices are paramount.

3. The global expansion of Marma Chikitsa necessitates the creation of a universal curriculum. What should be the primary focus while developing this curriculum to maintain its effectiveness across diverse cultural landscapes?
A) A. Focus exclusively on the technical aspects of Marma point application
B) B. Incorporate a variety of healing traditions and contemporary health sciences
C) C. Limit the curriculum to the regions where Marma Chikitsa originated
D) D. Develop the curriculum in one language to maintain its purity
Answer: B
Explanation: When developing a global curriculum for Marma Chikitsa, the primary focus should be on integrating a wide array of healing traditions and contemporary health science. This approach ensures that the curriculum is not only comprehensive but also adaptable to various cultural contexts, enhancing its global applicability. Including diverse healing traditions enriches the learning experience and leverages accumulated knowledge, while contemporary health sciences ensure the curriculum remains relevant and scientifically rigorous. Such an inclusive educational framework prepares practitioners to effectively apply Marma therapy across different cultural settings while maintaining technical proficiency.

4. With the advent of technology, online courses have become a crucial platform for teaching Marma Chikitsa. What key feature should these courses include to ensure effective learning and skill acquisition for distant learners?
A) A. Only provide theoretical knowledge through recorded lectures
B) B. Include interactive elements like webinars, virtual workshops, and real-time discussions
C) C. Use only traditional teaching methods such as direct apprenticeship
D) D. Limit access to courses to ensure exclusivity
Answer: B
Explanation: To ensure effective learning and skill acquisition in online Marma Chikitsa courses, including interactive elements such as webinars, virtual workshops, and real-time discussions is essential. These interactive modes of learning engage students more dynamically compared to passive listening and help simulate a classroom environment. They allow for real-time feedback, personal interaction with instructors, and the ability to address queries immediately, which are crucial for comprehensive understanding and effective learning.

5. In response to growing global interest, a university decides to host a series of workshops and seminars on Marma Chikitsa. What should be the primary focus of these events to foster a broader understanding and application of Marma practices?
A) A. Exclusively allow experienced Marma practitioners to attend
B) B. Focus solely on the revenue generation from these workshops
C) C. Facilitate diverse exchanges of ideas and practical demonstrations
D) D. Offer these sessions only in regions familiar with Marma Chikitsa
Answer: C
Explanation: The primary focus of hosting university-led workshops and seminars on Marma Chikitsa should be to facilitate a diverse exchange of ideas along with practical demonstrations. This approach ensures that participants from various backgrounds—whether they are seasoned practitioners or novices—can deepen their understanding and enhance their practical skills. It also promotes cultural exchange and adaptation of Marma Chikitsa into various medical practices, thereby supporting its integration into the broader medical community. Such interactive and inclusive events are crucial for fostering global comprehension and application of this ancient healing art.

CHAPTER THIRTEEN: Development and Evolution of Marma Chikitsa

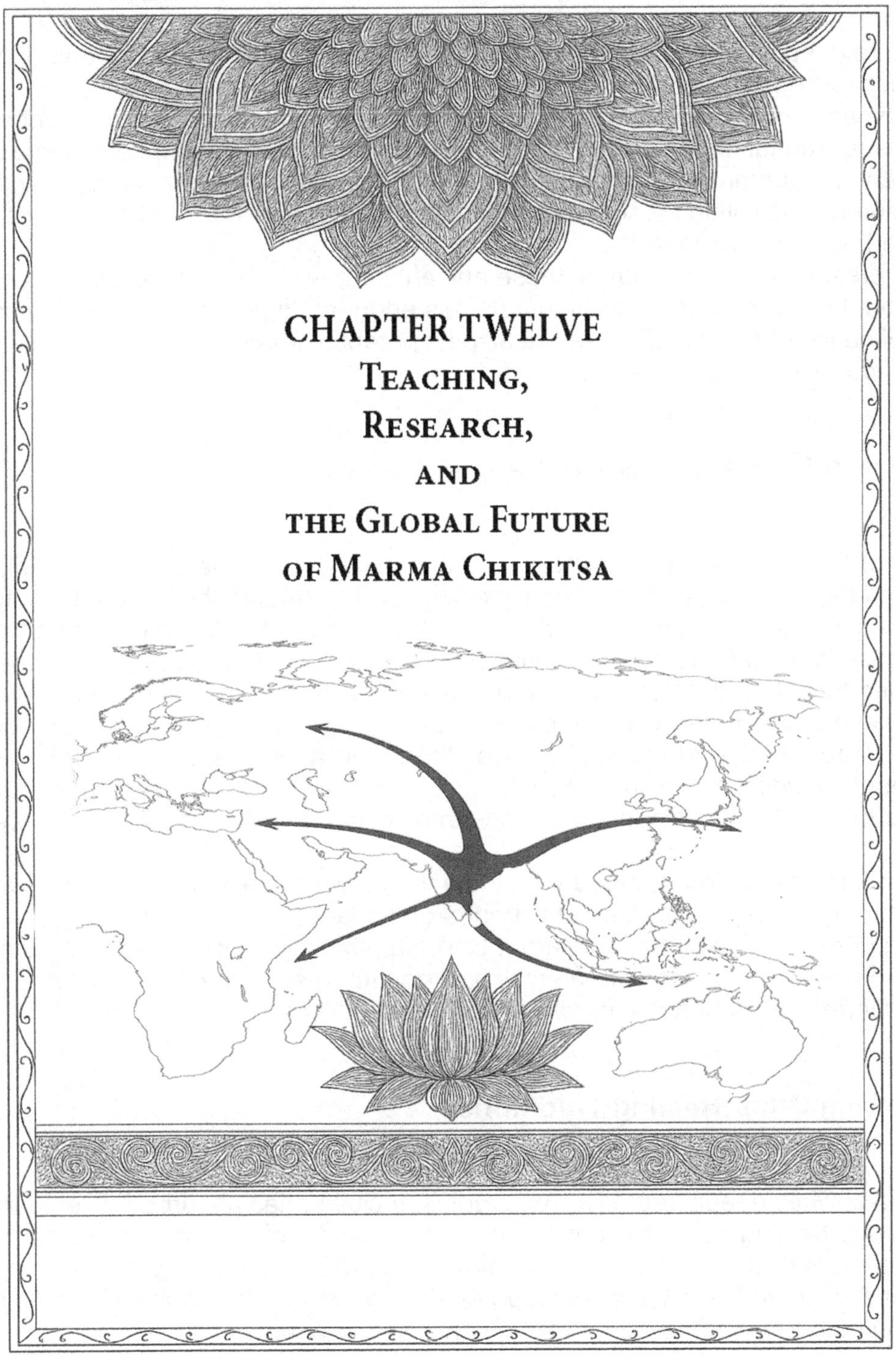

Early Foundations: Tracing Back to Ancient Scripts

The roots of Marma Chikitsa are deeply embedded in the ancient scriptures of Ayurveda, where the first notions of energy points on the human body were documented. These early texts, including the revered Charaka Samhita, elucidate the foundational concepts that underpin the practice, emphasizing its role in harmonizing the body's vital energies.

Scholars and sages of ancient times meticulously described the locations and attributes of marma points, essential for the flow of life force, or prana. These descriptions served as a guide for subsequent generations, shaping the early methodologies of Marma therapy. The integration of spiritual dimensions within these texts highlighted the belief in Marma Chikitsa's capacity to heal both the body and spirit.

Through the preservation and study of these ancient scripts, modern practitioners continue to refine and adapt these primordial techniques. This enduring legacy not only underscores the cultural significance of Marma Chikitsa but also its potential for contemporary relevance in holistic healing practices across Asia.

The First Practitioners: Profiles of Early Marma Healers

The genesis of Marma Chikitsa is anchored in the expertise of its inaugural practitioners, sages who discerned the subtle interplays of bodily energies. These early healers, often intertwined with the roles of spiritual guides, laid down the bedrock for this profound healing art through meticulous observation and experiential wisdom. Their deep understanding of life forces, or prana, enabled them to manipulate marma points for holistic healing and spiritual awakening.

Portraits of these pioneers, drawn from carvings and scriptures, depict them with tools that were rudimentary yet remarkably effective. Bamboo sticks, herbal pastes, and sanctified oils were their instruments, guiding the pranic currents to restore health and vitality. This illustration not only conveys their skills but also their revered status in communities as bearers of wellness and harmony.

As custodians of this sacred knowledge, their teachings were orally passed down, weaving a legacy that thrived through centuries. This unbroken lineage, enriched by each generation, ensured the survival and evolution of Marma Chikitsa, shaping it into a cornerstone of Ayurvedic medicine. The reverence for these healers is well documented in the classical texts, celebrating their contributions to ancient healthcare and spiritual practices.

Influences from Other Healing Traditions

Marma Chikitsa, while deeply rooted in Ayurvedic principles, has absorbed diverse influences from neighboring healing practices, enriching its scope and techniques over the centuries. The cross-pollination with traditional Chinese medicine, particularly the concepts like acupuncture, introduced new dimensions to the stimulation of Marma points, emphasizing energy pathways that complement the Ayurvedic focus on body energies or prana.

Interaction with Tibetan medicine also brought forth the incorporation of spiritual healing elements, using mantra and meditational techniques as adjuncts to physical point manipulation. These influences were adapted to suit the underlying philosophies of Marma Chikitsa, ensuring the integration maintained the essence of harnessing the body's innate healing capabilities.

Notably, the exchange with Greek medicine during the classical era introduced herbal poultices and oils that are now quintessential in Marma therapy. Each cultural interaction has left a lasting imprint, making Marma Chikitsa a holistic amalgam of global medicinal wisdom, continuously evolving with each new influence.

Cross-Cultural Exchanges in Marma Practices

The fabric of Marma Chikitsa is woven with myriad threads from various cultural tapestries, illustrating a rich history of cross-cultural exchanges. These interactions have infused Marma practices with a diverse palette of healing techniques, contributing significantly to its evolution and widespread acceptance. Each cultural intersection broadened the understanding and application of Marma points, harmonizing traditional Indian knowledge with insights from foreign lands.

The Silk Road, not just a conduit for trade but also for knowledge exchange, played a pivotal role. It facilitated the transmission of Marma practices into Central Asia and beyond, intertwining them with local medical practices. This blend enriched Marma Chikitsa, introducing new herbal remedies and massage techniques that were assimilated into the practice, enhancing its effectiveness and appeal.

Likewise, mariners and traders brought back concepts from Southeast Asia and the Middle East, which were seamlessly woven into Marma therapies. These contributions are evident in the adjusted manipulation techniques and expanded use of aromatic compounds in Marma therapy. Each cultural layer added through these exchanges has not only enriched the practice but also ensured its survival and relevance in the contemporary healing landscape.

Transmission of Knowledge: Oral and Written

The transmission of Marma Chikitsa knowledge played a crucial role in its preservation and evolution. Initially, the wisdom of Marma was imparted orally, a tradition rooted deeply in the guru-shishya parampara, where knowledge flowed from master to apprentice in an unbroken lineage. This oral method ensured that the subtleties and spiritual aspects of Marma therapy were conveyed with personal attention and deep understanding.

As the practice matured, the need for documentation became evident. Gradually, the ancient wisdom was encapsulated in manuscripts and later texts. These written records aimed to reach a wider audience, ensuring the dissemination of knowledge across different regions and generations. This shift marked a significant evolution in the educational tactics of Marma Chikitsa, from exclusively oral to a hybrid approach of oral and written transmission.

This transition not only democratized the knowledge but also facilitated a broader scholarly examination, enabling Marma Chikitsa to integrate scientifically with other traditional and modern medical practices. The amalgamation of oral wisdom with written documentation has crucially contributed to the robust scholarly and practical framework that supports Marma Chikitsa today.

Marma Chikitsa in Ancient Texts: A Literary Review

A profound exploration of ancient texts reveals the intricate tapestry of Marma Chikitsa, chronicled extensively in classical Ayurvedic literature. These texts serve as critical repositories, detailing the therapeutic manipulation of Marma points. Predominantly, the Sushruta Samhita elaborates on 107 Marma points, classifying them by their anatomical positions and potential impacts on health when treated.

This literary corpus illustrates how ancient scholars perceived the intersection of physical and etheric bodies through Marma points, aimed at achieving a balance that promotes healing and vitality. Moreover, the texts address the ensemble of tools and herbal concoctions used in early Marma practices, underlining the holistic approach embraced by practitioners of the time. Interwoven with philosophical underpinnings, these scriptures not only delineate practical aspects but also delve into the spiritual dimensions of Marma Chikitsa. Such integration highlights the dual objective of this ancient science—restoring physical health while fostering spiritual well-being, portraying a healing modality that transcends mere physical treatment.

Evolution of Tools and Techniques Over the Centuries

The transformation of tools and techniques in Marma Chikitsa demonstrates a riveting evolution, reflecting the broader shifts in Ayurvedic medicine. Initially, rudimentary implements like bamboo sticks and herbal concoctions were predominant, employed by early practitioners to manipulate vital points. As knowledge expanded, these tools were refined, incorporating metallurgy with the introduction of metallic probes, which offered more precision in treatment. Herbal pastes evolved into more sophisticated forms as botanic knowledge deepened. Ayurvedic oils, now integral, began to be tailored for specific doshic imbalances, enhancing the efficacy of Marma therapies. This period also saw the rise of specialized equipment designed to ensure more accurate application and reduction of practitioner fatigue, manifesting an intersection of ergonomic science with traditional practices.

As Marma Chikitsa entered contemporary times, technological integration became evident. Digital pressure instruments and anatomical software began assisting practitioners, ensuring treatments were both exact and deep-rooted in traditional efficacy. These advancements represent a bridge between ancient wisdom and modern practicality, continually shaping the future of Marma Chikitsa.

Integration of Marma with Other Ayurvedic Practices

The interweaving of Marma Chikitsa with other Ayurvedic practices showcases a symbiotic enhancement, vital for holistic healing. This fusion involves integrating Marma point stimulation with Ayurvedic diagnostics, enriching the treatment of doshic imbalances. Aligning Marma therapy with Panchakarma, for instance, enables a deeper purification process, where Marma aids in opening channels that facilitate the elimination of bodily toxins.

Furthermore, the adjunct use of Ayurvedic herbs, oils, and dietary recommendations with Marma treatments exemplifies a comprehensive approach, aiming at an all-encompassing restoration of health. These combinations cater to individual needs, tailoring therapies that address both physical and energetic imbalances. The synergy between Marma therapy and Ayurvedic lifestyle adjustments—like yoga and meditation—enhances overall vitality and

wellness, promoting a seamless integration of body, mind, and spirit.
By pulling together various threads of Ayurvedic wisdom, practitioners can offer more nuanced and effective therapies. This evolution of Marma Chikitsa reflects its adaptability and enduring relevance in the holistic health landscape, as it continually incorporates traditional insights with innovative approaches.

Milestones in Marma Chikitsa Development

Marma Chikitsa's development is marked by significant milestones that highlight its evolving influence and sophistication. The origins trace to the ancient Vedic texts, where preliminary concepts were recorded. This period heralded a foundational understanding, setting the stage for structured practices. Noteworthy is the 6th-century compilation of the Sushruta Samhita, which systematized Marma knowledge by cataloging 107 vital points. This era underscored a pivotal advance in medical texts, embedding Marma deeply within Ayurvedic traditions.
The adaptation of Marma techniques during the medieval period, especially with the influx of Islamic medical knowledge via the Mughal era, brought surgical and herbal enhancements that expanded its efficacy. Equally transformative was the 19th-century British colonial interest in Ayurveda, which introduced Marma Chikitsa to Western scholars, sparking a global curiosity that survives today.
In contemporary times, the establishment of dedicated institutions and formal courses for Marma Chikitsa around the late 20th century marks another critical milestone. These educational endeavors not only standardized the practice but also ensured its proliferation beyond traditional boundaries, fostering a modern renaissance in holistic healing that continues to grow.

Notable Practitioners and Their Contributions

The annals of Marma Chikitsa are illuminated by notable practitioners whose innovations and dedication have significantly shaped its course. Among these, Vagbhata and Sushruta stand out as pioneering figures. Vagbhata's contributions were crucial in systematizing the therapeutic approaches towards Marma, integrating it seamlessly with holistic Ayurvedic protocols. His texts serve as a bridge between ancient wisdom and contemporary practices.
Sushruta, often revered as the 'Father of Surgery', enriched Marma Chikitsa with his surgical precision and profound understanding of anatomy. His classifications of Marma points and detailed descriptions in the 'Sushruta Samhita' have been paramount in teaching generations of healers the critical intersections of energy and physiology.
In more recent times, practitioners like Krishnakumar from Kerala have revived traditional techniques that were on the verge of oblivion, innovating with modern tools while adhering to the spiritual essence of Marma. Their work not only maintains the integrity of Marma Chikitsa but also enhances its global relevance and adaptability.

Geographical Spread and Regional Variations of Marma Practice

The geographical spread of Marma Chikitsa, originally ingrained in the Indian subcontinent, has witnessed an expansive reach across diverse Asian territories, adjusting to varied cultural and medicinal landscapes. Over centuries, as these practices traversed through regions, distinct local adaptations emerged, reflecting the integrative essence of Marma Chikitsa with regional healing modalities.

In Sri Lanka, for instance, the practice incorporated elements of local ritual and folk medicine, becoming a staple in traditional Sri Lankan Ayurveda. Similar integrations can be observed in Tibetan healing practices, where Marma techniques blend seamlessly with Buddhist medicinal practices, highlighting a syncretic approach to health and spirituality.

Moreover, the assimilation of Marma therapy into Southeast Asian medical systems reflects a dynamic absorption of Ayurvedic principles fused with local herbal traditions. Countries such as Thailand and Indonesia have adapted Marma practices into their traditional massage therapies, crafting a unique hybrid that resonates with local health beliefs and practices. This geographical branching not only enriches Marma Chikitsa but also perpetuates its relevance in contemporary holistic health discourse.

The Renaissance of Marma in Modern Times

The modern renaissance of Marma Chikitsa marks a significant resurgence, reflecting both a revival of traditional practices and an embrace of new methodologies. As global interest in holistic and integrative medicine swells, Marma Chikitsa has regained prominence not just as an ancient art but as a relevant contemporary therapy. The dissemination of knowledge through digital platforms has played a pivotal role in this revival, enabling the widespread sharing and learning of Marma techniques across boundaries.

Educational programs in Ayurvedic colleges worldwide now frequently include Marma Chikitsa as a critical component of study, often coupled with modern anatomical sciences. This integration ensures practitioners are well-versed in both traditional techniques and modern medical understandings, broadening the appeal and applicability of Marma therapy.

Moreover, the renaissance encompasses a broader recognition of its efficacy in pain management and rehabilitation settings. Enhanced by scientific research validating its therapeutic claims, Marma Chikitsa continues to evolve, intertwining empirical evidence with centuries-old wisdom to meet the health demands of the modern era.

Shifts from Spiritual to More Clinical Approaches

The progression of Marma Chikitsa, historically rooted in spiritual practice, has witnessed a significant paradigm shift towards more clinical methodologies. Initially, this healing art emphasized the spiritual alignment and energy balance, deeply intertwined with religious rituals and meditative practices. However, with the advent of modern medicine and a growing demand for empirical validation, Marma Chikitsa began adopting a more evidence-based approach. This transition was catalyzed by increased scientific scrutiny and a global push towards standardizing alternative therapies. Clinical trials and anatomical studies started to dissect the mechanisms behind Marma points, striving to integrate them with contemporary medical understanding. This clinical perspective did not erase the spiritual roots but enhanced the

practice's credibility and facilitated its acceptance in medical communities.
Today, this synthesis of spiritual and clinical approaches enables Marma Chikitsa to offer a comprehensive treatment modality. It is now practiced in both holistic wellness centers and more conventional clinical settings, demonstrating its adaptability and sustained relevance in the field of integrative medicine.

Contemporary Adaptations in Marma Therapy

Contemporary adaptations in Marma therapy reflect its dynamic integration into the modern healthcare ecosystem. As holistic wellness garners mainstream appreciation, Marma Chikitsa has adapted significantly, mingling traditional practices with cutting-edge technology. Therapists now often use digital pressure mapping tools to precisely identify Marma points, enhancing treatment accuracy and effectiveness.
In cosmopolitan settings, Marma therapy has been sculpted to cater to the fast-paced lifestyle of urban dwellers. Shorter, more focused sessions designed to target specific ailments like stress and fatigue are becoming commonplace. Additionally, the inclusion of Marma principles in wellness programs at luxury spas and resorts exemplifies its broadening appeal, merging indulgence with health benefits.
Educational outreach and online tutorials have made Marma Chikitsa accessible to a global audience, furthering its reach beyond traditional boundaries. By embracing digital media, practitioners offer virtual consultations, extending the healing power of Marma globally. These adaptations ensure Marma Chikitsa remains a vital component of contemporary alternative medicine, bridging age-old traditions with modern-day health practices.

Influence of Modern Medicine on Marma Practices

The integration of modern medicine into Marma Chikitsa has ushered in a new era of validation and innovation for this ancient healing practice. Contemporary medical research has begun investigating the efficacy of Marma points, driving a deeper understanding and acceptance within the global medical community. This scientific engagement has not only extended the legitimacy of Marma therapy but also encouraged its incorporation into conventional treatment protocols.
Additionally, the advent of technology in healthcare has facilitated sophisticated diagnostic tools that aid in the precise identification and manipulation of Marma points. Innovations such as biofeedback mechanisms and imaging techniques have enhanced the accuracy of Marma applications, making treatments more targeted and effective.
Moreover, modern pharmacology has influenced Marma Chikitsa by integrating pharmaceutical agents with traditional remedies, creating hybrid therapeutic strategies that leverage the best of both worlds. As these interdisciplinary approaches gain traction, they bridge the gap between ancient wisdom and contemporary science, expanding the scope of Marma therapy in modern healthcare settings.

Revival of Esoteric Elements in Marma

The revival of esoteric elements within Marma Chikitsa heralds a fascinating confluence of age-old mysticism with contemporary healing practices. As modern medicine increasingly invites holistic approaches, there has been a rekindled interest in the more arcane aspects of Marma therapy. These elements, steeped in the spiritual traditions of ancient India, emphasize the subtle energies and spiritual dimensions that govern physical health.

Practitioners and scholars are revisiting ancient texts and practices, integrating rituals that were once sidelined by the clinical shift. This resurgence not only enriches the therapeutic landscape but also aligns with a global movement towards spiritual wellness. Workshops and courses focusing on these traditional techniques have sprouted, attracting both healers and those seeking deeper spiritual engagement with their health practices.

Consequently, this revival is not merely about bringing forgotten practices to light; it is a vibrant reintegration of spirituality into the healing arts, promising a more holistic approach to well-being in the modern era. With this, Marma Chikitsa continues to evolve, bridging the mystical with the empirical, offering profound therapeutic benefits that resonate across diverse global cultures.

Development of Educational Structures for Marma Practice

The educational frameworks for Marma Chikitsa have undergone significant transformations, aiming to create a robust academic infrastructure. Initially transmitted through master-disciple lineages, the formalization into structured curriculums began appearing as its therapeutic benefits gained widespread recognition. Notably, collaborations between traditional Ayurvedic universities and modern academic institutions have catalyzed the development of comprehensive educational programs that merge ancient Marma wisdom with scientific rigor.

Today, these programs offer rigorous coursework, practical workshops, and experiential learning opportunities to equip future practitioners with both theoretical knowledge and practical skills. Moreover, certification and degree programs specific to Marma Chikitsa have been instituted, setting professional standards and ensuring the consistency and quality of practice. These strides in educational development not only preserve the integrity of Marma teachings but also enhance their global accessibility and adoption.

As the practice continues to intersect with modern healthcare disciplines, ongoing educational enhancements reflect this convergence, promising a future where Marma Chikitsa's ancient techniques are perpetually rejuvenated through scholarly pursuit and research-oriented studies.

Legislation and Standardization in Modern Times

The modern era has seen significant strides in the legislative and standardization aspects of Marma Chikitsa, moments that heighten both its legitimacy and efficacy. Governments across Asia, recognizing the therapeutic values, began to integrate these ancient practices within their healthcare regulations. This formal recognition has facilitated an environment where standards could be implemented, ensuring that practitioners meet a universal criterion of knowledge and skill.

Standardization processes often involve certifying therapists and accrediting institutions that fulfill specific educational and ethical practices. Such measures have helped curb malpractices and maintain treatment integrity, increasing public trust and clinical acceptance. By setting

definitive guidelines for practice, Marma Chikitsa has embraced a new level of professional respect and accountability.
Moreover, legislative support has also paved the way for funding and research opportunities, fueling further exploration and understanding of Marma therapies. Overall, these legal frameworks serve not only to protect but also to propagate an informed, innovative, and culturally enriched practice, securing a place for Marma Chikitsa in both traditional and modern medical contexts.

Impact of Globalization on Marma Chikitsa

Globalization has heralded a new epoch for Marma Chikitsa, expanding its reach and transforming its practices. As the world becomes more interconnected, this ancient healing art has crossed its traditional boundaries, finding a place in healthcare settings around the globe. This widespread exposure has not only increased its visibility but also enhanced its credibility, attracting a worldwide clientele intrigued by its holistic appeal.
The dissemination of knowledge through global networks has introduced Marma Chikitsa to new audiences, fostering an integration of diverse healing techniques. Practitioners worldwide are now exchanging ideas, leading to innovative practices that blend Marma with other therapeutic traditions. Such synergies enrich the Marma protocol, making it more adaptable to varied health paradigms and increasing its efficacy.
Moreover, globalization has prompted the standardization of Marma Chikitsa practices to meet international quality standards. This ensures consistency and safety in its application, paving the way for its inclusion in global health platforms. Thus, globalization not only preserves Marma Chikitsa's rich legacy but also propels it into the future as a relevant and revered modality in the international wellness industry.

Recent Scientific Research and Its Implications

The landscape of Marma Chikitsa has been significantly influenced by recent scientific research, which has examined its methodologies through the prism of modern science. Studies focus on the physiological and psychological effects of pinpointing Marma points, establishing a scientific basis for the energy pathways long recognized by ancient practices.
These investigations not only substantiate the therapeutic claims associated with Marma Chikitsa but also encourage its integration within more conventional medical treatments. Research outcomes have led to broader acceptance and credibility among healthcare professionals globally, enhancing interdisciplinary approaches centered on patient wellness.
Furthermore, the findings have propelled advancements in training methods and the refinement of techniques ensuring greater efficacy and safety. Educational syllabi now incorporate these research-backed methodologies, marrying tradition with innovation. The ongoing research continues to unveil complex interactions within the human body, promising new frontiers in medical science and holistic health practices.

Technological Advancements in the Practice of Marma

The realm of Marma Chikitsa has been revolutionized by technological advancements, enhancing both the diagnostic precision and therapeutic efficacy of this ancient practice. Modern imaging technologies, such as MRI and thermal imaging, now allow practitioners to visualize Marma points and assess their bioenergetic status in real-time. This integration of technology facilitates a deeper understanding of the subtle energies that Marma therapy seeks to balance.

Furthermore, computerized pressure devices have been developed to standardize the application of pressure on Marma points, ensuring consistent and precise treatments across different sessions and practitioners. These devices, coupled with digital documentation systems, contribute to personalized patient management and follow-up, bridging traditional practices with contemporary clinical requirements.

On the educational front, virtual reality (VR) and augmented reality (AR) systems are being employed to train practitioners, simulating real-life scenarios that allow for immersive learning experiences. Such innovations not only preserve the integrity of Marma Chikitsa's techniques but also make the learning process more interactive and accessible. Through these technological integrations, Marma Chikitsa is set to reach unprecedented levels of efficacy and global adoption.

Adaptation of Marma Therapy in Non-Asian Contexts

As the practices of Marma Chikitsa spans continents, its integration into non-Asian contexts marks a significant evolution in its global journey. Predominantly rooted in India, the adaptation of this ancient therapeutic method in Western countries and beyond reflects a confluence of traditional wisdom and modern health sensibilities. Practitioners abroad are increasingly incorporating Marma techniques into holistic health regimes, often blending it with established modalities like massage therapy, acupuncture, and even psychotherapy to enhance its acceptance and applicability.

The nuanced application of Marma in these diverse settings also highlights cultural adaptability, where localized health beliefs and practices shape its integration. Training programs outside Asia have begun to include Marma courses, tailored to suit the regulatory and cultural landscapes of their countries. This not only fosters a broader understanding but also respects the integrity of Marma's methodologies.

Furthermore, international wellness conferences and symposiums now frequently feature Marma sessions, indicating its rising prominence. These platforms facilitate cross-disciplinary dialogues, enriching the practice with diverse therapeutic perspectives and research insights. As Marma Chikitsa grows in global stature, it continues to adapt, promising holistic health benefits to a wider audience.

Preservation Efforts and Cultural Heritage

The preservation of Marma Chikitsa is intrinsically tied to its cultural heritage, reflecting centuries of traditional wisdom and practices. As Marma therapy attracts global attention, preserving its authenticity becomes crucial. Various initiatives have been undertaken to maintain the integrity of its traditional methodologies, ensuring that Marma Chikitsa is not diluted by

modern interpretations or commercial exploitations.
Cultural heritage institutions and traditional Marma practitioners have collaborated in documenting the intricate techniques and philosophies associated with Marma therapy. This documentation helps in safeguarding the lore for future generations, facilitating educational programs that adhere closely to ancient practices. Moreover, cultural festivals and public workshops have become platforms for disseminating knowledge about Marma, enhancing public engagement and appreciation.
Furthermore, digital archives have been created, hosting vast amounts of data on Marma Chikitsa, accessible globally. These digital initiatives not only aid in the preservation of knowledge but also assist in the study and application of Marma across different cultural contexts, ensuring its survival and relevance in the modern era.

Looking to the Future: Emerging Trends in Marma Chikitsa

As we peer into the future of Marma Chikitsa, it is poised to undergo transformative shifts, integrating more deeply with modern healthcare frameworks while maintaining its ancient roots. Increased emphasis on evidence-based practices is catalysing new research initiatives that seek to solidify the efficacy of Marma points and techniques in clinical settings. These endeavors aim to weave Marma Chikitsa into the fabric of conventional medicine, potentially opening paths for holistic treatments within more rigid health systems.
Concurrently, digital technologies promise revolutionary changes, specifically through the development of AI-driven diagnostics and therapies that can interpret and apply Marma principles on a scale previously unimaginable. Such innovations could democratize Marma Chikitsa, making it accessible to remote areas where traditional practices are rare.
Sustainability in health practices is another emerging trend. As environmental concerns permeate all aspects of life, Marma Chikitsa is expected to spotlight eco-conscious and ethically sourced materials in its treatments, reinforcing the unity between human health and environmental vitality.

Summary

The chapter on the 'Development and Evolution of Marma Chikitsa' delves into the ancient origins and progressive maturation of Marma Chikitsa, a traditional Indian healing practice rooted in Ayurvedic medicine. It traces the beginnings of Marma Chikitsa to ancient scripts such as the Charaka Samhita and the Sushruta Samhita, which document the critical energy points in the human body known as marma points. These texts not only describe the physical locations but also the therapeutic significance of these points in maintaining health and energy flow, or prana. Early practitioners, revered as both healers and spiritual guides, employed rudimentary tools like bamboo sticks and herbal pastes, which were pivotal in the practice's initial methodology. Marma Chikitsa's evolution is further illustrated through its integration of influences from neighboring healing philosophies such as traditional Chinese medicine, which introduced acupuncture-like techniques, and Greek medicine, which contributed herbal oils and poultices. The chapter highlights how marma therapy was a cornerstone of cross-cultural exchanges along trade routes like the Silk Road, influencing and integrating diverse healing traditions. Educational transitions from oral transmission to formalized written texts are discussed, noting how this shift allowed for broader dissemination and preservation of knowledge. Noteworthy practitioners over the centuries are identified, marking significant developmental milestones. Furthermore, the narrative encapsulates the modern renaissance of

Marma Chikitsa, accentuated by a blending of traditional methods with scientific approaches and technological advancements, ensuring its relevance and application in contemporary therapeutic practices. In essence, this chapter thoroughly explores how Marma Chikitsa has sustained and evolved as a form of holistic treatment, emphasizing its potential in modern medicinal practices alongside a growing global recognition.

References

[1] Charaka Samhita. https://en.wikipedia.org/wiki/Charaka

[2] Sushruta Samhita. https://en.wikipedia.org/wiki/Sushruta_Samhita

[3] History of Ayurveda. https://www.ncbi.nlm.nih.gov/pmc/articles/PMC3218439/

[4] Marma Points of Ayurveda. https://www.ayurveda.com/pdf/marma_poster.pdf

[5] Therapeutic Potentials of Marma Therapy. https://www.researchgate.net/publication/311785290_Therapeutic_Potentials_of_Marma_Therapy

Case Study: Revitalizing Marma Chikitsa in Contemporary Healthcare

In the bustling city of Coimbatore, a clinic led by Dr. Ananya Joshi, a renowned specialist in Ayurvedic medicine, sought to integrate Marma Chikitsa into a multi-disciplinary healthcare setting. The aim was to enhance patient outcomes by incorporating this ancient practice into modern therapeutic regimens. This initiative was sparked by a notable increase in patients seeking holistic treatments that aligned more closely with natural healing processes, and an acknowledgment of the growing evidence supporting alternative therapies.

Dr. Joshi's clinic, which traditionally offered more conventional Ayurvedic treatments like Panchakarma and herbal remedies, faced challenges in adopting Marma Chikitsa. The primary obstacles included a lack of trained Marma specialists, skepticism from practitioners of conventional medicine, and the need to develop a curriculum that effectively combined scientific knowledge with traditional wisdom. To overcome these, Dr. Joshi initiated a training program for her staff, focusing on Marma point identification, therapeutic techniques, and the integration of these points with other treatment modalities.

As the program advanced, the inclusion of Marma Chikitsa exhibited promising results. Patients reported significant improvements in conditions such as chronic pain, anxiety, and post-surgical recovery. The clinic documented these outcomes, contributing to a growing database of clinical evidence supporting Marma therapy. Furthermore, the integration of digital pressure mapping tools enhanced treatment precision, generating broader acceptance among the medical staff.

The case of Dr. Joshi's clinic illustrates the potential for Marma Chikitsa to adapt within modern healthcare frameworks, highlighting how ancient practices can be revitalized to meet contemporary health demands. The successful incorporation of Marma therapy in a multi-disciplinary setting not only elevated patient care but also set a precedent for future integrative healthcare models.

Case Study: Marma Chikitsa's Role in Combating Lifestyle Diseases in Urban Populations

In a sprawling urban center like Mumbai, known for its high-stress lifestyle and prevalence of lifestyle diseases such as diabetes and hypertension, the traditional healing practice of Marma Chikitsa presented a natural intervention attracting the attention of both healthcare professionals and the public. Dr. Priya Mehta, an experienced Ayurvedic consultant, introduced a comprehensive Marma therapy program tailored specifically to address these contemporary health issues.

Dr. Mehta's clinic, situated in the heart of Mumbai, was initially geared towards providing generic Ayurvedic treatments. However, observing the increasing number of urban dwellers suffering from stress-related ailments and chronic pain, she envisaged a specialized approach using Marma Chikitsa. The methodology was to integrate it seamlessly with lifestyle alterations, dietary changes, and regular counseling sessions.

The challenge was significant—as Marma Chikitsa required precise knowledge and skill in identifying and stimulating Marma points effectively, and skepticism about its benefits compared to established medical treatments was prevalent. To combat these challenges, Dr. Mehta began a series of workshops and seminars aimed at educating her patients and the community about the benefits of Marma Chikitsa. She partnered with local yoga studios and dietitians to provide a holistic health service.

The program started showing positive results within a few months. Patients who participated reported not only a reduction in symptoms of their chronic ailments but also a noticeable improvement in overall wellness and energy levels. The success stories were documented and analyzed to provide empirical data supporting the efficacy of Marma Chikitsa in the treatment of lifestyle diseases. Moreover, Dr. Mehta utilized innovative tools like biofeedback devices to track the improvements in patients' prana alignment after Marma therapy sessions, further validating the technique's effectiveness.

This case study represents an important instance of how traditional practices like Marma Chikitsa can be effectively adapted to solve modern health crises, making a compelling argument for the integration of ancient wisdom in urban healthcare strategies.

Case Study: Innovative Integration of Marma Chikitsa in Pediatric Care

In the scenic, yet bustling town of Shimla, Dr. Veena Sandhu spearheaded an innovative project aimed at integrating Marma Chikitsa into pediatric care, a novel approach especially in a region where conventional medicine predominates in treating children. The project began at the Himalayan Integrative Medical Center, a facility renowned for combining Ayurvedic practices with modern medicine to provide holistic care.

The initiative was motivated by the increasing incidence of behavioral and developmental disorders such as ADHD and autism in children, which often do not respond optimally to conventional treatments alone. Dr. Sandhu, known for her pioneering work in integrative medicine, viewed Marma Chikitsa as a potential complementary therapy that could be tuned specifically to cater to the physiological and energy meridians more sensitive in children.

One of the primary challenges was adapting Marma therapy for young patients, who are often more sensitive to touch and uneasy with new experiences. Dr. Sandhu and her team initiated a detailed study on the adapted methods for children, incorporating gentle touch techniques and integrating playful interaction to keep the children engaged and comfortable. Each treatment was also shorter in duration than those typically administered to adults, emphasizing less intrusion and more swift, visible outcomes.

The training of pediatric care staff was pivotal. It entailed not just the technical aspects of identifying and stimulating Marma points, but also behavioral management skills tailored to young children's needs. As the initiative progressed, reported outcomes included improved attention spans, better sleep patterns, and a reduction in anxiety among treated children. These observations were systematically documented and analyzed, contributing significant findings to the field of pediatric integrative medicine.

Dr. Sandhu's efforts transcended beyond treatment; they augmented the educational tapestry of Marma Chikitsa by highlighting its adaptability and efficacy in pediatric care. This case not only supports the relevance of traditional practices within modern therapeutic regimens but also pioneers a path for broader integration of Marma Chikitsa in child healthcare, potentially resetting therapeutic standards in pediatric medicine.

Case Study: Expanding Marma Chikitsa Through Telemedicine: A Case Study in Rural Outreach

In the remote village of Bhinder in Rajasthan, access to comprehensive healthcare has historically been a significant challenge due to geographic isolation and limited medical resources. This scenario provided a unique opportunity for the implementation of Marma Chikitsa via telemedicine - an approach under-represented in the realm of traditional therapies but promising in extending healthcare reach. Spearheaded by Dr. Lalit Mohan, an Ayurvedic practitioner with a deep interest in rural health improvement, this project combined the ancient wisdom of Marma Chikitsa with modern technology to address rural health disparities.

Dr. Mohan's initiative began with establishing a telemedicine center equipped with the latest communication technologies. A local healthcare worker trained in basic Marma therapy under Dr. Mohan's supervision served as the intermediary, facilitating real-time interactions between Dr. Mohan and patients. Despite initial skepticism, the simplicity and non-invasiveness of Marma Chikitsa made it a suitable candidate for teleconsultations, where Dr. Mohan guided the application of Marma techniques for various ailments like chronic pain, digestive issues, and stress-related disorders.

One of the significant challenges was educating rural populations about Marma Chikitsa's benefits. Dr. Mohan conducted virtual workshops and distributed educational materials developed in local languages. These resources elaborated on the science behind Marma points, their role in maintaining health, and self-applicable techniques for minor ailments. Over time, his approach witnessed a gradual acceptance, marked by increasing patient engagement and reported improvements in health conditions.

The pilot phase outcomes included enhanced patient satisfaction, reduced travel time for medical consultations, and, importantly, an increased interest in traditional practices. Documenting these results has been crucial in promoting telemedicine-based Marma Chikitsa to other rural areas, showcasing a scalable model for traditional therapy integration into modern telehealth frameworks.

Case Study: Enhancing Sports Rehabilitation with Marma Chikitsa: A Case Study

In the sports-centric city of Pune, renowned for fostering numerous athletic talents, the integration of Marma Chikitsa into sports rehabilitation presented an innovative approach at the Rising Star Sports Academy. Dr. Niharika Patel, a specialist in sports medicine and trained in Ayurvedic practices, spearheaded this initiative. The objective was to harness the therapeutic benefits of Marma Chikitsa to expedite recovery and enhance performance amongst injured athletes. This case study examines the implementation, challenges, and outcomes of this fusion in a high-performance sports environment.

The academy initially faced resistance from traditional sports therapists and athletes, skeptical of integrating a traditional healing technique into a scientifically dominated field. Dr. Patel began by conducting educational sessions, presenting empirical data and case studies that highlighted Marma Chikitsa's efficacy in pain management and tissue healing. Recognizing the necessity for a customized approach, she developed a Marma therapy protocol adapted specifically for athletic injuries, focusing on points that corresponded to common sports injuries.

A pilot program was launched with a group of athletes suffering from conditions like tendonitis, sprains, and muscle strains. The Marma treatment was integrated with conventional rehabilitation practices like physiotherapy and strength training. Each athlete's progress was meticulously documented, noting improvements not only in injury recovery times but also in their overall agility and performance levels.

Challenges included adapting Marma techniques to different body types and sports-specific stress areas, and ensuring the athletes adhered consistently to the treatment protocol. Overcoming these, the pilot study produced compelling results. Athletes reported decreased pain levels and increased range of motion, with most returning to their sports activities quicker than with conventional treatment alone.

These findings led to broader acceptance of Marma Chikitsa within the academy, inspiring further research and development of sport-specific Marma protocols. Dr. Patel's work not only broadened the scope of sports rehabilitation but also set a precedent for the integration of traditional healing arts into modern athletic healthcare practices.

Case Study: Integrating Marma Chikitsa into Geriatric Wellness Programs

In the serene town of Haridwar, nestled by the Ganges, an innovative approach to elder care was unfolding at the Anandam Senior Living Facility. Spearheaded by Dr. Aparna Singh, a seasoned practitioner of Ayurvedic medicine with a special interest in geriatric care, the initiative aimed to integrate Marma Chikitsa into routine wellness programs for the elderly. The objective was to address common age-related issues such as arthritis, insomnia, and decreased mobility, enhancing overall life quality for the facility's residents.

Dr. Singh noticed that while conventional medications were effective in managing symptoms, they often came with side effects that affected the seniors' quality of life. Believing in the holistic benefits of Marma Chikitsa, she proposed a pilot project to integrate these ancient techniques into the care regimen. The project began with training the facility's caregivers and therapists in the basics of Marma therapy, focusing on points that target joint health, sleep enhancement, and energy rejuvenation.

Implementing the program, however, came with its challenges. Many residents were skeptical of this non-conventional method, and their families were concerned about the adequacy of such treatments compared to modern medicine. To address these concerns, Dr. Singh organized seminars with the residents and their families, explaining the benefits of Marma Chikitsa and showcasing success stories from other regions.

The program started showing positive results within a few months. Residents participating in the Marma sessions reported better sleep patterns, reduced pain in joints, and a general feeling of wellbeing. The caregivers also noted easier mobility among the seniors and a decreased need for pain medications. These observations were systematically documented, analyzed, and presented at healthcare conferences to provide empirical data supporting the efficacy of Marma Chikitsa in geriatric care.

This case illustrates the potential for ancient practices like Marma Chikitsa to be integrated effectively into modern geriatric healthcare. The success of the program at Anandam has not only improved the residents' quality of life but has also paved the way for similar integrative health initiatives in senior care facilities nationwide.

Case Study: Reviving Traditional Healing with Modern Science: The Case of Alpana Ayurveda Clinic

In the tranquil outskirts of Bangalore, India, the Alpana Ayurveda Clinic, under the leadership of Dr. Radhika Krishnan, embarked on an ambitious initiative to integrate Marma Chikitsa into a comprehensive treatment protocol for autoimmune diseases, with a special focus on Rheumatoid Arthritis (RA). This clinic, known for blending traditional Ayurvedic practices with modern diagnostics, observed an increasing demand for holistic approaches to complex health conditions.

The clinic's staff, initially trained in general Ayurvedic treatments, required intensive training in Marma Chikitsa. The challenge was twofold: they needed to assure that Marma treatments could be scientifically validated, and they needed to train practitioners in these methods in a rigorous, medically informed manner. Dr. Krishnan collaborated with local universities to develop a data-backed training program that included both hands-on practice and theoretical learning, focusing particularly on the relationship between Marma points and immune modulation.

As the advanced training progressed, the clinic introduced pilot sessions specifically designed for RA patients. These sessions incorporated Marma Chikitsa alongside regular rheumatologic treatments. Each session aimed to restore balance to the doshas (body energies according to Ayurveda) and improve pranic flow through specific Marma points, theoretically reducing inflammation and pain. This holistic approach was cautiously optimized, with continuous adjustments based on patient feedback and clinical observations.

Patient outcomes from these pilot sessions were meticulously recorded and analyzed. Remarkably, patients reported improvements in pain management and mobility. Furthermore, biomarkers associated with inflammation, routinely measured through blood tests, showed notable improvements. These outcomes contributed to a preliminary clinical study that advocated for integrating Marma Chikitsa into standard RA management protocols.

This case from the Alpana Ayurveda Clinic demonstrates how ancient healing techniques, when underpinned by modern scientific research and methodical validation, can be effectively utilized to enhance contemporary medical practices, offering new avenues for treating chronic diseases that challenge conventional medical solutions.

Case Study: Revival of Marma Chikitsa for Mental Health in Urban India

In the fast-paced urban environment of Bangalore, India, a unique integrative health care model was developed at the Vedic Harmony Center to address mental health challenges like anxiety, depression, and stress-related disorders, leveraging the ancient practice of Marma Chikitsa. The project was led by Dr. Kavita Rao, a practitioner of Ayurvedic medicine with extensive experience in mental wellness. Dr. Rao observed a growing need for holistic treatment options that go beyond pharmacological interventions to manage symptoms, providing sustainable and natural wellness solutions.

The center initially faced challenges including skepticism from patients accustomed to conventional psychiatric treatments, a general lack of awareness about the benefits of Marma Chikitsa, and the need for practitioners skilled in both mental health care and Ayurvedic practices. To address these barriers, Dr. Rao spearheaded a comprehensive educational program for both her team and the patients. The program emphasized the connections between mental health and energy channels in the body, explained through Marma Chikitsa principles.

As the program advanced, practitioners trained under this initiative started integrating Marma therapy with cognitive behavioral therapies, creating a multifaceted treatment approach. Patients underwent sessions where Marma points associated with relaxation and mental clarity were stimulated to enhance psychological therapy outcomes. The integration also included meditation sessions and Ayurvedic nutrition, forming a 360-degree approach to mental health.

The results from the initial cohorts were encouraging. Patients reported improvements in symptoms of depression and anxiety, enhanced mood stability, and reduced stress levels. These improvements were not only based on self-reported assessments but were also supported by reduced cortisol levels checked before and after the treatment cycles. Vedic Harmony Center's approach provided a groundbreaking model for addressing urban mental health challenges, showcasing how traditional practices can be symbiotically combined with contemporary psychological treatments to enhance patient well-being.

Case Study: Harnessing Marma Chikitsa for Occupational Health in the Tech Industry

In the heart of Silicon Valley, a progressive tech company, Innovatech, embarked on a pioneering wellness initiative aimed at addressing the occupational health challenges prevalent in high-stress tech environments. Spearheaded by Dr. Maya Desai, a wellness consultant specialized in Ayurvedic practices, the program sought to integrate Marma Chikitsa into the daily routine of software developers and engineers who experienced high levels of stress and associated musculoskeletal disorders from prolonged periods of sitting and intense computer work.

Dr. Desai's approach was multi-faceted; recognizing that the rigorous demands of tech jobs often lead to chronic pain, fatigue, and burnout, she proposed that Marma Chikitsa could offer a preventive and therapeutic benefit by enhancing energy flow and reducing stress. Initial challenges were significant, including skepticism from employees accustomed to conventional medical treatments, and logistical issues in integrating these sessions into the fast-paced corporate schedule. To tackle these, Dr. Desai introduced brief, regular Marma therapy sessions scheduled throughout the workday as a start. These sessions focused on key Marma points that are believed to boost mental clarity and alleviate physical strain, particularly in the neck, back, and wrists.

As the program unrolled, the company noted a decline in complaints about physical ailments and a marked improvement in employee productivity and overall satisfaction. Dr. Desai used a robust tracking method to monitor the health outcomes and gathered substantial empirical data which highlighted reduced rates of absenteeism and a decline in the usage of standard pain management medications among the participating employees.

This case study from Innovatech serves as an inspiring illustration of how ancient techniques like Marma Chikitsa can be seamlessly integrated into modern occupational health strategies. It opens avenues for further research and application in various professional settings, emphasizing the adaptability and effectiveness of Marma Chikitsa in fostering a healthier, more productive workforce in high-stress environments.

Case Study: Reviving Ancient Practices in Modern Veterinary Care: Marma Chikitsa for Animal Treatment

In the vibrant city of Hyderabad, India, a unique initiative called VetAyurveda was introduced by Dr. Varun Sharma, a pioneering veterinarian and a passionate proponent of integrating traditional Ayurvedic practices, including Marma Chikitsa, into veterinary medicine. This initiative aimed to offer alternative healing options for animals, particularly those not responding well to conventional treatments. The use of Marma Chikitsa in animal care presented an innovative approach to enhancing animal wellness and recovery, addressing a significant gap in veterinary care practices.

Dr. Sharma's clinic initially encountered several obstacles. The primary challenge was the adaptation of Marma therapy from human to animal use, requiring meticulous study and modifications. Special training for veterinary practitioners was essential to accurately identify and stimulate Marma points on different animal species, which possess anatomical and physiological differences from humans. Another significant hurdle was skepticism from pet owners and fellow veterinarians who were unfamiliar with or doubtful about the efficacy of these ancient techniques on animals.

To overcome these challenges, Dr. Sharma organized workshops and seminars to educate pet owners and veterinary professionals about the practical applications and benefits of Marma Chikitsa in treating animals. Live demonstrations and pilot treatment sessions showcased significant improvements in chronic conditions such as arthritis, digestive upset, and anxiety-related disorders in pets, which bolstered its acceptance.

As VetAyurveda's practices gained traction, more veterinary professionals were trained, and the scope of treatments expanded. Systematic documentation of treatment protocols, outcomes, and case studies further validated the effectiveness of Marma Chikitsa. By integrating these ancient practices into veterinary medicine, Dr. Sharma not only enhanced treatment options for animals but also carved a niche for alternative veterinary care in the modern healthcare landscape. This case exemplifies a remarkable exploration into the adaptability and relevance of traditional healing practices in contemporary veterinary medicine, inspiring similar integrations worldwide.

Review Questions

1. A 56-year-old male with chronic lower back pain, refractory to conventional treatments, consults an Ayurvedic practitioner. The practitioner suggests Marma Chikitsa focusing on specific energy points. Which of the following Marma points is primarily targeted for alleviating lower back pain?

A) A. Janu Marma
B) B. Kati Marma
C) C. Hridaya Marma
D) D. Gandha Marma

Answer: B

Explanation: Kati Marma points are in the lower back region and are associated with alleviating pain in the lumbar and sacral areas. Targeting these points in Marma Chikitsa helps release pranic blockages specifically in the lower back, which can significantly reduce pain and improve mobility. Unlike Janu Marma, which relates to the knee, and Hridaya Marma which is associated with the heart region, Kati Marma directly addresses the common sites of discomfort in cases of lower back issues.

2. During a session of Marma Chikitsa, a practitioner focuses on activating Urah Marma points on a patient suffering from asthma. What is the primary benefit of stimulating Urah Marma in individuals with respiratory issues?

A) A. It enhances digestive function
B) B. It stabilizes emotional disturbances
C) C. It improves respiratory efficiency
D) D. It alleviates skin irritation

Answer: C

Explanation: Urah Marma points are situated in the chest region and are pivotal in managing respiratory conditions such as asthma. Activation of these points is believed to enhance prana distribution throughout the respiratory system, thereby improving lung capacity, easing breathing, and reducing asthma symptoms. Unlike digestive or skin conditions, respiratory efficiency is directly influenced by the manipulation of Urah Marma points.

3. A patient experiencing severe migraines is recommended Marma therapy. Which Marma points would be most likely targeted by the practitioner for effective relief?

A) A. Sthapani and Adhipati Marma
B) B. Kurcha and Kshipra Marma
C) C. Kati and Nitamba Marma
D) D. Indrabasti and Janu Marma

Answer: A

Explanation: For migraines, Sthapani and Adhipati Marma, located on the head, are emphasized in Marma Chikitsa. These points are strategically used to regulate the flow of pranic energy in areas typically affected by migraine pain, such as the frontal and temporal regions of the skull. The stimulation of these points helps in reducing the intensity and frequency of migraine attacks, offering a holistic approach to pain management.

4. A 34-year-old woman with PCOS (Polycystic Ovary Syndrome) seeks alternative treatments. The Ayurvedic practitioner decides to use Marma Chikitsa. Which Marma points are appropriate for addressing symptoms of PCOS?

A) A. Guda and Basti Marma
B) B. Hridaya and Talahridaya Marma
C) C. Sthapani and Urvi Marma
D) D. Nabhi and Parsruti Marma

Answer: A

Explanation: Guda Marma (located near the anal region) and Basti Marma (related to the urinary and reproductive organs) are critically relevant in treating reproductive health conditions like PCOS. These points help in balancing the reproductive energies and regulating hormonal function, which can alleviate symptoms such as menstrual irregularities and hormonal imbalances associated with PCOS. The focused treatment on these Marmas supports overall pelvic health and enhances fertility.

5. An elderly patient suffering from knee osteoarthritis approaches for Marma Chikitsa. The practitioner plans to stimulate specific Marma points to relieve joint pain. Which set of Marma points is directly involved in alleviating knee issues?

A) A. Janu and Indrabasti Marma
B) B. Kati and Nitamba Marma
C) C. Gandha and Talahridaya Marma
D) D. Urah and Kurchasira Marma

Answer: A

Explanation: Janu Marma, located around the knee joint, and Indrabasti Marma, positioned above the knee, are specifically effective in managing knee pain and conditions like osteoarthritis. The stimulation of these points helps to improve circulation, reduce pain, and enhance mobility in the affected areas. These points are crucial in the context of Ayurvedic therapy for patients suffering from joint-related ailments, particularly in the knees.

CHAPTER FOURTEEN: Contemporary Practice and Legal Aspects of Marma Chikitsa

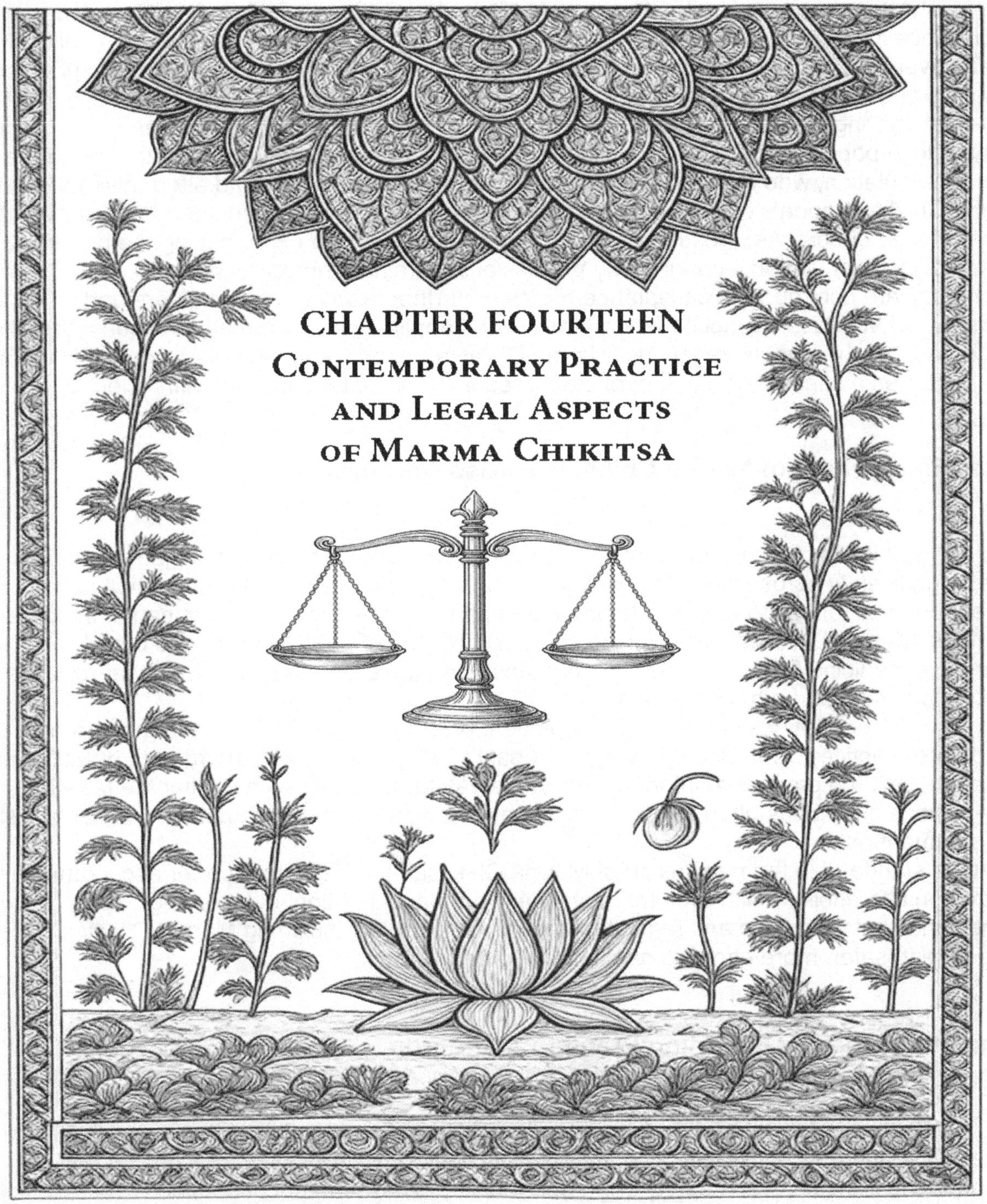

Current Marma Practice Trends in the Healthcare Industry

Marma Chikitsa, once confined primarily to traditional practitioners in Asia, is now seeing a renaissance in the global healthcare industry. Driven by a growing body of research validating its effectiveness, this ancient form of healing is being integrated into modern medical practices. Hospitals and wellness centers worldwide are beginning to incorporate Marma therapy into their treatment offerings, particularly for pain management and psychological well-being.

This surge in popularity is also encouraged by a more holistic approach to health among the general population, who are increasingly seeking out complementary and alternative medicines. Marma Chikitsa appeals to this audience with its non-invasive techniques and the promise of no chemical side effects. As a result, a broader demographic is now experiencing the benefits of Marma points stimulation, supported by professionally trained therapists.

The healthcare community's acceptance has been further facilitated by seminars and workshops that educate practitioners on the correct application of Marma techniques. With its integration into therapeutic regimens, Marma Chikitsa not only enriches our therapeutic tools but also illustrates a successful blend of ancient wisdom with contemporary health science.

Legal Recognition of Marma Chikitsa Across Countries

As Marma Chikitsa gains prominence in the realm of alternative medicine, its legal standing varies significantly across countries. Nations vary in their recognition and regulation of this ancient practice, affecting both practitioners and patients seeking these treatments. In some countries, Marma Chikitsa is recognized as a distinct form of therapy within the broader alternative medicine framework. These countries often have specific guidelines that regulate training, practice, and ethical standards.

Conversely, other nations lack formal recognition, placing Marma Chikitsa in a grey area of healthcare practices. This discrepancy can impact the legal protection afforded to practitioners and might limit the practice to informal settings, away from mainstream healthcare facilities. Patients in such regions often turn to Marma Chikitsa as a last resort rather than a viable first-line treatment option.

Efforts to standardize the recognition of Marma Chikitsa could lead to broader acceptance and integration into public health systems, potentially enhancing patient outcomes globally. Legal frameworks that recognize and regulate alternative therapies, including Marma Chikitsa, contribute to safer, more effective health service delivery.

Regulatory Bodies Governing Practice Standards

The governance of Marma Chikitsa is underpinned by various regulatory bodies dedicated to establishing and maintaining practice standards. These organizations play a crucial role in safeguarding the quality and safety of Marma therapy. They set educational and professional requirements that practitioners must meet to ensure a consistent level of competency and care. These bodies also issue guidelines on the ethical practice of Marma Chikitsa, aiming to protect both the practitioner and client. Standards cover diverse aspects from treatment protocols and patient confidentiality to professional conduct in practice. National and international certifications may be required, depending on the region, which serves as a benchmark for proficiency in this specialized field.

Moreover, these regulatory authorities conduct periodic reviews and updates of their standards to adapt to new research and clinical findings, ensuring that Marma practice remains scientifically valid and effective. Their oversight is essential for integrating Marma Chikitsa into broader healthcare systems, providing a structured path for its acceptance and application.

Certification and Licensing Requirements for Practitioners

The pathway to becoming a certified Marma Chikitsa practitioner intertwines stringent educational and licensing thresholds, ensuring that only proficient individuals administer this ancient therapeutic art. Candidates must complete accredited training programs, which include theoretical knowledge of Ayurvedic principles and practical skills in identifying and stimulating Marma points. These programs are often followed by rigorous examinations to assess the practitioner's competence and understanding.

Upon passing these examinations, practitioners are required to obtain licenses from recognized regulatory bodies. These licenses are not static; they necessitate continual professional development to align with evolving practices and research in Marma Chikitsa. This ensures that practitioners remain adept at employing current methodologies effectively and safely.

Furthermore, as Marma Chikitsa garners global recognition, international certification becomes crucial for practitioners wishing to operate across geographical boundaries. This certification supports uniform standards of practice worldwide, fostering trust and consistency in Marma Chikitsa treatments administered internationally.

Practice Guidelines and Standard Operating Procedures

Developing and adhering to robust practice guidelines and standard operating procedures (SOPs) is vital in Marma Chikitsa, ensuring uniformity and safety in treatments. These guidelines encapsulate critical points ranging from patient assessment to post-treatment care, structured to maximize therapeutic efficacy and minimize risks. Each step is meticulously outlined to uphold the integrity of the practice and ensure that practitioners can deliver consistent care across diverse settings.

Notably, SOPs in Marma Chikitsa are designed to integrate seamlessly with both traditional Ayurvedic principles and modern medical protocols. This integration supports practitioners in navigating complex cases where Marma Chikitsa is employed alongside conventional treatments. By formalizing these procedures, the practice gains legitimacy and reliability, which are essential for wider acceptance within medical communities.

Furthermore, continuous updates to these guidelines reflect ongoing research and technological advancements. Such evolution in SOPs is critical to adapt to new insights and maintain relevance in a rapidly changing healthcare landscape, thereby fostering enhanced patient outcomes and practitioner expertise.

Risk Management and Malpractice in Marma Therapy

Navigating the intricacies of risk management in Marma Chikitsa is crucial given the therapy's increasing incorporation into modern healthcare. As with any medical practice, there exists a potential for malpractice, necessitating robust preventative strategies. Firstly, thorough training and a deep understanding of Marma points are imperative for minimizing risks. Practitioners must possess the competence to avoid unintended harm, such as aggravating existing conditions, which underscores the importance of rigorous certification and the adherence to the guidelines outlined by regulatory bodies.

Furthermore, clear communication with clients about the therapy's benefits and potential risks is essential. Consent forms should meticulously document these discussions, ensuring informed decisions by clients. This transparency not only builds trust but also legally protects practitioners and their practices.

Lastly, having adequate malpractice insurance is advisable, serving as a safeguard against legal and financial repercussions. This element of risk management is critical in fostering a resilient operational framework for Marma therapy, ensuring its ethical and safe application in varying healthcare settings.

Insurance Coverage and Reimbursement Scenarios

The financial aspects of Marma Chikitsa, particularly concerning insurance coverage and reimbursement, are pivotal for both practitioners and patients. Insurance policies that embrace alternative medicine, including Marma therapies, vary significantly. In regions where Marma Chikitsa is legally recognized and regulated, insurers are more likely to provide coverage. This inclusion empowers patients to opt for Marma Chikitsa without bearing the full cost out-of-pocket, enhancing accessibility to traditional healing methods.

However, the reimbursement process can be intricate. It demands precise documentation and often, evidence of the efficacy of Marma Chikitsa for specific ailments, which can pose a challenge due to the traditional nature of the practice. Practitioners need to navigate these requirements carefully to ensure that patients can claim their treatments. Establishing standardized protocols and robust outcome reporting can streamline this process, fostering broader acceptance by insurance entities.

Looking ahead, the evolution of healthcare policies will likely influence insurance scenarios for Marma Chikitsa. Advocacy by professional associations and integration of Marma with conventional treatments can enhance its credibility, encouraging more insurers to recognize and cover these therapeutic practices extensively.

Ethical Marketing and Promotion of Marma Services

The ethical marketing and promotion of Marma Chikitsa are pivotal to maintaining the integrity and trustworthiness of this ancient healing practice. Marketing strategies must not only attract clients but also respectfully convey the true essence and scientific backing of Marma therapy. Practitioners are encouraged to adopt honest, accurate advertising that clearly outlines the potential benefits without making unfounded claims. This approach helps in preserving the credibility and authentic tradition of Marma Chikitsa.

Furthermore, promotional activities should be inclusive, aiming to educate the public about the holistic and therapeutic values of Marma rather than merely driving service sales. Collaborative engagements, such as workshops and seminars, can serve as ethical platforms for raising awareness and fostering deeper understanding.

Lastly, it is crucial for practitioners to adhere to ethical guidelines issued by regulatory bodies. These guidelines often include stipulations for protecting consumer rights and ensuring transparency, which are essential in building long-term trust with clients. In an era where misinformation can spread quickly, maintaining high ethical standards in marketing will safeguard both practitioners and consumers.

Data Privacy Issues in Client Management

In the realm of Marma Chikitsa, the management of client data presents unique challenges and essential privacy considerations. This ancient practice requires the collection and handling of sensitive personal health information, which mandates stringent data protection measures. As practitioners integrate technology into client management, they must navigate adherence to local and international laws on data privacy, such as GDPR in Europe and HIPAA in the United States, ensuring that client confidences are securely maintained.

The necessity for robust encryption and secure storage systems cannot be overstated. Any breach of data can severely undermine client trust and the viability of a Marma practice. Moreover, specialists must be vigilant in training staff on privacy policies and protocols, emphasizing the ethical responsibility to protect patient information.

Additionally, as telemedicine becomes prevalent in Marma therapy, concerns about data security in digital communication channels also escalate. Practitioners are, therefore, tasked with continually updating their data protection strategies to counter new cyber threats, thus assuring clients of their commitment to confidentiality and trust.

Integration of Marma with Conventional Medical Treatments

The integration of Marma Chikitsa with conventional medical treatments presents a promising frontier in the healthcare domain. This synthesis combines the holistic touch of ancient Ayurvedic techniques with the precision of modern medicine, offering a comprehensive treatment protocol that caters to both physical ailments and subtler energetic imbalances.

A pivotal aspect of this integration involves cross-disciplinary training where medical doctors and Marma practitioners share knowledge and skills, ensuring treatments are both safe and synergistic. Crucially, such integrative approaches require clear regulatory frameworks to maintain high standards of practice and patient safety.

Aligning with current medical protocols, Marma treatments can be structured to complement surgical procedures and pharmacotherapy, potentially reducing recovery times and enhancing overall therapeutic outcomes. This collaborative model does not merely juxtapose two methods but interweaves them to create enriched, patient-centered healthcare experiences.

Ultimately, successful integration hinges on continuous research, legal clearances, and educational collaborations, fostering a harmonious marriage between time-tested wisdom and contemporary clinical practices.

Professional Associations and Their Role in Advocacy

Professional associations play a pivotal role in the advocacy and progression of Marma Chikitsa within the broader healthcare framework. These organizations serve as crucial conduits for the dissemination of knowledge, upholding the tradition and integrity of Marma Chikitsa. They organize training sessions, conferences, and seminars that facilitate ongoing education and

networking among practitioners.
Moreover, professional associations are instrumental in lobbying for legal recognition and support for Marma Chikitsa. They advocate for policies that recognize and integrate Marma into mainstream healthcare systems, thereby enhancing its legitimacy and accessibility. Their efforts ensure that Marma Chikitsa receives a fair evaluation and incorporation into health insurance schemes, which is vital for patient access and practitioner sustainability.
Finally, these associations maintain practice standards and ethical guidelines that bolster the credibility of Marma Chikitsa. They address public and legal questions, protecting practitioners and clients while promoting an environment of trust and professional integrity. Through their advocacy, professional associations underpin the evolution and modern relevance of Marma Chikitsa.

Interdisciplinary Collaboration in Clinical Settings

Interdisciplinary collaboration in clinical settings marks a cornerstone of modern Marma Chikitsa practice, bridging the gap between traditional Ayurvedic healing and contemporary medical science. By fostering a cooperative environment, practitioners of Marma can work alongside physicians, physical therapists, and other healthcare professionals to provide a holistic approach to patient care. This synergy not only enhances treatment efficacy but also facilitates a broader understanding and acceptance of Marma Chikitsa within the health community.
Key to this collaboration is the shared goal of patient-centric care, where diverse medical perspectives converge to tailor treatments that address both physical and energetic health dimensions. Regular interdisciplinary meetings and case discussions help ensure that all therapeutic angles are considered, promoting comprehensive and integrated care plans.
Such collaborations are also instrumental in advancing Marma Chikitsa research, combining rigorous scientific methodologies with rich traditional insights to explore new therapeutic potentials. As these partnerships flourish, they pave the way for innovative treatment protocols that could significantly transform patient outcomes in diverse clinical environments.

Impact of Legal Regulations on Marma Research

The terrain of Marma Chikitsa research is intricately shaped by legal regulations, which play a pivotal role in defining the scope and protocol of studies conducted in this ancient therapeutic field. Legal frameworks help ensure that research on Marma Chikitsa adheres to ethical standards, protecting both the subjects involved and the authenticity of the data collected. These regulations often require researchers to undergo rigorous approval processes before experiments can commence, emphasizing the importance of compliance with both national and international ethical standards.
Moreover, legal constraints influence the dissemination and application of research findings. Intellectual property laws, for instance, can impact the sharing of new Marma techniques and therapies, affecting how widely such innovations can be adopted and implemented. Also, the mandatory registration of clinical trials and results publication helps maintain transparency and boosts public and medical confidence in Marma Chikitsa.
Ultimately, while sometimes viewed as restrictive, these legalities are crucial for advancing Marma Chikitsa. They ensure that research is conducted responsibly, fostering an environment where scientific inquiry can flourish within established legal and ethical bounds. This nurtures a credible, scientifically sound foundation for future innovations in Marma therapy.

Practitioner Rights and Responsibilities

In the realm of Marma Chikitsa, practitioners' shoulder significant responsibilities while also being granted specific rights that ensure the integrity and ethical conduct of their practice. As healthcare providers, they are obligated to maintain a high standard of care, adhering strictly to established guidelines and the ethical principles of Ayurveda. This includes continuously updating their skills and knowledge through mandatory continuing education to remain abreast of advancements and changes in practice protocols.

On the rights side, practitioners are entitled to work within environments that respect their professional judgment and provide opportunities for career growth and exploration. They hold the right to advocate for the integration of Marma Chikitsa into broader healthcare settings, contributing to policy development processes that affect their practice. Moreover, they are protected under laws that recognize their unique skills, provided they meet licensing requirements which underscore their legitimacy as health care providers.

Finally, balancing these rights, they must also comply with data protection regulations, ensuring patient confidentiality and security is never compromised. This dual framework of rights and responsibilities not only guides Marma practitioners but also ensures that patient care remains the focal point of all therapeutic engagements.

Consent Protocols for Sensitive Demographics

Addressing sensitive demographics in Marma Chikitsa necessitates rigorous consent protocols to ensure ethical treatment and respect for the vulnerabilities of specific patient groups. These protocols are designed not only to fulfill legal obligations but also to foster trust and transparency between practitioners and patients. Particularly, this involves clear communication about the nature of Marma therapies, potential risks, and expected outcomes.

Consent forms must be meticulously tailored to accommodate the unique needs of sensitive groups such as minors, the elderly, and those with cognitive impairments. This includes using language that is easily understandable and offering additional support for decision-making, such as involving caregivers or legal guardians in the consent process. Ensuring voluntariness in these scenarios is crucial, and undue influence must be vigilantly avoided.

Furthermore, digital consent options are being considered to enhance accessibility and maintain records efficiently. However, these digital methods come with the requisite responsibility of safeguarding personal health information, adhering to stringent data privacy laws. The adoption of such advanced consent procedures underlines Marma Chikitsa's commitment to ethical standards and patient-centered care.

Healthcare Equality and Accessibility in Marma Practice

Healthcare equality in Marma Chikitsa lies at the intersection of legal, ethical, and social considerations. Ensuring equal access to this traditional form of medicine is vital for its integration into global health systems. This involves addressing disparities in healthcare provision and promoting inclusivity across different demographics, including socio-economic statuses and geographies.

Legal frameworks governing Marma Chikitsa must mandate equitable access as part of licensing requirements for practitioners. Policies should outline clear paths for underserved communities to receive Marma treatments under health coverage schemes. Moreover, training programs need to emphasize culturally competent care, enabling practitioners to effectively serve diverse populations.

In regions where Marma Chikitsa is less recognized, partnerships with local health authorities can facilitate workshops and awareness campaigns to educate the public on its benefits. Ensuring accessibility also means investing in research and infrastructure that support remote and rural healthcare delivery, leveraging technology to reach broader audiences.

Through these measures, Marma Chikitsa can achieve true healthcare equality, offering a holistic and integrated approach that respects and rejuvenates all individuals, regardless of their background.

Intellectual Property Issues in Marma Methodologies

Intellectual property (IP) issues present unique challenges in the domain of Marma Chikitsa, where ancient wisdom meets modern practice. Protecting these methodologies while encouraging innovation demands delicate handling to avoid stifling the broader dissemination and evolution of knowledge. For practitioners, the delineation between traditional knowledge and proprietary techniques becomes a critical concern.

Registration and protection of IP are intricate, given that Marma techniques are deeply rooted in cultural heritage. Legal frameworks struggle with the dual need to preserve this as public domain knowledge while also recognizing individual or institutional innovations. This tension often leads to debates on whether and how Marma methodologies can be patented or trademarked under current IP laws.

Furthermore, the global nature of Marma Chikitsa complicates IP protection across different legal jurisdictions, potentially leading to inconsistent rights enforcement. Practitioners seeking to navigate this complex landscape must be well-informed about international IP law variations, ensuring their practices do not inadvertently infringe on existing protections or neglect potential IP opportunities. As such, ongoing legal education and consultancy with IP experts become paramount for maintaining ethical and legal adherence in Marma practice.

Public Health Implications of Widespread Marma Adoption

The widespread adoption of Marma Chikitsa across various populations presents potential transformative implications for public health systems. As this ancient practice gains traction, its integrative approach could significantly reduce the reliance on pharmaceutical interventions, promoting natural, preventive health measures. This shift could lead to decreased healthcare costs and improve long-term outcomes by addressing the root causes of ailments rather than just symptoms.

Moreover, comprehensive implementation of Marma Chikitsa could enhance general wellness, reducing the incidence of chronic diseases prevalent in modern societies. Such a holistic health framework encourages lifestyle changes that contribute not only to physical health but also to mental and emotional well-being. Public health initiatives may leverage these benefits to bolster community health resilience and reduce disparities.

However, the integration of Marma into public health requires careful consideration of resource allocation and practitioner training to ensure equitable access. Establishing standard protocols and ensuring consistent quality of care are paramount to harnessing Marma's full potential at the community and national levels.

Safeguarding Traditional Knowledge and Cultural Heritage

Safeguarding the traditional knowledge and cultural heritage embedded in Marma Chikitsa is essential as this ancient practice undergoes globalization. Recognizing and protecting these intangible assets involves legal mechanisms that prevent unauthorized appropriation and commercial exploitation. Laws must support the preservation of Marma's methodologies not just as therapeutic practices, but as cultural treasures linked to the identity and history of its origins. Efforts to document and archive the traditional wisdom of Marma are critical. This ensures that the practice's roots and authenticity are maintained, even as it evolves in modern therapeutic contexts. Intellectual property laws play a crucial role here by defining frameworks that respect the collective heritage while fostering educational and therapeutic applications.

Governments and international bodies can aid in these efforts by formulating policies that acknowledge the value of traditional knowledge. This not only protects but also promotes the use of Marma Chikitsa within and beyond its traditional boundaries, ensuring that this venerable practice continues to benefit future generations worldwide.

Legal Challenges in Cross-Border Practice

Navigating the legal terrain of cross-border Marma Chikitsa poses distinct challenges, primarily due to variations in international healthcare regulations. Practitioners must adeptly balance respect for local medical practices with adherence to their home country's standards, often leading to a complex mesh of legal considerations. For instance, certain therapies accepted in one country may be restricted or considered alternative in another, complicating the provision of consistent care.

Moreover, issues such as licensing foreign practitioners or verifying their credentials across borders add another layer of complexity. Practitioners are required to obtain multiple accreditations or undergo specific training tailored to regional legal requirements. This not only increases the administrative burden but also impacts the timeliness and accessibility of Marma therapy.

The enforcement of patient privacy and data security laws across different jurisdictions further complicates these practices. With varying standards on patient data handling, practitioners must ensure robust compliance to avoid legal repercussions. Therefore, strategic legal planning and international cooperation are crucial for the seamless continuation of Marma Chikitsa across borders, ensuring that legal barriers do not hinder the healing potential of this ancient practice.

Continuing Education Requirements for License Renewal

The dynamic landscape of Marma Chikitsa mandates continual learning for practitioners, a critical factor addressed by continuing education requirements essential for license renewal. These stipulations are integral to ensure that practitioners remain abreast of the latest advancements and methodologies in Marma therapy. Typically, these requirements include a specified number of training hours within a renewal cycle, focusing on both theoretical knowledge and practical skills.

Educational programs for license renewal aim to deepen the practitioners' understanding of new research and its implications for treatment. This ongoing education is crucial not only for enhancing treatment efficacy but also for maintaining ethical standards and patient safety.

Regulatory bodies often coordinate with professional associations to develop relevant courses that reflect current trends and legal standards in healthcare.
Ultimately, by fulfilling these continuing education requirements, Marma practitioners reinforce their commitment to professional integrity and patient care excellence. The process ensures that practitioners are not just recertifying their credentials but are genuinely enhancing their therapeutic capabilities to serve their patients better.

Updates and Changes in Global Marma Practice Laws

The landscape of global Marma practice laws is continuously evolving, reflecting broader trends in healthcare regulation and the increasing recognition of alternative therapies. Recent updates have focused on enhancing the legitimacy and safety of Marma therapies by establishing more rigorous requirements for practitioners. This shift aims to harmonize standards across borders, ensuring that Marma Chikitsa retains robust efficacy and safety profiles irrespective of geographic location.
In countries where Marma was previously unregulated, new laws now mandate specific educational qualifications and adherence to ethical practices. These changes are designed to protect patients and promote high standards in Marma therapy. For instance, some regions have introduced licensing exams that include both theoretical and practical assessments of Marma techniques, alongside ongoing professional development requirements.
Moreover, changes in global practice laws make it imperative for practitioners to stay informed. Regular seminars and workshops, often sponsored by professional associations, provide insights into legal requirements and updates. By engaging with these educational opportunities, Marma therapists can ensure their practices align with international standards, enhancing the credibility of Marma Chikitsa as a respected therapeutic option worldwide.

Telemedicine and Remote Marma Services: Legal Implications

The expansion of Marma Chikitsa into telemedicine introduces a complex web of legal considerations, pivotal for practitioners and recipients alike. This digital transition necessitates strict adherence to telehealth regulations which vary significantly across regions. Key concerns include ensuring confidentiality and security in digital communications, critical to preserving client trust and complying with medical privacy laws.
Moreover, licensure poses a formidable challenge; practitioners must navigate jurisdictional boundaries where telemedicine might be tightly regulated. Cross-border practice, especially, demands knowledge of both sources and destination legal frameworks, often requiring multiple accreditations. Consequently, the scalability of remote Marma services might be tempered by significant legal overheads.
Additionally, Internet-based practices invite scrutiny over practitioner qualifications and the authenticity of virtual consultations. Implementing standard operational protocols and acquiring relevant certifications becomes indispensable. These legal precautions assure clients of the credibility and legal sanctity of receiving Marma therapy remotely, thereby fostering its growth in the digital healthcare landscape.

Future Legal Trends and Predictions for Marma Chikitsa

As Marma Chikitsa gains widespread recognition, future legal frameworks are expected to evolve significantly. The burgeoning interest in this ancient therapy will likely prompt stricter regulations to ensure practice standards and patient safety. Advancements in related legal stipulations will focus on integrating Marma's traditional aspects with contemporary health laws to foster its global acceptance and implementation.

One anticipated shift is the development of international agreements and standards, facilitating smoother cross-border practices. Such legal harmonization will address previous inconsistencies and reduce barriers to entry, enabling practitioners to offer services more freely across nations. This will also likely include more rigorous credentialing processes to maintain high treatment standards universally.

Further, legal protections concerning intellectual property, particularly in preserving proprietary methodologies of Marma Chikitsa, will be emphasized. Enhanced rights for practitioners and stricter penalties for unauthorized practices are expected as part of these changes. Engaging with these future legal trends will be crucial for the stakeholders to navigate the expanded landscape of Marma Chikitsa effectively.

Summary

The chapter 'Contemporary Practice and Legal Aspects of Marma Chikitsa' provides a comprehensive overview of the current trends, legal challenges, and regulatory frameworks surrounding the practice of Marma Chikitsa, a traditional form of Ayurvedic therapy. The practice is gaining international acclaim due to its non-invasive nature and effectiveness, especially in pain management and psychological well-being, leading to its integration into modern healthcare systems globally. As Marma Chikitsa grows in popularity, it faces diverse legal recognitions and regulations that vary significantly across countries, affecting the licensure, scope of practice, and rights of practitioners and patients alike. Regulatory bodies set specific practice standards to ensure safety and efficacy, ensuring practitioners are well-trained and adhere to ethical guidelines. The chapter also highlights the requirement for practitioners to undergo rigorous certification and licensing processes, which include continuous professional development to keep up with advancements in the field. Standard Operating Procedures (SOPs) are detailed, emphasizing the integration of Marma practices within traditional and modern medical protocols, thereby enhancing legitimacy and acceptance within medical communities. Moreover, issues of risk management, insurance coverage, ethical marketing, data privacy, and integration with conventional medical treatments are meticulously discussed, showcasing how Marma Chikitsa is becoming a part of integrated healthcare solutions. The segment on professional and interdisciplinary collaborations further elaborates on the role of professional associations in advocacy and setting standard practices that encourage a safe and ethical practice environment. Finally, the chapter considers the challenges involved in protecting the intellectual property of Marma methodologies, the importance of continuous education for practitioners, the impact of global legal changes on practice, and the potential of telemedicine in expanding the reach of Marma Chikitsa.

References

[1] Satyapriya, M., Nagendra, H. R., Nagarathna, R., Padmalatha, V. 'Effect of integrated yoga on stress and heart rate variability in pregnant women.', International Journal of Gynaecology and Obstetrics, March 2009. https://www.ncbi.nlm.nih.gov/pubmed/19171361

[2] Patwardhan, B., 'Bridging Ayurveda with evidence-based scientific approaches in medicine.', EPMA Journal, December 2014. https://www.ncbi.nlm.nih.gov/pmc/articles/PMC4259414/

[3] Warnock, C., McBean, D., Suter, E., Tan, J., Whelan, J. 'Effectiveness of a novel integrative online treatment for depression: Randomized controlled trial', BMC Psychiatry, October 2014. https://bmcpsychiatry.biomedcentral.com/articles/10.1186/s12888-014-0286-0

[4] Furst, D. E., Venkatraman, M. M., McGann, M., Manohar, P. R., Booth-LaForce, C., Sarin, R. 'Double-blind, randomized, controlled, pilot study comparing classic Ayurvedic medicine, methotrexate, and their combination in rheumatoid arthritis', Journal of Clinical Rheumatology, June 2011. https://journals.lww.com/jclinrheum/pages/default.aspx

Case Study: Integrating Marma Chikitsa in a Western Clinic: Challenges and Innovations

In the bustling urban center of Vancouver, Dr. Emily Robertson decided to integrate Marma Chikitsa into her established western medical practice, aiming to offer holistic treatment options to her patients. Understanding the benefits of this traditional Indian therapy, especially for chronic pain and mental health, Dr. Robertson faced several challenges in integration, including legal regulations, practitioner training, and patient acceptance.

Initially, Dr. Robertson had to navigate complex legal terrains. The Canadian health regulations were stringent with non-conventional medical practices. She embarked on a meticulous process of obtaining the necessary certifications and licenses required by provincial health authorities. This involved engaging with professional associations both locally and internationally to ensure her practice met all necessary standards while respecting the traditional roots of Marma Chikitsa.

Clear communication with her patients was paramount; she had to educate them about the benefits and methodologies of Marma Chikitsa. By conducting workshops and seminars, she gradually built a clientele who were keen on exploring these alternative therapies alongside conventional medical treatments. However, maintaining transparency about the scope and limitations of Marma therapy was vital to gain trust.

Embracing technology was another significant step; Dr. Robertson integrated telemedicine services to provide Marma Chikitsa, aligning with legal standards for privacy and data protection. Despite the hurdles, the positive outcomes witnessed in her patients' health reflected the potential of integrating such traditional practices into Western medicine; it reduced the reliance on pharmaceutical treatments and promoted holistic wellness.

Case Study: Navigating Legal and Educational Barriers in Marma Chikitsa Globalization

The case involves Dr. Anita Desai, a seasoned practitioner of Marma Chikitsa, who embarked on an ambitious project to globalize this traditional Indian therapeutic practice, with a focus on establishing training centers across Europe and America. Her goal was to bridge the gap between Eastern and Western healing methodologies, providing comprehensive Marma therapies that cater to both physical and psychological ailments within diverse populations.

Dr. Desai's first challenge was the varying legal regulations concerning alternative medicine practice in different countries. In the United States, she encountered stringent licensure and certification requirements that differed markedly from those in India. Each state had its protocol, requiring Dr. Desai to navigate a maze of bureaucratic processes to legally establish her training centers. She engaged with local legal experts and professional healthcare consultants to adapt her business model in compliance with regional healthcare laws, ensuring that her practice conformed to local standards without diluting the essence and effectiveness of Marma Chikitsa.

Furthermore, Dr. Desai grappled with the educational aspect of her mission. Not only did she need to educate potential practitioners about the benefits and techniques of Marma Chikitsa, but she also faced skepticism from the western medical community used to evidence-based practices. To address this, Dr. Desai developed a curriculum that included both theoretical knowledge and hands-on practice, supplemented with clinical research data illustrating the efficacy of Marma points in treatment protocols. She hosted cross-disciplinary workshops that allowed western doctors to directly experience and evaluate the effects of Marma therapy, which slowly built a supportive network of healthcare professionals advocating for its integration into conventional treatment plans.

Despite these strides, Dr. Desai recognized the ongoing need for advocacy and adaptation. She actively contributed to discussions on regulatory changes, pushing for more inclusive health policies that acknowledged and facilitated the practice of holistic and integrative medicine such as Marma Chikitsa. Her efforts highlighted the significance of combining traditional wisdom with contemporary medical practices, paving the way for a more diversified, effective healthcare system globally.

Case Study: Implementing Marma Chikitsa in Remote Areas: A Technological and Ethical Approach

To enhance healthcare accessibility in remote areas, a non-profit organization, Global Health Initiatives (GHI), launched a pilot project aimed at the introduction and integration of Marma Chikitsa into local healthcare practices in rural Nepal. The project was spearheaded by Dr. Lisa Nguyen, who saw the potential for Marma Chikitsa to alleviate common ailments in regions with limited access to conventional medical resources.

The initiative faced multifaceted challenges including the scarcity of trained practitioners, ethical considerations regarding patient consent and understanding, and logistical hurdles in delivering consistent care. To tackle these issues, GHI employed a blended approach. Firstly, they utilized telemedicine technologies to bridge the gap between skilled practitioners and remote patients. They provided training sessions via video conferencing tools, ensuring practitioners could learn and consult experts despite geographical barriers.

Ethically, GHI placed a strong emphasis on patient education and informed consent. Understanding that Marma Chikitsa was unfamiliar to many locals, Dr. Nguyen and her team developed multilingual educational materials, which detailed treatment processes and potential outcomes in layman's terms. They held community meetings to discuss these treatments, ensuring a transparent dialogue about the benefits and limitations of Marma Chikitsa.

Another significant concern was the integration of traditional practices with the existing healthcare framework. GHI worked alongside local health authorities to ensure that the introduction of Marma Chikitsa complemented existing medical practices rather than substituting critical medical care. This cooperation also facilitated a smoother navigation through legal and ethical approvals required for such integrative health services.

Throughout the project, the feedback from the community was overwhelmingly positive, with many reporting improved wellbeing and decreased reliance on over-the-counter medications. The success prompted GHI to consider expanding similar models to other underserved areas, thereby broadening the reach of holistic and accessible healthcare solutions.

Case Study: Revolutionizing Pain Management in Sports Medicine with Marma Chikitsa

The integration of Marma Chikitsa into the sports medicine program at the Elite Sports Academy in Texas presents a unique case of traditional techniques transforming modern health practices. The program, initiated by Dr. Aaron Spencer, a sports medicine specialist, sought to incorporate Marma Chikitsa to enhance recovery processes and prevent injuries in elite athletes. This approach was driven by the need to offer non-pharmacological alternatives for pain management and rehabilitation.

Dr. Spencer faced significant challenges at the onset. The first was the skepticism from other medical staff and athletes accustomed to conventional treatment methods. To address this, he organized several in-depth training sessions and seminars featuring experts in Marma Chikitsa, explaining its benefits and scientific underpinnings. These sessions helped in gradually shifting perceptions and gaining buy-in from the academy's staff and athletes.

Moreover, Dr. Spencer navigated through regulatory hurdles that involved integrating a non-Western medical practice into a conventional sports medicine framework. Collaborating closely with legal advisers and medical boards, he established guidelines that complied with national sports medicine regulations while incorporating Marma Chikitsa. An adaptive training regime for therapists focusing on athlete anatomy and injury types was also instituted to ensure the effectiveness and safety of treatments.

The implementation phase saw individualized treatment plans for athletes, incorporating specific Marma points tailored to the athlete's sport and physical conditions. The results were positive, with many athletes experiencing quicker recovery times, improved flexibility, and a significant reduction in pain recurrence. The success story of a star quarterback who credited Marma Chikitsa for his swift return post-injury particularly bolstered the academy's confidence in this integrative approach.

Given the success at the Elite Sports Academy, Dr. Spencer has advocated for more widespread use of Marma Chikitsa in sports medicine. The establishment of a continued education program for sports therapists interested in Marma techniques underscored the academy's commitment to this innovative approach, suggesting a potential shift in how sports injuries could be managed in the future.

Case Study: Establishing Marma Chikitsa in Corporate Wellness Programs

In a strategic initiative to enhance employee well-being and reduce healthcare costs, BlueTech, a leading software company in Silicon Valley, incorporated Marma Chikitsa into its corporate wellness program. Spearheaded by the Chief Human Resources Officer, Janet Lee, the program aimed to address the high stress and burnout rates among its employees through this traditional Indian healing practice.

Janet faced numerous challenges initially, ranging from skepticism about the efficacy of Marma Chikitsa to logistical issues in integrating this ancient practice with modern corporate culture. To begin, she organized educational sessions for employees to introduce the concept and benefits of Marma Chikitsa, specifically highlighting its effectiveness in managing stress and enhancing mental clarity. She collaborated with expert Marma practitioners to tailor sessions that suited a corporate environment, focusing on Marma techniques that could be applied even in an office setting.

To address legal and regulatory concerns, Janet consulted with healthcare compliance experts to ensure that the program adhered to all national health regulations and corporate wellness guidelines. She also set up a pilot project to monitor the outcomes of this initiative and gather data on its impact on employee productivity and job satisfaction. The pilot involved voluntary participation from employees, with pre- and post-intervention assessments to gauge the effectiveness of the treatments.

The results were overwhelmingly positive. Employees who participated reported significant improvements in their stress levels and overall job satisfaction. This led to increased productivity and a noticeable decrease in sick leaves. Encouraged by the success of the pilot, Janet expanded the program to include regular Marma Chikitsa sessions, making them a core component of the company's health benefits.

Janet's approach not only transformed employee wellness at BlueTech but also set a precedent in the tech industry. The case of BlueTech serves as an influential model, demonstrating the potential of integrating traditional wellness practices like Marma Chikitsa into contemporary work environments. It highlighted the importance of strategic planning, legal compliance, and effective communication in successfully implementing unconventional health practices in corporate settings.

Case Study: Overcoming Legal Hurdles for Marma Chikitsa in Healthcare Integration

The scenario revolves around Dr. Sara Ming, a practitioner of both Western medicine and Marma Chikitsa, who aimed to formally integrate Marma Chikitsa into the health services provided at a prominent wellness center in Melbourne, Australia. Her primary goal was to create a holistic treatment option for patients suffering from chronic illnesses and stress-related disorders where

Marma Chikitsa would be offered alongside conventional medical treatments. Dr. Ming also envisioned training other health professionals within the center to use Marma therapies as a complement to their traditional medical practices.

Dr. Ming's journey began with a thorough investigation into the legal status of Marma Chikitsa in Australia. She discovered that while recognized as a form of complementary medicine, there were no clear regulations that governed its practice within a clinical setting, creating a gray area for healthcare providers. This prompted her to work closely with healthcare attorneys and local Marma Chikitsa associations to propose new regulatory guidelines that would ensure the safety and efficacy of the treatments and protect practitioners legally.

After much deliberation, Dr. Ming set up a professional development program for other medical professionals at the wellness center, ensuring that they received accredited training in Marma Chikitsa. This included the physiological theories behind Marma points, techniques for their stimulation, and education on the potential mental and physical health benefits. Her efforts culminated in the integration of standard operating procedures and practice guidelines for Marma Chikitsa within the wellness center to ensure consistency and safety in treatments.

As a result of these steps, the wellness center not only saw an uptick in patient interest and satisfaction but helped set a precedent for the legal and professional integration of Marma Chikitsa in healthcare institutions across Australia. Dr. Ming's case became a cornerstone discussion in various professional seminars and contributed significantly to the broader acceptance and understanding of Marma Chikitsa in Western healthcare settings.

Case Study: Advancing Marma Chikitsa through Interdisciplinary Research Collaborations

In the renowned health sciences university in Toronto, Canada, Dr. Helen Cartwright, a leading researcher in complementary and alternative medicines, embarked on a ground-breaking project to study the physiological effects of Marma Chikitsa on chronic pain management. Dr. Cartwright's interest in Marma Chikitsa stemmed from observing the limitations of conventional pain management therapies, particularly in patients with chronic conditions. Her objective was to explore the interconnection between Marma Chikitsa and neurological responses to pain, aiming to integrate these findings into broader pain management programs.

To accomplish this, Dr. Cartwright formed an interdisciplinary research team consisting of neurologists, pain management specialists, and seasoned Marma Chikitsa practitioners. The team designed a comprehensive study to measure real-time changes in neurological activity as Marma points were stimulated. Additionally, they utilized advanced imaging techniques and biometric analysis to observe the physiological responses in subjects under controlled and blinded study conditions.

The research faced multiple challenges right from the outset, including securing ethical approval, and ensuring rigorous controls to meet scientific standards. Dr. Cartwright and her team spent considerable time designing the study to address potential criticisms regarding the validity of alternative medical practices. This involved creating stringent protocols for data collection and analysis to ensure that the outcomes could withstand peer scrutiny.

The results were eye-opening; preliminary data indicated significant reduction in pain markers and increased pain threshold in subjects receiving Marma Chikitsa compared to the control group. These findings prompted further studies funded by national health bodies, aimed at integrating these methods into clinical practice.

Dr. Cartwright's research not only helped in advancing the understanding and acceptance of Marma Chikitsa in the scientific community but also paved the way for potential policy changes in pain management protocols. The success of this interdisciplinary approach emphasized the value of combining traditional wisdom with modern scientific techniques, providing a holistic path to patient care that could influence future healthcare strategies globally

Case Study: Expanding Marma Chikitsa in Emerging Markets: Strategies and Outcomes

Amid the surge in popularity of alternative medicine, the expansion of Marma Chikitsa into emerging markets presents a unique case of strategic healthcare integration. The focus of this case study is on Global Wellness Corp (GWC), a multinational health corporation, which spearheaded an initiative to introduce Marma Chikitsa in Southeast Asia, specifically targeting health-conscious populations in urban Thailand, Indonesia, and the Philippines.

The strategic intention behind GWC's initiative was multifaceted. Firstly, it aimed to tap into the growing demand for holistic and non-invasive treatments prevalent in these culturally rich regions where traditional medicine still holds significant sway. Secondly, it sought to provide a legitimate and scientifically backed alternative therapy option that could be integrated with existing wellness programs and medical treatments.

GWC's approach involved several critical steps. Initially, they conducted extensive market research to understand the cultural inclinations and healthcare needs of target demographics. They collaborated with local healthcare providers and traditional medicine practitioners to gain insights and foster partnerships. Legal and regulatory compliances were meticulously navigated to align Marma Chikitsa's offerings with local healthcare laws, which varied significantly across countries.

To build credibility and ensure high standards of practice, GWC established training centers offering accredited courses in Marma Chikitsa. These centers served not only as educational hubs but also facilitated research and development. GWC managed to integrate modern scientific validation with traditional knowledge, a move that significantly heightened local practitioner and consumer trust.

Implementation involved rolling out pilot wellness programs that incorporated Marma therapy with conventional treatments, monitored for efficacy and patient satisfaction. Success in early implementations led to broader acceptance, with subsequent phases seeing incorporation into more mainstream healthcare services. Reflecting on strategic challenges and achievements, GWC's initiative showcases the potential for Marma Chikitsa's growth in global healthcare, provided that thoughtful integration, legal clarity, and educational empowerment are prioritized.

Case Study: Standardizing Marma Chikitsa Practice in Multinational Healthcare

The case study explores the challenges and strategies involved in standardizing Marma Chikitsa across a multinational healthcare corporation, United Health Consortium (UHC), which operates in over twenty countries. UHC aimed to integrate Marma Chikitsa into its diverse array of health services, focusing on standardization to ensure uniformity in the quality of care, adherence to international healthcare guidelines, and culturally sensitive implementations across its global operations.

The initiative began with UHC forming a special task force comprising of senior healthcare administrators, legal experts, local cultural advisors, and Marma Chikitsa specialists. The primary objective was to define a unified set of practice standards that would be applicable and adaptable in different countries, taking into consideration the local legal and cultural nuances. This involved extensive consultation with international regulatory bodies and alignment with global health safety standards.

Key challenges emerged in regions where Marma Chikitsa was relatively unknown or where local regulations did not formally recognize it as a legitimate medical practice. In such areas, UHC worked tirelessly with local healthcare officials and legal advisors to advocate for Marma Chikitsa's acknowledgment and inclusion in the national list of approved complementary therapies. They provided evidence-based research data and documented case studies demonstrating the efficacy and safety of Marma Chikitsa.

Simultaneously, the task force developed comprehensive educational programs for UHC's healthcare providers, ensuring they were well-versed in the theoretical knowledge and practical application of Marma techniques. This training was supplemented with regular workshops, live demonstrations, and annual refresher courses to maintain a high standard of practice.

An integral component of the standardization process was the development of a robust quality assurance system. This system included periodic audits, patient feedback mechanisms, and compliance checks to ensure that every UHC facility adhered to the set standards. The health outcomes from various centers were meticulously tracked and analyzed, with findings used to further refine and optimize Marma Chikitsa protocols.

Case Study: Legal Reform and Marma Chikitsa Integration into National Healthcare

In the European nation of Bellaria, a landmark initiative was launched to integrate Marma Chikitsa into its national healthcare system, fueled by its growing popularity and recognized therapeutic benefits. Dr. Johan Schmidt, a prominent advocate for holistic health practices and a leading Ayurvedic practitioner, spearheaded this initiative, aiming to bridge traditional Marma therapies with modern medical treatments for comprehensive patient care.

Dr. Schmidt faced several complex challenges, the most significant being the existing legal framework that did not recognize Marma Chikitsa as a formal medical practice. His first step involved collaborating with national healthcare policymakers to educate them about the benefits and scientific evidence supporting Marma therapy. By organizing symposiums with health experts and showcasing detailed case studies from global practices, Dr. Schmidt provided substantial backing for his advocacy.

To pave the way for legal reforms, Dr. Schmidt proposed specific guidelines for practicing Marma Chikitsa safely within hospitals and clinics. This included rigorous practitioner certification standards and operational protocols that aligned with the country's health regulations. The proposal suggested the formation of a new regulatory body to oversee Marma practices, ensuring consistent quality and safety of treatments across healthcare settings.

The negotiations with healthcare authorities and legal experts spanned over two years, featuring extensive discussions on integrating these traditional practices without compromising the integrity and standards of existing medical systems. The breakthrough came when a pilot program, sanctioned by the health ministry, was successfully implemented in three state hospitals, leading to noticeable improvements in patient recovery rates and satisfaction.

This pilot not only demonstrated Marma Chikitsa's efficacy but also its potential to lessen the burden on the conventional healthcare system by providing cost-effective, non-invasive treatment alternatives. Following the pilot's success, a national legislative amendment was passed, officially recognizing Marma Chikitsa as a complementary therapy in Bellaria. Dr. Schmidt's efforts culminated in the establishment of training centers across the nation, fostering a new generation of certified Marma therapists.

Review Questions

1. Dr. Alice, a medical practitioner in a multicultural urban hospital, recently integrated Marma Chikitsa into her practice for pain management after attending several workshops. One of her patients, Mr. John, a 58-year-old male with chronic lower back pain not responsive to conventional treatments, is skeptical about Marma Chikitsa. Dr. Alice decides to use a non-invasive Marma therapy technique. Which of the following techniques is she most likely to start with, based on the information on practice trends?
A) A rigorous regimen of invasive needles at Marma points
B) Non-invasive stimulation of Marma points using hand pressure
C) A combination of aggressive pharmaceutical treatments with Marma therapy
D) Referral to a traditional practitioner without trying Marma therapy
Answer: B
Explanation: Given the non-invasive nature of Marma Chikitsa and its appeal for providing pain management without chemical side effects, Dr. Alice would most likely start with non-invasive stimulation of Marma points using hand pressure. This method aligns with modern integration trends of Marma therapy into conventional medical practices, as it is gentle and less likely to be met with resistance from skeptical patients like Mr. John. It introduces the patient to the therapeutic effects of Marma Chikitsa without the discomfort potential of invasive techniques.

2. Considering the case of a country where Marma Chikitsa is in a legal grey area, what potential legal challenges could Marma practitioners face in such countries, according to the latest trends discussed?
A) Practitioners could practice freely without any legal constraints
B) Practitioners may face challenges in obtaining malpractice insurance
C) There are no legal challenges since Marma Chikitsa is not regulated
D) Practitioners might receive government support regardless of the legal standing
Answer: B

Explanation: In countries where Marma Chikitsa lacks formal recognition and thus remains in a legal grey area, practitioners might face significant challenges, including difficulty in obtaining malpractice insurance. This lack of legal clarity could limit the degree of protection afforded to practitioners and make it harder for them to obtain the necessary insurance to safeguard against potential lawsuits, thus impacting their practice stability.

3. A new regulatory body is formed to govern Marma Chikitsa where Dr. Susan, a seasoned practitioner, operates. What could be the most likely initial requirement from this regulatory body for existing practitioners like Dr. Susan?
A) Immediate cessation of practice until further notice
B) Participation in an introductory seminar on Marma Chikitsa
C) Submission of detailed records of past Marma sessions for review
D) Undergoing a certification exam to validate competency in Marma techniques
Answer: D
Explanation: With the formation of a new regulatory body governing Marma Chikitsa, it is likely that existing practitioners like Dr. Susan would be required to undergo a certification exam. This step ensures that all practitioners meet a standardized level of competency and knowledge in Marma techniques, aligning with the regulatory body's aim to safeguard quality and safety in Marma therapy practice. Such measures support the integration of Marma Chikitsa into broader healthcare systems with validated and trustworthy practices.

4. A health clinic in a region where Marma Chikitsa is well recognized legally plans to incorporate it into its services. What is one critical step they must take to comply with standard legal and professional practice?
A) Hiring practitioners without any specific Marma training
B) Implementing robust practice guidelines and standard operating procedures (SOPs)
C) Ignoring guidelines on ethical Marma practice to reduce operational costs
D) Focusing solely on marketing without setting up any formal patient care protocols
Answer: B
Explanation: For a health clinic planning to incorporate Marma Chikitsa into its services in a region where it is legally recognized, implementing robust practice guidelines and standard operating procedures (SOPs) is a critical compliance step. These guidelines ensure that the treatment offered meets the regional legal standards and maintains patient safety and care quality. Such formal protocols are vital for integrating Marma Chikitsa seamlessly and ethically into conventional healthcare settings, ensuring consistency in practitioner performance and patient experience.

CHAPTER FIFTEEN: The Way Forward: Innovations and Ethical Practices in Marma Chikitsa

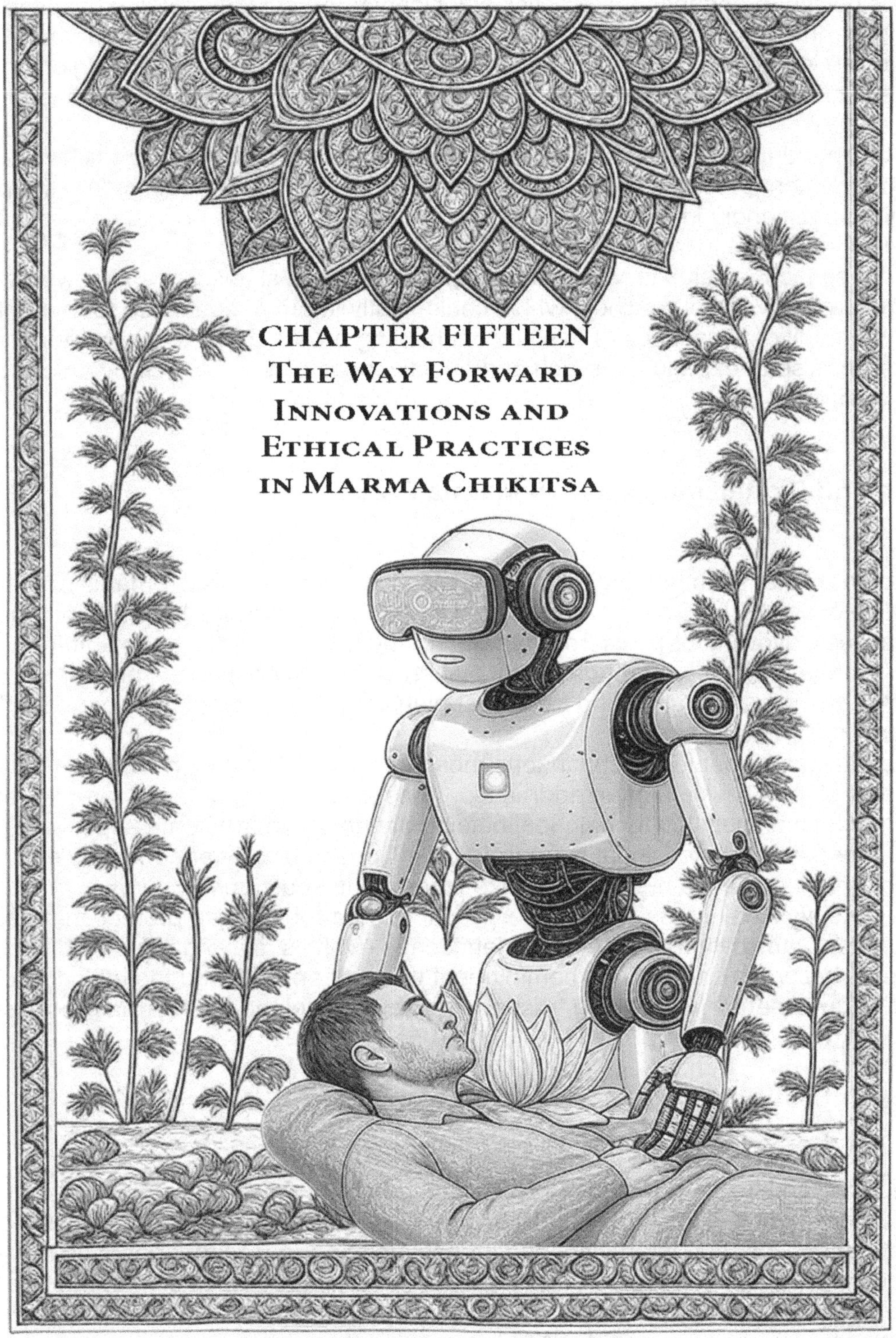

Emerging Technologies in Marma Therapy

The field of Marma Chikitsa is on the brink of technological revolution, with emerging technologies poised to enhance the practice significantly. Advancements such as biometric sensors and AI-driven diagnostic tools are beginning to integrate into Marma therapy, allowing for more precise identification and stimulation of Marma points. These technologies not only improve the accuracy of treatments but also enable personalized therapy plans based on real-time data.

Moreover, the introduction of augmented reality (AR) offers transformative possibilities for both training and treatment processes. AR applications can project Marma points onto the patient's body, guiding practitioners in real-time during therapy sessions. This not only reduces the risk of errors but also enhances learning curves for novice therapists.

The use of these technologies in Marma Chikitsa represents a significant shift towards more scientific and data-driven approaches, which could vastly improve outcomes for patients while preserving the traditional essence of this ancient healing art. As these technologies continue to evolve, they promise to expand the reach and effectiveness of Marma therapy across global healthcare settings.

Telehealth and Digital Integration in Marma Practice

The integration of telehealth and digital technologies into Marma Chikitsa marks a transformative phase in this ancient medicinal practice. The digital era brings with it the potential to expand access, allowing patients from remote or underserved areas to benefit from specialized Marma therapies. Through digital platforms, practitioners can conduct virtual consultations, providing guidance and treatment plans that were traditionally bounded by geographical constraints.

Moreover, digital tools enable the continuous monitoring of patient progress, essential in chronic conditions that Marma Chikitsa often addresses. Apps and online platforms can offer step-by-step Marma point manipulation techniques, helping patients perform some aspects of the therapy at home, under professional supervision. This does not only enhance patient engagement and compliance but also optimizes therapeutic outcomes.

Addressing potential challenges, practitioners must ensure robust data protection measures to safeguard patient information. As the digital landscape evolves, staying abreast of cybersecurity advancements becomes crucial. This commitment to confidentiality and the ethical use of technology is fundamental in nurturing trust and reliability in telehealth Marma practices.

Innovative Educational Tools for Teaching Marma

The pedagogical landscape of Marma Chikitsa is undergoing a dynamic transformation with the introduction of innovative educational tools. These tools are designed to transcend traditional learning boundaries, offering interactive and immersive experiences that enhance the comprehension of complex Marma therapies. Virtual Reality (VR) and Augmented Reality (AR) technologies have emerged at the forefront, enabling students to visualize and interact with Marma points in a 3D space, which drastically improves their practical understanding and precision in locating these critical points.

Additionally, online platforms have revolutionized the accessibility of Marma education, allowing for a broader reach across different geographical locations. These platforms integrate multimedia resources, such as video tutorials and live webinars, which provide real-time interaction with seasoned practitioners. This not only boosts learner engagement but also facilitates immediate feedback, a crucial element in mastering the intricate techniques of Marma Chikitsa.

The fusion of gamification strategies with conventional teaching methods is another significant advancement. By incorporating game-design elements into the curriculum, educators can induce a motivational learning environment that fosters continuous learning and skill enhancement. This approach not only makes learning more enjoyable but also encourages deeper engagement with the material, setting a solid foundation for aspiring Marma therapists.

Sustainable Practices in Marma Chikitsa

Sustainable practices in Marma Chikitsa underscore an essential shift towards an environmentally conscious healing approach. By incorporating biodegradable and recyclable materials into tools and equipment, practitioners are minimizing ecological impact. Utilization of organic oils and sustainably sourced herbs in therapy further aligns with green principles, ensuring that treatments respect both patient health and our planet.

Moreover, energy conservation strategies are being adopted in clinical settings. Practices such as optimizing natural light and using energy-efficient devices help reduce the carbon footprint of Marma centers. This integration of sustainability into daily operations not only serves environmental goals but also exemplifies ethical practice standards that resonate with patients increasingly concerned about ecological issues.

Lastly, the digitalization of Marma training and resources reduces physical waste and increases accessibility. Providing digital copies of manuals and employing virtual reality for practitioner training conserves resources while maintaining educational efficacy. These advancements exemplify how traditional practices can evolve with modern environmental ethics, setting Marma Chikitsa as a leader in sustainable medical practices.

Collaborations between Biotech Companies and Marma Researchers

The intersection of biotechnology and Marma Chikitsa presents a fertile ground for transformative advancements in healthcare. By partnering with biotech companies, Marma researchers can harness cutting-edge scientific tools and methodologies. These collaborations facilitate the development of more precise diagnostic devices which are vital for accurately pinpointing Marma points, thus enhancing treatment efficacy.

Moreover, these partnerships often provide Marma practices with access to molecular biology expertise and advanced imaging technologies. This synergy helps in the deeper understanding of the physiological and biochemical impacts of Marma therapy at a cellular level. Researchers can explore tailored therapeutic approaches that align with individual genetic profiles, potentially ushering in a new era of personalized Marma therapy plans.

Biotech companies benefit from these collaborations by venturing into the previously unexplored market of traditional healing arts, adding value to their portfolio and broadening the scope of applications for their technologies. Both fields contribute uniquely to these partnerships, driving innovation while respecting the ancient wisdom of Marma Chikitsa.

Development of Patented Marma Devices and Tools

In the burgeoning field of Marma Chikitsa, the development of patented devices and tools signifies a major innovation, safeguarding not only intellectual property but also promoting standardized therapeutic practices. These patented devices are ingeniously designed to accurately identify and activate Marma points, which are crucial for effective therapy. By ensuring consistency in the application of Marma techniques, these tools help in minimizing variability in treatment outcomes, thus elevating the overall credibility of Marma practices.
Moreover, the development of such tools involves rigorous scientific research and testing to meet global medical standards. This not only enhances the therapeutic accuracy but also instills trust among practitioners and patients alike. By integrating modern engineering with traditional knowledge, these devices offer a blend of authenticity and innovation.
As patents protect these innovations, they encourage further research and development within the Marma community. This is vital for the evolutionary growth of Marma Chikitsa, allowing it to flourish globally while maintaining its unique therapeutic identity.

Social Media as a Platform for Marma Education and Awareness

Leveraging social media as a platform for Marma education and awareness heralds a significant expansion in disseminating this ancient knowledge. Platforms like Instagram, Facebook, and YouTube have become vital in reaching a global audience, elucidating Marma Chikitsa's principles, techniques, and benefits. Through curated posts, detailed infographics, and interactive live sessions, practitioners can engage with both novices and seasoned enthusiasts, fostering a broader understanding and appreciation of this healing art.
Moreover, social media facilitates community building among followers of Marma therapy, enabling the exchange of testimonials and tips. This peer-to-peer interaction enhances credibility and encourages a proactive approach to health management. With user-generated content, individuals share their personal experiences, making Marma more accessible and relatable to a diverse audience.
From an ethical standpoint, practitioners using social media must navigate potential misinformation by ensuring content accuracy and adherence to professional standards. This responsibility underscores the need for certified Marma therapists to guide public discourse, solidifying trust and authenticity in the digital realm.

Artificial Intelligence for Predictive Analysis in Marma Practice

Artificial Intelligence (AI) is revolutionizing Marma Chikitsa, offering unprecedented predictive capabilities that enhance treatment precision and effectiveness. By analyzing vast datasets of patient histories and treatment outcomes, AI algorithms can identify patterns and predict the most efficacious Marma points for individual patients. This tailored approach not only improves patient outcomes but also accelerates the healing process.
Furthermore, AI supports continuous learning in Marma practices. It enables practitioners to update their knowledge base with the latest findings from global research, integrating these insights into their therapeutic strategies. The AI systems also facilitate the monitoring of therapy effectiveness in real-time, providing practitioners with instant feedback that can be used to adjust treatment plans on the fly.

The ethical integration of AI in Marma Chikitsa also raises important considerations. Practitioners must ensure that AI tools are used responsibly, maintaining patient confidentiality and adhering to medical ethics. Regular audits and updates of AI systems are crucial to mitigate biases and ensure equitable treatment across diverse patient populations. This careful oversight will safeguard the integrity of Marma Chikitsa and its foundational principles.

Blockchain Technology for Securing Marma Therapy Data

Blockchain technology offers a groundbreaking solution for securing sensitive Marma therapy data. By utilizing this decentralized digital ledger system, Marma practices can ensure the integrity and privacy of patient information. Each transaction recorded on a blockchain is timestamped and encrypted, forming a chain of inalterable records that protect against unauthorized modifications and cyber threats.

Implementing blockchain technology in Marma Chikitsa also enhances transparency and trust among patients and practitioners. Patients gain access to their treatment histories and can verify the security protocols in place, fostering a deeper sense of security and compliance with medical regulations. For practitioners, the ability to track every detail of treatment securely simplifies data management and supports the accurate reporting of therapeutic outcomes.

Moreover, blockchain can facilitate the sharing of anonymous treatment data for research without compromising patient privacy. Researchers can analyze large volumes of secure data to uncover insights and trends, potentially driving innovations in Marma therapy practices. The convergence of blockchain technology and Marma Chikitsa not only empowers practitioners but also contributes significantly to the evolution of holistic health care.

Virtual Reality Simulations for Marma Training

The application of Virtual Reality (VR) technology in Marma Chikitsa training offers an innovative leap towards immersive learning environments. By employing VR, practitioners can experience a three-dimensional simulation of Marma point locations and techniques, enhance their precision and understand. This hands-on virtual experience is particularly beneficial for beginners, providing a risk-free platform to practice and refine their skills before applying them in real patient scenarios.

Moreover, VR simulations can replicate a variety of patient cases, allowing practitioners to prepare for diverse clinical situations. This dynamic form of training aids in advancing their diagnostic and therapeutic abilities without the need for physical patient presence, which is crucial in times of limited access or during pandemics.

The ethical use of VR in training also demands rigorous standards to ensure the simulations are accurate and representative of genuine Marma practice. It must incorporate feedback from experienced practitioners to continually improve the VR training modules, adhering to the traditional authenticity and efficacy of Marma Chikitsa.

Nanotechnology and Its Potential in Marma Point Activation

Integrating nanotechnology into Marma Chikitsa heralds a transformative era in energy healing, enabling precision at the molecular level in activating Marma points. Microscopic nanoparticles, engineered to target specific Marma points, can potentially enhance the pinpoint accuracy and effectiveness of energy transfer. This innovative approach could dramatically refine how therapies are administered, focusing on minute physiological responses to achieve significant health outcomes.

Envision nanoparticles programmed to release therapeutic substances directly at Marma points under certain physiological conditions. This could allow for sustained and controlled treatment, reducing systemic side effects and increasing therapeutic efficacy. By aligning with the natural biochemical pathways, such nanoparticles could bolster the body's innate healing processes, making treatments not only more efficient but also more aligned with the holistic principles of Marma Chikitsa.

However, the incorporation of nanotechnology raises crucial ethical questions, particularly concerning patient safety and long-term impacts. Rigorous testing and clear regulatory guidelines will be essential to ensure that these advanced technologies benefit patients without compromising traditional ethical standards of care.

Genomics and Personalized Marma Therapy Plans

The integration of genomics into Marma Chikitsa marks a groundbreaking shift towards personalized energy healing. By mapping an individual's genetic profile, practitioners can devise Marma therapy plans that are finely tuned to each person's unique biological makeup. Tailoring these ancient techniques to one's genetic predispositions empowers practitioners to target underlying health issues more effectively, enhancing both efficacy and safety.

Moreover, personalized Marma plans have the potential to revolutionize preventive health care. With insights from a patient's genomic data, therapists can anticipate potential health issues and intervene early with customized Marma therapies. This proactive approach promotes long-term wellness and minimizes the reliance on more invasive medical interventions later.

However, the use of genomics in Marma Chikitsa raises ethical considerations about privacy and data handling. Ensuring the confidentiality of genetic information and gaining informed consent are paramount. Ethical deployment of these personalized plans will require strict adherence to medical ethics and regulatory guidelines, safeguarding patient rights while embracing these innovative therapeutic strategies.

3D Printing of Customized Tools for Marma Practice

The advent of 3D printing technology has opened new vistas in Marma Chikitsa by enabling the creation of highly customized tools tailored to individual therapeutic needs. This innovation allows for the precise replication of anatomical models and therapy instruments, ensuring a perfect fit for each practitioner's unique approach and each patient's specific physiological requirements.

With 3D printing, the design and production of Marma tools can be adapted quickly to accommodate new research findings or address specific patient anomalies. This flexibility enhances the effectiveness of treatments and accelerates the development cycle of new therapy techniques. Moreover, such customization ensures that practitioners can work with tools that are ideally suited to trigger Marma points with unprecedented accuracy, thereby increasing the therapeutic impact.

However, the integration of 3D printing into Marma Chikitsa also necessitates stringent ethical standards, particularly concerning material safety and device efficacy. Regulatory oversight is essential to ensure that these tools are both effective and safe for clinical use, maintaining the integrity of Marma practice while embracing technological advancements.

Wearable Devices for Monitoring Effects of Marma Therapy

The integration of wearable technology into Marma Chikitsa offers a promising frontier for real-time, continuous monitoring of therapy effects. These devices, equipped with sensors, can track physiological responses to Marma point stimulation, providing invaluable data on patient outcomes. Wearables enable practitioners to assess the immediate and long-term effects of treatments, adjusting techniques to optimize therapeutic results.

Moreover, the data collected from wearable devices can be analyzed to personalize patient care. By understanding individual responses to various Marma points, therapists can tailor interventions more precisely, enhancing both the impact and efficiency of treatments. This approach not only fosters a deeper understanding of Marma therapy's efficacy but also supports clinicians in their ongoing practice development.

Nevertheless, integrating wearable technology into Marma Chikitsa raises significant ethical considerations. Ensuring data privacy and security is paramount, as is maintaining the traditional integrity of Marma practices. Rigorous standards and clear guidelines will be essential to navigate these challenges, ensuring that technological advancements augment rather than undermine the holistic ethos of Marma therapy.

Ethical Guidelines for New Technologies in Marma Practice

As Marma Chikitsa embraces cutting-edge technologies, establishing ethical guidelines becomes paramount to ensure the integrity and trustworthiness of these practices. The primary concern lies in maintaining the authenticity of traditional methods while integrating novel tools like AI, blockchain, and nanotechnology. Ethical standards must address both the efficacy and safety of these technologies, ensuring they do not compromise the holistic essence of Marma therapy.

Confidentiality and informed consent are at the core of ethical practices in Marma Chikitsa. As new technologies facilitate deeper data integration and patient monitoring, practitioners must safeguard patient data against misuse. This includes stringent data protection measures and transparent patient communication about how their information is used and stored. Furthermore, it is crucial to obtain informed consent, particularly when incorporating genomics or AI that may predict patient health trajectories.

Lastly, ethical guidelines should encourage ongoing education and certification for practitioners. This ensures they remain proficient in both traditional Marma techniques and new technological advancements, fostering a balanced approach that respects the ancient wisdom while innovating responsibly.

Privacy and Data Security Concerns in Digital Marma Platforms

As Marma Chikitsa ventures into the digital realm, safeguarding personal health data becomes crucial. The implementation of digital platforms entails a risk of data breaches, which could compromise patient privacy. Ensuring robust cybersecurity measures and compliance with

international data protection regulations, such as GDPR and HIPAA, is indispensable. Data encryption, secure channels for data transfer, and regular security audits are essential to protect sensitive information.
In addition, the ethical handling of data in Marma platforms requires transparent policies regarding data usage. Patients must be informed about how their data is collected, used, and shared. Building a trust-based relationship encourages patient participation and boosts the credibility of digital Marma services. This also involves implementing strict access controls and ensuring that only authorized personnel can view sensitive data to minimize the risk of internal breaches.
Moreover, as technology evolves, so do the threats to data security. Continuous monitoring and updating of security protocols are vital to stay ahead of potential cyber threats. Engaging cybersecurity experts to oversee the safety of digital platforms ensures that Marma Chikitsa adheres to the highest standards of data privacy, maintaining the integrity and confidentiality essential to the therapeutic bond.

Impact of Global Health Trends on Marma Practices

Global health trends significantly influence the practices and adoption of Marma Chikitsa, linking traditional healing with modern health priorities. As the world grapples with chronic diseases and a surge in mental health issues, Marma Chikitsa's non-invasive techniques align well with the growing demand for holistic and preventive healthcare solutions.
Awareness and integration of global wellness movements also enhance the credibility and interest in Marma therapies. These include practices that emphasize the reduction of pharmaceutical dependencies and a shift towards natural, side-effect-free medical alternatives. Marma Chikitsa's potential in pain management and mental wellness positions it favorably within such trends, driving both community-based initiatives and individual health choices.
Furthermore, accessibility concerns (highlighted by global health policies emphasizing healthcare equity) propel innovations in Marma training and dissemination. Online platforms and certifications expand reach and engage younger audiences, while ongoing research into its efficacy helps Marma therapy to resonate with scientific communities and healthcare providers, fostering broader acceptance and integration into conventional health regimes.

Cross-disciplinary Approaches to Marma Therapy

The dynamic realm of Marma Chikitsa is increasingly witnessing the infusion of cross-disciplinary approaches, enhancing therapeutic strategies through collaboration and integration of diverse scientific fields. Leveraging insights from neuroscience, physiology, and biomechanics, Marma therapy is evolving into a more precise and evidence-based practice, offering holistic interventions tailored to the intricate human body systems.
Integration with digital health technology exemplifies cross-disciplinary innovation, where biomechanical sensors and analytical software transform the way Marma points are stimulated and monitored. This convergence not only streamlines the therapy process but also augments its efficacy, facilitating personalized treatment plans that are scientifically sound and verifiable.
Furthermore, the collaboration with psychological sciences enriches Marma practice by embedding stress reduction and emotional well-being into the core therapy protocols. This holistic inclusion is vital as it acknowledges the interdependency of physical and mental health, driving the effectiveness of Marma therapy in contemporary therapeutic landscapes.

Robotics and Automation in Marma Point Stimulation

The integration of robotics and automation within Marma Chikitsa heralds a groundbreaking paradigm for precision in alternative medicine. These technologies facilitate the exact stimulation of Marma points, transcending the limitations of human error and inconsistency. Robotic arms, equipped with sensors and detailed anatomical data, can identify and manipulate specific points with a precision unachievable by human hands.

This advancement not only enhances the efficacy of treatments but also democratizes Marma Chikitsa, making sophisticated therapies accessible in remote areas. Automation in scheduling and treatment personalization further streamlines the therapeutic process, allowing practitioners to focus on holistic patient care. Moreover, these technologies foster consistency in treatment outcomes, critical for the broader acceptance and validation of Marma therapy in scientific and medical communities.

Despite these advances, the integration of robotics raises ethical and practical considerations. Preserving the empathetic and intuitive aspects of Marma Chikitsa, traditionally passed through generations, challenges practitioners to balance technology with tradition. As such, ongoing dialogue and guidelines are crucial to ensure these innovations enhance rather than dilute the essence of Marma therapy.

Ethical Marketing Strategies in the Marma Industry

Ethical marketing in the Marma Chikitsa industry involves strategies that respect both cultural traditions and consumer rights while promoting health therapies. It is crucial to convey the effectiveness of Marma techniques honestly, without exaggerating outcomes or understating potential risks. Marketing materials should be transparent, educational, and backed by scientific research, reflecting Marma's holistic values.

In the digital age, online advertising platforms present both opportunities and challenges for ethical marketing. Advertisers must ensure that digital campaigns do not exploit consumers' data or infringe on privacy. Additionally, diversity in marketing approaches is essential to address a global audience sensitively, acknowledging cultural differences in health perceptions and practices.

Furthermore, collaborations with healthcare professionals can enhance credibility and ensure that marketing claims are substantiated. Ethical partnerships help maintain the integrity of Marma Chikitsa while expanding its reach. Ultimately, fostering trust through ethical marketing will drive the sustainable growth of Marma practices worldwide.

Cultural Competence and Sensitivity in Global Marma Practice

As Marma Chikitsa broadens its reach globally, the imperative of cultural competence and sensitivity becomes crucial. Practitioners must understand and respect the diverse cultural contexts in which they operate, ensuring that Marma therapies are adapted sensitively and appropriately. This not only enhances therapeutic efficacy but also builds trust and respect between practitioners and patients from different cultural backgrounds.

Education and training in cultural competence should be integral to Marma Chikitsa curriculums.

This involves learning about cultural beliefs, values, and practices related to health and healing. By fostering an environment of respect and understanding, practitioners can avoid cultural insensitivity that might otherwise alienate or harm patients.
Moreover, culturally tailored communication strategies in Marma practice can significantly enhance patient engagement and therapeutic outcomes. Employing interpreters or culturally knowledgeable assistants can bridge language and cultural gaps, making treatments more accessible and effective. Implementing these strategies ensures that Marma Chikitsa not only heals physically but also respects and honors the cultural identities of those it serves.

Patent Law and Intellectual Property in Marma Innovations

As Marma Chikitsa integrates more deeply with modern technology, issues concerning patent law and intellectual property (IP) have grown increasingly significant. Innovations such as robotic devices for Marma point stimulation or AI-driven diagnostic tools involve considerable investment and intellectual effort, necessitating proper IP management to safeguard inventors' rights and stimulate further innovation.
The registration of patents provides a protective boundary that can promote a healthy competitive environment while ensuring that inventors can reap financial benefits. This is crucial for funding ongoing research and supporting the infrastructure behind the development of Marma devices and methodologies. However, this can also lead to monopolies, potentially making these innovations less accessible to marginalized communities or smaller practitioners. Balancing these interests requires thoughtful legislation and ethical guidelines. By encouraging ethical licensing models and cross-sector partnerships, the field of Marma Chikitsa can continue to grow, ensuring that these profound healing practices are preserved and propagated responsibly across global communities.

Future Challenges in Marma Chikitsa Research and Practice

As Marma Chikitsa strides into the future, several formidable challenges lie ahead. Firstly, bridging the gap between traditional knowledge and modern scientific validation remains critical. Though strides have been made, much of Marma therapy still requires empirical research to integrate fully into conventional medical protocols, increasing its acceptance across broader healthcare systems. Furthermore, the incorporation of advanced technologies raises concerns about the standardization of techniques, where variability in applications could affect outcomes and replicability of results.
The industry also faces the challenge of training practitioners who can adeptly combine ancient wisdom with modern technology. Developing standardized, rigorous training programs that are accessible worldwide will be essential to maintain the integrity and efficacy of Marma Chikitsa. Moreover, the rising interest might strain the limited resources that teach and propagate these ancient techniques, risking dilution of the practice.
Lastly, ethical dilemmas abound as commercial interests in Marma grow. Ensuring that these developments benefit patients without succumbing to commercial pressures will require robust ethical frameworks and regulatory oversight, ensuring Marma Chikitsa's expansion is both responsible and patient centric.

The Role of Marma in Global Health Initiatives

Marma Chikitsa is poised to redefine global health paradigms by integrating traditional insights with contemporary health strategies. This holistic modality focuses on activating body points that regulate physical, mental, and energetic health, offering profound implications for preventive and therapeutic measures worldwide.

In global health initiatives, Marma can serve as a bridge between conventional medical practices and traditional healing wisdom, especially in regions where access to modern healthcare is limited. Its non-invasive nature makes it an appealing option for primary care and chronic disease management, thus supporting sustainable health infrastructure in underserved areas.

Moreover, integrating Marma into international health policies could enhance the cultural sensitivity of these programs, aligning treatments with local traditions and beliefs. Collaboration with global health bodies to standardize and research Marma practices can further establish its credibility, ensuring that these ancient techniques contribute effectively to contemporary health challenges.

The potential of Marma Chikitsa in global health circles invites a deeper exploration of its capacity to not only heal but also harmonize the diverse health landscapes across cultures.

Summary

The chapter explores technological and ethical advancements in Marma Chikitsa, highlighting the integration of modern tools and technologies that augment the traditional practice. Emerging technologies like biometric sensors, AI-driven diagnostic tools, and augmented reality (AR) are revolutionizing the identification and stimulation of Marma points, enhancing the precision and personalization of treatments. These technologies support more data-driven approaches, potentially improving patient outcomes while maintaining the essence of this ancient healing art. Telehealth and digital platforms are expanding access to Marma therapy, allowing patients in remote areas to receive care and enabling practitioners to monitor progress effectively. Innovative educational techniques, including virtual reality (VR) and gamification, are transforming Marma education by facilitating interactive learning experiences. The chapter also discusses the integration of sustainability in practice by using biodegradable materials and energy conservation methods, thus aligning with modern environmental ethics. Collaborations between Marma researchers and biotech companies are fostering developments in diagnostic tools and personalized therapy plans, leveraging molecular biology and advanced imaging technologies. Patented tools are being developed to standardize Marma application techniques, enhancing consistency and credibility. Moreover, social media platforms are utilized to increase awareness and educate the public, enhancing community engagement. The ethical use of AI in predictive analysis, the benefits of blockchain for data security, and the potential of nanotechnology in precision therapy are explored. Concerns about privacy and data security in digital platforms are addressed, emphasizing the importance of robust protections and ethical guidelines to safeguard patient information. The chapter touches on the global impact of Marma Chikitsa, its role in cross-disciplinary approaches, and the challenges facing its research and practice, stressing the need for ethical guidelines to navigate integrating new technologies while preserving traditional values of Marma therapy.

References

[1] Emerging Trends in Holistic Health: The Role of Marma Chikitsa and Technology Integration. https://www.holistichealthtrends.com/marma-and-technology

[2] Technological Advancements in Traditional Medicine Practices. https://www.traditionalmedtech.com

[3] Ethical Considerations in Integrating Digital Health Solutions. https://www.digitalhealthethics.com

[4] Innovative Educational Strategies in Traditional Medicine. https://www.educationinmedicine.com/traditional-strategies

[5] Sustainable Practices in Healthcare. https://www.sustainablehealthcarepractices.com

Case Study: Revolutionizing Marma Therapy with AI and AR Technologies

In the evolving field of Marma Chikitsa, a new technological breakthrough has emerged, a specialized clinic in Bangalore has successfully integrated Artificial Intelligence (AI) and Augmented Reality (AR) technologies to enhance the traditional practice. This integration began when the clinic partnered with a tech startup to develop an AI-driven diagnostic system that analyzes patient data to predict the most effective Marma points for individual treatment plans. Simultaneously, they introduced an AR application designed for both practitioners and patients that visually maps Marma points onto the body in real time. The case study examines the experiences of two primary users: Dr. Aarav, a seasoned Marma therapist, and his patient, Rhea, who suffers from chronic back pain. Dr. Aarav utilizes the AR app during sessions, which overlays digital images of Marma points over Rhea's body scanned through a tablet. This visual aid helps him to accurately locate and stimulate the correct points, reducing the room for error and enhancing the treatment's precision. The AI system analyses Rhea's feedback post-treatment, adjusting future sessions based on her progress and responses. Over several sessions, Rhea reports a significant decrease in pain and an improvement in mobility. The clinic has noted increased patient satisfaction and higher precision in therapy application since integrating these technologies. However, challenges arose, including initial resistance from traditional practitioners concerned about the integrity of conventional methods and patient data security issues posed by incorporating AI and digital tools. The clinic addressed these by conducting comprehensive training for its staff, focusing on the synergy between technology and tradition, and implementing robust cybersecurity measures to protect patient data.

Case Study: Enhancing Marma Therapy Access Through Telehealth Innovations

To make Marma Chikitsa more accessible to patients in remote areas, a clinic in Kerala has embarked on integrating telehealth technologies into their practice. This initiative, spearheaded by Dr. Kavya, a renowned Marma practitioner, aims to bridge the geographical divide, bringing specialized Marma therapy to the underserved populations. The program utilizes a secure telehealth platform, which allows patients to consult with therapists via video calls. A case in point is Geetha, a patient suffering from rheumatoid arthritis, who lives in a rural part of Kerala with limited access to specialized healthcare. Through the digital platform, Geetha connects with Dr. Kavya for weekly sessions, during which Dr. Kavya guides her through the stimulation of Marma points, meticulously explaining the process and observing Geetha's technique through the camera. The platform also enables Dr. Kavya to track Geetha's progress remotely by analyzing data fed into the system from wearables that monitor physiological responses to the therapy. Over several months, Geetha reports significant improvements in her condition, with reduced pain and increased joint mobility. The therapy's success in Geetha's case boosts the clinic's reputation and paves the way for a broader telehealth adoption among Marma therapy providers. Additionally, the clinic starts an online training module for new patients, preparing them on how to use the digital tools effectively before starting the treatment. However, the program faces challenges, particularly concerning the digital literacy of older patients and the initial skepticism about the efficacy of remote Marma therapy. Overcoming these involves structured digital education sessions and incorporating interactive 3D models that visually demonstrate the techniques being taught. The clinic continuously adapts their approach based on user feedback, improving both the technological interface and the educational tools

Case Study: Navigating Ethical Challenges with Blockchain in Marma Therapy

The integration of blockchain technology in Marma Chikitsa introduced a novel approach to managing patient data with enhanced security and trust. A pioneering case emerged with the introduction of this technology at a holistic wellness center in Mumbai, which aimed to overhaul its data management systems by implementing a blockchain-based solution. The center, which traditionally relied on paper-based records and basic digital entries, faced challenges with data breaches and inefficiencies in handling patient information securely.

Dr. Meera, a lead Marma therapist at the center, collaborated with a technology firm specializing in healthcare blockchain applications. Their goal was to create a decentralized ledger that records all patient interactions and treatments, ensuring data immutability and traceability. The initial phase involved entering historical patient data into the blockchain, followed by real-time updates during and after every therapy session. This system allowed patients to access their treatment histories securely and gave therapists a comprehensive view of each patient's treatment progression.

However, the migration to blockchain was met with several challenges. Firstly, there was a significant learning curve for the staff at the wellness center. Many practitioners, accustomed to traditional record-keeping, found the new system complex. To address this, the center organized intensive training sessions, focusing on the benefits and operational knowledge of blockchain technology. Secondly, ethical concerns arose regarding patient consent and the transparency of how their data would be stored and used. Dr. Meera and her team developed clear consent forms explaining the technology and implemented strict access controls to protect patient information.

Over time, the blockchain system proved beneficial. Instances of unauthorized data access were eliminated, and efficiency in managing patient records increased significantly. Patient trust also grew as they could see the tangible benefits of secure and private access to their treatment details. Nonetheless, continuous evaluation of ethical considerations remains crucial, ensuring that technological advancements serve both the interests of the therapy and the well-being of the patients.

Case Study: Innovating Patient Education and Engagement Through Augmented Reality in Marma Therapy

In a bid to enhance patient understanding and involvement in Marma Chikitsa, a longstanding Marma therapy clinic in Chennai embarked on an innovative journey by integrating Augmented Reality (AR) technology into their educational and treatment protocols. The project's idea initiated by Dr. Priya, a distinguished Marma therapist, aimed to demystify the intricate concepts of Marma points to patients, thus enhancing their active participation in their own therapy sessions.

The clinic launched an AR-driven software which overlays interactive, educational content about Marma points directly onto the user's body through a smartphone app. This technology allows patients to visually identify and learn about the specific Marma points that their therapy would target, guiding them on how their self-administered home routines should be accurately performed. One notable case involved Rajan, a middle-aged man with chronic neck pain who struggled with understanding and adhering to his prescribed home therapy regimen. Upon introduction to the AR app, Rajan could visualize and stimulate correct Marma points on his neck, which significantly increased his comfort and compliance, leading to improved therapeutic outcomes.

However, this technological integration was not devoid of challenges. The initial phase saw significant reluctance from older patients, who were overwhelmed by the digital interface. This called for the development of a user-friendly design and hands-on demonstrations during clinic visits. Moreover, ensuring the accuracy of the AR overlay on diverse body types required continuous algorithm adjustments to ensure inclusivity and precision across all patient physiologies.

The case study's findings suggest that integrated AR applications could well represent the future of patient education in traditional therapies like Marma Chikitsa. Feedback indicated a marked improvement in patient engagement and a deeper understanding of the therapy process. The next steps involved evaluating long-term patient outcomes to fine-tune the application and planning for a broader rollout. Nevertheless, the clinic continues to balance technology with the traditional tactile essence of Marma Chikitsa, ensuring that augmented reality complements rather than replaces the hands-on healing experience.

Case Study: Integrating Wearable Technology in Marma Chikitsa for Chronic Disease Management

The adoption of wearable technology in Marma Chikitsa was pioneered by a holistic health clinic in Pune, aiming to advance the management of chronic diseases through continuous monitoring. The clinic, renowned for its integrative approach to traditional and modern medicine, embarked on a project to enhance Marma therapy for patients with chronic conditions such as diabetes and hypertension. The case study focuses on the clinic's collaboration with a tech company specializing in medical-grade wearables. The joint venture led to the development of a specialized device that patients wore, which was capable of monitoring physiological responses and the effectiveness of Marma point stimulation in real-time.

The first phase of integration saw the participation of Sanjay, a long-term hypertension patient. Sanjay was equipped with a wearable device that tracked his cardiovascular responses, including heart rate variability and blood pressure, before, during, and after therapy sessions. The data was synchronized with a cloud-based platform accessible by his Marma therapist, Dr. Lakshmi. This allowed for tailored therapy sessions focused on specific Marma points believed to regulate blood pressure. Over several months, Sanjay's readings showed noticeable improvements, correlating with periods following intense Marma sessions.

Despite the promising outcomes, the clinic faced challenges including technical glitches with data synchronization and initial patient skepticism about wearing devices continuously. Resolving these issues required iterative feedback loops with the tech provider and extensive patient education on the benefits and operation of the wearables. Additionally, concerns about data privacy and the ethical use of personal health data were addressed through stringent data protection protocols and transparent patient communication.

This innovative application of wearable technology in Marma Chikitsa not only demonstrated a potential increase in the efficacy of traditional practices but also established a new model for patient monitoring and management in the realm of alternative medicine. The clinic plans to expand this approach to other chronic conditions, constantly refining the technology based on ongoing research and patient feedback.

Case Study: Empowering Global Marma Therapy with Cross-disciplinary Research

In a pioneering initiative to elevate Marma Chikitsa on a global scale, a collaboration was formed between a prominent Marma therapy institute in New Delhi, India, and a leading European university specializing in biomechanics and neurology. This unique partnership aimed to integrate the knowledge of Marma points with scientific insights into human biomechanics and neurological pathways to create more effective, personalized therapy protocols.

The collaboration began with a comprehensive study involving a diverse group of patients suffering from neurological disorders, including chronic migraines and post-stroke motor deficits. The institute provided expertise in Marma therapy, while the university contributed advanced diagnostic tools and research methodologies. A customized software was developed to map the neurological responses of patients during Marma therapy, using sensors to monitor neuromuscular activity and neural pathways stimulation. The patients, hailing from varied ethnic backgrounds, were closely monitored throughout the therapy sessions, with all data being rigorously analyzed to identify patterns and outcomes.

One case was that of Anjali, a 45-year-old woman suffering from chronic migraines. Anjali had been refractory to conventional treatments and was selected to undergo the newly developed Marma-neurological protocol. During the sessions, real-time data displayed how specific Marma points influenced her neural activity, noticeably reducing migraine intensity after just a few sessions. Success stories such as Anjali's brought to light how integrating Marma Chikitsa with neurological research could significantly enhance therapeutic outcomes.

Despite the promising results, challenges such as cultural differences in treatment perception, language barriers, and differing regulatory standards posed substantial hurdles. The teams addressed these by organizing cross-cultural workshops, developing multilingual treatment guides, and working closely with regulatory bodies to align the therapy protocols with international healthcare standards. The ongoing collaboration continues to refine their approaches based on detailed feedback from a growing database of international case studies, paving the way for a new era in holistic healthcare.

Case Study: Advanced Genomics in Personalizing Marma Therapy Treatments

The integration of genomics into Marma Chikitsa has begun transforming personalized medicine landscapes. A notable healthcare facility in Hyderabad, known for pioneering integrative medicine, embarked on a groundbreaking project incorporating genomic data to tailor Marma therapy treatments to individual genetic profiles. The project launched with a pilot study involving fifty patients with diverse chronic conditions, such as fibromyalgia and autoimmune diseases, to explore personalized Marma therapy's efficacy.

The initiative involved collecting and analyzing patients' DNA samples to identify genetic markers that influence response to Marma therapy, such as pain sensitivity and inflammatory responses. Dr. Nisha, the lead Marma therapist, collaborated with geneticists to develop customized treatment plans that targeted specific Marma points linked to these genetic markers. For instance, one patient, Mr. Aravind, exhibited a genetic predisposition to heightened pain sensitivity. Based on his genomic analysis, Dr. Nisha adjusted the stimulation of Marma points known to modulate pain perception, achieving significantly improved outcomes compared to standard Marma therapy.

However, the integration of these advanced techniques was not devoid of challenges. Ethical concerns about genetic privacy, potential discrimination, and the psychological impact of genetic knowledge needed careful management. The facility addressed these by implementing stringent data protection protocols and mandatory counseling sessions for patients regarding the implications of genomic information.

Despite initial ethical and technical hurdles, the outcomes were profound. Patients reported better-managed symptoms, and there was a marked decrease in adverse reactions often associated with generalized treatments. The detailed feedback and clinical data further refined the genomic correlations with therapy responses, enhancing the precision of Marma therapy protocols. The success of this pilot project has set a precedent, and the facility is planning a larger-scale implementation to validate and standardize genomics-integrated Marma therapy across broader clinical settings.

Case Study: Expanding Digital Marma Therapy Through a Global Online Platform

The recent establishment of a comprehensive online platform for Marma therapy marks a significant expansion in its global outreach and accessibility. The platform, conceived by a consortium of leading Marma practitioners from India, developed in collaboration with a Silicon Valley tech firm, seeks to offer a standardized, easily accessible form of Marma Chikitsa to a worldwide audience. This case study explores the development, deployment, and outcomes of this ambitious project, especially focusing on a case involving Maya, a middle-aged woman from South Africa suffering from chronic stress and sleep disorders.

The platform, named 'Global Marma Online', provides live video consultations, virtual workshops, and a rich library of resources including detailed tutorials and interactive anatomical guides on Marma points. Maya, intrigued by the non-invasive nature of Marma therapy, registered for a personalized consultation session. Her therapy was facilitated by Dr. Sunil, a seasoned Marma therapist based in Mumbai, who conducted an initial assessment through a secure video call.

Utilizing high-definition visuals from the platform's resources, he guided Maya in identifying her critical Marma points related to alleviating stress and improving sleep quality.

Despite the benefits observed, several challenges emerged. The significant time zone differences necessitated 24/7 availability of therapists, pushing the platform's scheduling flexibility to its limits. Additionally, variations in internet connectivity posed intermittent disruptions during live sessions, impacting the learning and therapy process. The platform's management responded by deploying AI-driven chatbots to offer basic guidance during off-hours and enhanced their servers to ensure smoother streaming of live sessions.

This online platform's impact on Marma therapy's global outreach was profound, boosting international interest and participation in Marma Chikitsa. It allowed practitioners to cater to a broader demographic, transcending geographical and cultural boundaries, while patients like Maya benefitted from accessing these specialized treatments without the need for physical travel. The platform continues to evolve, integrating user feedback to refine its offerings and address the challenging aspects of delivering holistic health services digitally.

Case Study: Innovative Integration of Virtual Reality for Marma Therapy Training

A health institute in Toronto, Canada, spearheaded a revolutionary project to integrate Virtual Reality (VR) technology into Marma Therapy training. This initiative aimed to overcome the limitations of conventional training methods by providing an immersive and interactive learning environment. The project commenced with the creation of a comprehensive VR curriculum, developed in collaboration with experts in Marma Chikitsa and VR software developers.

One key module was a VR simulation that allowed users to interact with a 3D model of the human body, highlighting Marma points. This module was designed to help students identify and simulate treatment on these points with greater accuracy. For instance, during the pilot phase of the project, trainee therapist Sarah had the opportunity to practice on virtual patients with various health conditions. The VR system provided instant feedback on her technique, accuracy, and timing, enabling rapid learning and adaptation. Sarah mentioned that the haptic feedback feature, which mimicked the sensation of touching human skin, significantly enhanced her understanding and comfort level with placing pressure on Marma points.

Despite the advanced technology, the institute faced several challenges. Firstly, the high cost of VR equipment limited the number of students who could access the training simultaneously. Secondly, some students experienced motion sickness while using the VR headsets, which distracted from the learning experience. To address these issues, the institute initiated a scholarship program to acquire more equipment and adjusted the VR headset display settings to reduce motion blur and sickness.

As the project evolved, feedback from students like Sarah helped refine the system, making it more user-friendly and effective. The success of this VR training module not only enhanced the skills of Marma practitioners but also set a precedent in medical education, demonstrating the potential for wider application in other areas of traditional medicine. The long-term effectiveness of this training approach is continuously monitored, with ongoing modifications based on student performance and technological advancements.

Case Study: Advancing Marma Therapy with Nanotechnology for Targeted Treatment

The progressive integration of nanotechnology in Marma Chikitsa has initiated a groundbreaking approach to precise, targeted therapies in a clinical setting in Hyderabad, focusing particularly on chronic inflammation disorders such as arthritis and fibromyalgia. Leveraging the microscopic scale of nanotechnology, the clinic piloted a program involving the creation of nanoscale devices designed to act at specific Marma points to modulate pain and inflammation more effectively.

The clinical trial featured thirty patients with a history of inadequate responses to conventional treatments. Each patient received nanodevices specifically engineered to target Marma points associated with their condition. These devices were programmed to release anti-inflammatory agents directly at the Marma points upon detecting certain biochemical signals, a method thought to enhance the therapeutic effect while minimizing side effects typically associated with systemic medications.

The trial's primary subject, Mrs. Anjali Rao, a 58-year-old arthritis patient, experienced a significant reduction in joint pain and improved mobility within weeks of starting the treatment. Continuous monitoring via embedded sensors in the nanodevices allowed for real-time adjustments in treatment protocols, establishing a dynamic therapeutic process that adapted to immediate physiological responses.

However, this pioneering application of nanotechnology in Marma Chikitsa was not without challenges. Ethical and safety concerns regarding long-term effects and biocompatibility of nanomaterials were prominent. The clinic addressed these through rigorous pre-trial safety assessments and ongoing monitoring, supplemented by detailed informed consent processes that ensured patients were fully aware of the treatment's novel nature.

The case study endeavors to highlight the interaction between ancient therapeutic techniques and cutting-edge technology, underscoring the balance between innovation and tradition in modern healthcare. Long-term follow-up of the trial subjects and scaled-up studies are planned to further validate the efficacy and safety of nanotechnology-enhanced Marma therapy.

Review Questions

1. Dr. Anand, a practitioner of Marma Chikitsa, recently integrated AI-driven diagnostic tools into his practice. He is examining a patient, Mr. Sharma, who suffers from chronic back pain. After collecting real-time data through biometric sensors located on various Marma points, the AI tool suggests several points for acute pain relief. Which of the following Marma points could be suggested by the AI for optimal pain management in Mr. Sharma's condition?

A) Kati Marma
B) Hridaya Marma
C) Sthapani Marma
D) Talahridaya Marma

Answer: A

Explanation: In the scenario provided, the AI tool integrated into Dr. Anand's Marma therapy practice likely suggests the Kati Marma point for treating Mr. Sharma's chronic back pain. Kati Marma points are in the lower back and are often targeted in Marma Chikitsa for alleviating pain in this area. The inclusion of AI-driven diagnostic tools helps to identify the most effective

Marma points based on real-time physiological data, ensuring a precise and personalized treatment approach.

2. A Marma therapist, Ms. Patel, is using augmented reality (AR) to train new therapists in identifying Marma points on patients effectively. During a training session, a novice therapist uses AR glasses to locate Marma points on a volunteer. If the training focuses on headache relief, which Marma points are the therapists most likely taught to identify?
A) Shankha and Sthapani Marma
B) Kati and Ani Marma
C) Hridaya and Nabhi Marma
D) Ani and Talahridaya Marma
Answer: A
Explanation: For headache relief, identifying the Shankha and Sthapani Marma points would be crucial in the training session led by Ms. Patel using AR technology. Shankha Marma is located around the temporal region, which is often associated with relieving temporal headaches, while Sthapani Marma, located at the center of the forehead, is targeted for frontal headaches and sinus relief. The use of AR in training helps in precisely locating these points, potentially reducing errors and enhancing therapeutic effectiveness in novice therapists.

3. A new telehealth platform for Marma Chikitsa has been launched to reach patients in remote areas. Dr. Rao, a Marma practitioner, conducts a virtual consultation with a patient experiencing digestive issues. Utilizing the digital tools, which Marma points might Dr. Rao suggest the patient stimulate at home for alleviating their condition?
A) Parsvadhara and Nabhi Marma
B) Guda and Basti Marma
C) Hridaya and Kshipra Marma
D) Apana and Prana Marma
Answer: B
Explanation: For a patient experiencing digestive issues, Dr. Rao would likely suggest stimulation of Guda and Basti Marma points. Guda Marma is associated with the rectal area and can help in regulating bowel movements and alleviating constipation, while Basti Marma is related to the urinary and reproductive organs and can help in balancing the excretory functions, which indirectly affect digestion. The telehealth platform enables Dr. Rao to guide the patient on how to locate and stimulate these points accurately for relief.

4. During an advanced training workshop on Marma Chikitsa, the instructor introduces an innovative educational tool incorporating Virtual Reality (VR). The session focuses on identifying and stimulating Marma points for cardiovascular health. Which Marma points are the participants most likely to practice on using VR tools for promoting heart health?
A) Hridaya and Kukundara Marma
B) Hridaya and Prana Marma
C) Kukundara and Guda Marma
D) Prana and Anahata Marma
Answer: B
Explanation: In the VR-based training session focusing on cardiovascular health, participants would most likely practice identifying and stimulating the Hridaya (heart) and Prana (chest) Marma points. Hridaya Marma is directly associated with the heart, vital for regulating cardiac functions, while Prana Marma located in the chest aids in improving respiratory functions and overall energy flow, which are crucial for cardiovascular health. The VR tools provide a three-dimensional interactive experience, allowing for accurate location and stimulation practices without physical risk to a patient.

Epilogue

As we conclude this extensive exploration of Marma Chikitsa in 'MARMA CHIKITSA™: The Hidden Science of Ayurvedic Energy Healing for Pain Relief, Disease Reversal, and Vitality Restoration Across Asia', it becomes clear that this ancient tradition holds profound relevance in today's world, offering deep insights into holistic healing practices. The journey through the chapters not only highlights the therapeutic potential of Marma points but also underscores the interconnectivity of body, mind, and spirit as recognized in traditional Ayurvedic wisdom. Across Asia, the regional practices and adaptations of Marma Chikitsa remind us of the rich tapestry of cultural wisdom that supports and enhances the universal principles of Ayurveda. Through understanding the detailed anatomy and physiology of Marma points, we can approach health and disease from a truly integrative perspective. The philosophical and esoteric foundations discussed facilitate a deeper engagement with the spiritual aspects of healing, broadening the scope of Marma Chikitsa beyond mere physical relief. By engaging with the tools, oils, and therapeutic techniques described, practitioners are equipped not only with knowledge but also with the practical tools necessary to implement Marma Chikitsa effectively.

This book has also provided a platform to share the significant clinical applications that showcase the potential of Marma Chikitsa in managing chronic diseases, mental and emotional disorders, and achieving overall well-being. Furthermore, our discussion on the integration of this discipline with yoga, Ayurveda, and other traditional and modern health systems reinforces its versatility and capacity for inclusiveness in integrated health practices. As we step forward, the global future of Marma Chikitsa is not only promising but essential.

We must continue to uphold the rigorous standards of education, research, and practice while adapting to technological advances and evolving health paradigms. To our readers - practitioners, students, and enthusiasts of Ayurvedic medicine - we hope this book serves as both a comprehensive guide and a constant companion in your pursuit of knowledge and mastery in Marma Chikitsa. Let us progress with respect for ancient wisdom and a commitment to ethical practice, ensuring the vitality of Marma Chikitsa for generations to come.

Educational Resources:

The **American College of Natural Medicine** in Brooksville, FL. USA offer several college degrees in Ministry, Holistic, Natural and Integrative medicine based on Ayurveda and Marma Chikitsa, Live and Online. Visit https://naic-edu.org

The **Thai Yoga Center**: Brooksville, FL USA has been offering professional certification programs in Traditional Thai Medicine, SomaVeda® style, "Traditional Thai Yoga Therapy" (Traditional Thai Medical Massage) Since 1983. TYC offer five certification courses and programs from introductory-beginner practitioner to the SomaVeda® Teacher Certification Program. All professional programs are nationally and internally accredited. Visit https://ThaiYogaCenter.com

The **Tayapro Mediverse** offers premiere education and Medical technologies education for a discerning international medical community. https://Tayapro.com

Made in United States
North Haven, CT
12 November 2026

22198997R00176